Pediatric Sports Medicine

Essentials for Office Evaluation

Edited by

Chris Koutures, MD, FA
Pediatric and Sports Medicine Specialist
Gladstien & Koutures
Anaheim Hills, California
Team Physician, USA Volleyball and Cal State Fullerton
Fullerton, California

Valarie Wong, MD, FAAP
Assistant Professor, Pediatrics and Sports Medicine
Loma Linda University, School of Medicine
Loma Linda, California

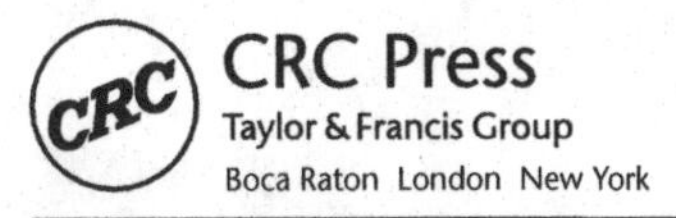

CRC Press is an imprint of the
Taylor & Francis Group, an **informa** business

First published 2014 by SLACK Incorporated

Published 2024 by CRC Press
2385 NW Executive Center Drive, Suite 320, Boca Raton FL 33431

and by CRC Press
4 Park Square, Milton Park, Abingdon, Oxon, OX14 4RN

CRC Press is an imprint of Taylor & Francis Group, LLC

Library of Congress Cataloging-in-Publication Data

Pediatric sports medicine (Slack Incorporated)
Pediatric sports medicine : essentials for office evaluation / [edited by] Chris Koutures, Valarie Wong.
p. ; cm.
Includes bibliographical references and index.
ISBN 978-1-61711-052-8 (alk. paper)
I. Koutures, Chris, editor of compilation. II. Wong, Valarie, editor of compilation. III. Title.
[DNLM: 1. Athletic Injuries--diagnosis. 2. Adolescent. 3. Child. 4. Physical Examination--methods. 5. Sports Medicine--methods. QT 261]
RC1218.C45
617.1'027083--dc23

2013022989

ISBN: 9781617110528 (pbk)
ISBN: 9781003525561 (ebk)

DOI: 10.1201/9781003525561

Dedication

This book is dedicated to the mentors who have guided us with their knowledge and wisdom through the years, and the parents who have entrusted us with the care of their children. These young athletes continue to expand our clinical knowledge and teach us daily with their injuries and stories.

Contents

Acknowledgments

I am humbled by the opportunity to participate in the creation of this textbook, and I wish to thank SLACK Incorporated for reaching out to us and putting its confidence in our work. I am sincerely grateful for the opportunity to work with my wonderful coeditor, colleague, and trusted friend, Valarie Wong. This project has been fueled by the contribution of many close colleagues in the pediatric sports medicine field; there is no way it could have been finished without their expertise and insight. A special thanks to Rebecca Demorest for her creative thoughts and guidance during the early planning stages of this book, and to Cora Maglaya for her amazing artwork. I am also indebted to my patients and mentors who have enlightened me with personal tales and practical pearls that continue to shape my clinical and teaching styles. My career in pediatric sports medicine would not be possible without the love and dedication of my mother, Maria, and my late father, George, who unfortunately passed away during the writing of this book. Finally, my heartfelt love to my wife, Niki, my daughter, Mary, and my sons, Luke and Greg, for all of their support and willingness to share family time with the production of this book; and to occasionally pose for important pictures along the way.

Chris Koutures, MD, FAAP

I am very honored that my colleague and coeditor, Chris Koutures, asked me to come on this adventure with him, and I cherish the friendship that has emerged from our collaboration on this project. I also want to acknowledge and thank SLACK Incorporated for the wonderful opportunity to participate in the creation of this book. A special thank you goes out to Rebecca Demorest for her contribution in formulating the foundation of this book and to Cora Maglaya for graciously lending her artistic talents to many of our illustrations. Further, this book could not have come to fruition without the hard work, dedication, and collective efforts of all of our authors and friends within the field of sports medicine. Finally, I am most thankful for my parents, Allen and Rosemay, my sister, Roxanne, and my close friends, Colin, Kathy, and Daphne. As any author and editor knows, writing and editing a book while juggling other work and family responsibilities is always a challenge. My family and friends have always been there for me, offering their constant love and support for my life's endeavors. I could not accomplish anything if I did not have all of you by my side. Thank you from the bottom of my heart!

Valarie Wong, MD, FAAP

About the Editors

Chris Koutures, MD, FAAP is American Board of Pediatrics certified in both pediatrics and sports medicine and practices both specialties at Gladstien & Koutures in Anaheim Hills, California. He received an undergraduate degree in kinesiology at the University of California, Los Angeles before finishing both medical school and his pediatric residency at the University of Wisconsin. He then completed a sports medicine fellowship with the University of California, San Diego. He is the medical team physician for the USA Volleyball Men's and Women's National Teams and attended the 2008 Beijing Olympics. He is also the team physician for California State University, Fullerton Intercollegiate Athletics, Orange Lutheran High School, and Chapman University Dance Department. He recently completed a 6-year elected term on the Executive Committee of the American Academy of Pediatrics Council on Sports Medicine and Fitness. Dr. Koutures regularly mentors and teaches pediatric residents, medical students, and athletic training students along with speaking at regional and national conferences on sports medicine topics.

Valarie Wong, MD, FAAP is currently an assistant professor at Loma Linda University in Southern California. Her practice consists of both sports medicine as well as general pediatric patients. Dr. Wong is American Board of Pediatrics certified in pediatrics and sports medicine. She completed her sports medicine fellowship at Jersey Shore Medical Center and Rutgers University. Dr. Wong received her medical degree from Baylor College of Medicine and finished her pediatric residency at the University of California, Los Angeles. She obtained her undergraduate degree in biochemistry and cell biology at the University of California, San Diego. Along with teaching medical students, residents, nursing and physical therapy students, she has been the team physician for the Inland 66er's, a minor league baseball team in San Bernardino, for many years. Dr. Wong also provides medical coverage for local community sports events.

Contributing Authors

Suraj Achar, MD, FAAFP (Chapter 15)
Professor, Family and Preventive Medicine
Associate Director of Sports Medicine
University of California at San Diego School of Medicine
San Diego, California

Suriti Kundu Achar, MD (Chapter 15)
Staff Physician
Chase Avenue Family Health Center
El Cajon, California

Holly J. Benjamin, MD, FAAP, FACSM (Chapter 13)
The University of Chicago
Comer Children's Hospital
Primary Care Sports Medicine
Chicago, Illinois

David T. Bernhardt, MD (Chapter 5)
University of Wisconsin
School of Medicine and Public Health
General Pediatrics and Sports Medicine
Madison, Wisconsin

Kate E. Berz, DO (Chapter 17)
Assistant Professor of Pediatrics
Division of Sports Medicine
University of Cincinnati College of Medicine
Cincinnati Children's Hospital Medical Center
Cincinnati, Ohio

Terra Blatnik, MD, FAAP (Chapter 11)
Pediatric Staff Physician
Cleveland Clinic Foundation
Cleveland, Ohio

Joel S. Brenner, MD, MPH, FAAP (Chapters 6, 31)
Director, Sports Medicine and Adolescent Medicine
Children's Hospital of The King's Daughters
Associate Professor of Pediatrics
Eastern Virginia Medical School
Norfolk, Virginia

Susannah Briskin, MD, FAAP (Chapter 11)
Assistant Professor of Pediatrics
Assistant Director, Primary Care Sports Medicine Fellowship
Rainbow Babies and Children's Hospital/ University Hospitals Case Medical Center
Cleveland, Ohio

Paul D. Brydon, DO (Chapter 3)
Fellow
UCSD Sports Medicine
San Diego, California

Monique S. Burton, MD (Chapter 43)
Seattle Children's Hospital
Department of Orthopedics and Sports Medicine
Department of Pediatrics
Seattle, Washington

Kelly Chain, MD (Chapter 21)
Pediatric Resident
CHOC Children's Hospital
Orange, California

Philip J. Cohen, MD (Chapter 32)
Internal Medicine and Sports Medicine
Staff Physician
Hurtado and Busch-Livingston Health Centers
Rutgers University
New Brunswick, New Jersey

Yasmin D. Deliz, DO (Chapter 19)
Pediatric Sports Medicine Fellow (2011 to 2012)
Jersey Shore University Medical Center
Neptune, New Jersey
Pediatrician
The Children's Hospital of Philadelphia Care Network/Harborview Pediatrics
Somers Point, New Jersey

Rebecca A. Demorest, MD, FAAP (Chapter 38)
Pediatric and Young Adult Sports Medicine
Webster Orthopedics
Team Physician, US Rowing
Dublin, California

Emanuel Elias, MD (Chapter 4)
University of California, Irvine
Family Medicine Residency Program
Orange, California

Emelynn J. Fajardo, DO (Chapter 19)
Pediatric Sports Medicine Fellow (2012 to 2013)
Jersey Shore University Medical Center
Neptune, New Jersey
Advocare, The Orthopedic Center
Cedar Knolls, New Jersey

Kenton H. Fibel, MD (Chapter 42)
Resident Physician
University of California, San Diego
Scripps Ranch Family Medicine
San Diego, California

Katherine M. Fox, MD (Chapter 13)
Advocate Medical Group
MyMD Family and Sports Medicine
The Center for Health and Nutrition
Oak Brook, Illinois

Matthew Grady, MD, FAAP (Chapters 14, 39)
Fellowship Director, Primary Care Sports Medicine
Assistant Professor of Clinical Pediatrics
University of Pennsylvania Perelman School of Medicine
Pediatric and Adolescent Sports Medicine
Department of Orthopedic Surgery
Children's Hospital of Philadelphia
Philadelphia, Pennsylvania

Andrew J.M. Gregory, MD, FAAP, FACSM (Chapter 1)
Associate Professor
Orthopedics and Pediatrics
Vanderbilt University School of Medicine
Nashville, Tennessee

Mark Halstead, MD (Chapter 16)
Assistant Professor
Departments of Pediatrics and Orthopedics
Washington University
St. Louis, Missouri

Tho Brian Hang, MD (Chapter 40)
Clinical Instructor
Division of Emergency Medicine
Northwestern University's Feinberg School of Medicine
Division of Orthopaedic Surgery and Sports Medicine
Ann & Robert H. Lurie Children's Hospital of Chicago
Chicago, Illinois

Quynh B. Hoang, MD (Chapter 20)
Pediatric Primary Care Sports Medicine
Assistant Professor, Department of Orthopedics
Children's Hospital Colorado/University of Colorado Health Sciences Center
Denver, Colorado

T.J. Howell, MD (Chapter 36)
Loma Linda University
Private Practice
Elk Grove, California

Mary M. Hung, DO, MS (Chapter 25)
Department of Pediatrics
Loma Linda University
Loma Linda, California

Phuong N. Huynh, MD (Chapter 26)
Driscoll Children's Hospital
Corpus Christi, Texas

Amanda Weiss Kelly, MD (Chapter 26)
Rainbow Babies and Children's Hospital
University Hospitals of Cleveland
Case Western Reserve University
Cleveland, Ohio

Austin Krohn, MD (Chapter 33)
Broadway Family Medicine
Minneapolis, Minnesota

David Kruse, MD (Chapters 4, 27)
Orthopaedic Specialty Institute
Orange, California

Cynthia R. LaBella, MD (Chapter 40)
Medical Director
Institute for Sports Medicine
Ann & Robert H. Lurie Children's Hospital of Chicago
Associate Professor of Pediatrics
Northwestern University's Feinberg School of Medicine
Chicago, Illinois

Michele LaBotz, MD, FAAP, CAQSM (Chapter 12)
InterMed Sports Medicine
South Portland, Maine

Greg Landry, MD (Foreword, Chapter 30)
Professor of Pediatrics and Orthopedics
University of Wisconsin School of Medicine and Public Health
Head Medical Team Physician
University of Wisconsin-Madison Athletic Teams
Madison, Wisconsin

Christopher Lynch, MD (Chapter 35)
Pediatric Resident at CHOC/UCI
University of California Davis School of Medicine
Orange, California

Teri M. McCambridge, MD, FAAP (Chapters 17, 44)
Division Director, Sports Medicine Biodynamics Center
Associate Professor of Pediatrics and Orthopedics
University of Cincinnati College of Medicine
Cincinnati Children's Hospital Medical Center
Cincinnati, Ohio

Megan Groh Miller, MD (Chapter 7)
Primary Care Sports Medicine Physician
Tri-Rivers Surgical Associates
Pittsburgh, Pennsylvania

Rob Monaco, MD (Chapter 7)
Director of Sports Medicine
Rutgers University
Piscataway, New Jersey

Mohammed Mortazavi, MD (Chapter 20)
Department of Pediatrics/Department of Sports Medicine
Davis Medical Center
University of California
Sacramento, California

Kirk Mulgrew, MD (Chapter 9)
Fellow, Primary Care Sports Medicine
University of Washington/Seattle Children's Hospital
Seattle, Washington

Kyle B. Nagle, MD, MPH (Chapter 5)
University of Wisconsin
School of Medicine and Public Health
General Pediatrics and Sports Medicine
Madison, Wisconsin

Jeremy Ng, MD (Chapters 14, 39)
Attending Physician, Primary Care Sports Medicine
Coastal Orthopedics
Bradenton, Florida

David Olson, MD (Chapter 33)
University of Minnesota
Department of Family Medicine and Community Health
Roseville, Minnesota

Kentaro Onishi, DO (Chapter 27)
University of California Irvine Medical Center
Department of Physical Medicine and Rehabilitation
Orange, California

Neesheet Parikh, DO (Chapter 24)
South Bay Sports and Preventive Medicine Associates
San Jose, California

Byron Patterson, MD (Chapter 8)
Primary Care Sports Medicine
Encino, California

Miriam G.S. Reece, MD, CAQSM (Chapter 42)
Highlands Family Medicine
Denver, Colorado
Formerly UCSD Sports Medicine Fellow
La Jolla Family and Sports Medicine
San Diego, California

Stephen G. Rice, MD, PhD, MPH, FAAP, FACSM (Chapter 19)
Program Director, Pediatric Sports Medicine Fellowship
Director, Jersey Shore Sports Medicine Center
Jersey Shore University Medical Center
Neptune, New Jersey
Clinical Professor of Pediatrics
UMDNJ-Robert Wood Johnson Medical School
New Brunswick, New Jersey

William O. Roberts, MD, MS, FACSM (Chapter 10)
Professor
Department of Family Medicine and Community Health
University of Minnesota
Minneapolis, Minnesota
Program Director
University of Minnesota St. John's Family Medicine Program
St. Paul, Minnesota

Anthony Saglimbeni, MD (Chapter 24)
Head Team Physician, San Francisco Giants
Team Physician, Bellarmine College Preparation High School
President of South Bay Sports and Preventive Medicine Associates
San Jose, California

John A. Schlechter, DO (Chapters 28, 29)
Pediatric Orthopedic and Sports Medicine Surgical Specialist
Children's Hospital of Orange County
Orange, California

Charmaine Sekona, MD (Chapter 18)
Department of Internal Medicine and Department of Pediatrics
Loma Linda University
Loma Linda, California

Robby S. Sikka, MD (Chapter 33)
TRIA Orthopaedic Center
Bloomington, Minnesota

David V. Smith, MD, FAAP (Chapters 6, 31)
Pediatrics and Sports Medicine
Children's Hospital of the King's Daughters
Eastern Virginia Medical School
Norfolk, Virginia

Paul R. Stricker, MD, FAAP (Chapter 41)
Scripps Clinic Sports Medicine
San Diego, California

Alysha Taxter, MD (Chapter 44)
Fellow, Division of Pediatric Rheumatology
Children's Hospital of Philadelphia
Philadelphia, Pennsylvania

Kenneth S. Taylor, MD (Chapters 3, 42)
Director, UCSD Sports Medicine
La Jolla Family and Sports Medicine
San Diego, California

Nate Waibel, MD (Chapter 10)
University of Minnesota St. John's Family Medicine Program
St. Paul, Minnesota

David Wang, MD (Chapters 3, 15)
Resident
Family Medicine
UCSD School of Medicine
San Diego, California

Tracy L. Zaslow, MD, FAAP, CAQSM (Chapters 23, 34)
Assistant Professor of Orthopaedic Surgery
University of Southern California
Medical Director, Sports Medicine Program
Director, Sports Concussion Program
Children's Orthopaedic Center
Children's Hospital Los Angeles
Los Angeles, California

Foreword

I am pleased to have been asked to write a foreword to *Pediatric Sports Medicine: Essentials for Office Evaluation*. I have known the authors since their residency training, knowing at that time that they were 2 rising stars in the field of pediatric sports medicine. As fellowship-trained sports medicine specialists with over 26 years of combined experience, they are well equipped to edit this textbook.

Although exercise recommendations are universal and the number of children participating in organized sports continues to rise, the medical and musculoskeletal issues related to sports and exercise do not receive much attention in pediatric training. This leaves many trainees and practitioners alike in need of a readily accessible and applicable resource for managing sports medicine issues in the outpatient setting. To that end, Drs. Koutures and Wong have assembled an impressive list of contributing authors. Most are very well known as established experts in the field of pediatric sports medicine. I am pleased that the authors chose to cover both musculoskeletal problems as well as medical issues as this is what is needed for most practitioners and learners interested in sports medicine. The question and answer format makes the book user friendly and easy to read. The authors clearly knew the clinically relevant questions for each topic. This well organized book is loaded with practical advice on a myriad of sports medicine issues. The tables and illustrations are nicely done and clarify the teaching points. Finally, this textbook offers important information on several unique topics. The chapters on Sports Lingo and the ABCs of Bracing and Taping in particular are quite useful and not found in other sports medicine textbooks.

I am often asked by medical students and residents, "What book would you recommend for sports medicine?" Now I have an easy answer. This book will serve as an excellent reference for anyone in training as well as anyone practicing primary care medicine. I have been practicing pediatric sports medicine and teaching medical students and residents since 1984. I only wish this book was available when I started.

Greg Landry, MD
University of Wisconsin School of Medicine and Public Health
Head Medical Team Physician, UW Madison Athletic Teams
Madison, Wisconsin

Introduction

On more than one occasion, we have been asked to recommend a practical, quick reference book for pediatric sports medicine that can be used in the office setting. This became the seed for our creation, which is now in your hands. We envisioned a busy practitioner appreciating a set-up that allowed for rapid reference on a subject; therefore, a question and answer format emerged.

This book can be read from cover to cover, or used as a quick "look-up" for topics of interest. When certain subjects of controversy are discussed, we attempt to give the reader educated, evidence-based information from multiple viewpoints so that they may make the best personalized management decisions for the patient. In each chapter, we explore the most common questions pertaining to pediatric sports medicine.

This text provides the most up-to-date information on sports medicine at the time of printing to health care professionals who take care of pediatric and young adult athletes. This would include primary care physicians, nurse practitioners, physical therapists, athletic trainers, chiropractors, and those in these respective fields that may be in training. It will also provide educational benefit to interested coaches, mothers and fathers, and perhaps the athletes themselves.

Section I

General Information

1 Sports Lingo
Musculoskeletal Terms

Andrew J.M. Gregory, MD, FAAP, FACSM

Much like in other areas of medicine, sports medicine has unique terminology—proper knowledge of anatomy and relevant terms is vital to the performance of a proper musculoskeletal examination and the successful documentation and communication of the findings to others. This may require you to refer back to your basic anatomy text, which you may not have opened since your first year of medical school! Unfortunately in orthopedics we have historically given classification systems, anatomic features, and physical examination tests the names of doctors (eg, Salter-Harris fracture classification, Gerdy's tubercle, Thompson's test), which make them much harder to remember than if anatomic terms (eg, greater trochanter) and descriptive test names (eg, apprehension test) were used. We will try to refrain from the overuse of doctors' names in this chapter as much as possible; however, some of these terms are very important to know for the physical examination and will therefore be discussed.[1]

1. What Are Some Key Anatomic Terms to Remember?

Anatomic terminology is used to be very specific in the description of the physical examination. One should be familiar with this type of terminology and use it in clinic notes whenever possible. Most of the terms refer to the body in what is called the *anatomic position* with the body in the standing position, the head in a neutral position, the arms and legs extended, and the palms facing up.[1]

- *Distal/proximal*—Distal refers to the part of the structure (bone) that is further away from the head in the anatomic position. Conversely, proximal refers to the part of the structure (bone) that is closer to the head in the anatomic position.
- *Medial/lateral*—Medial refers to a part of the structure that is closer to the midline in the anatomic position; whereas, lateral refers to the part of the structure that is further away from the midline in the anatomic position.
- *Cephalad/caudal*—Cephalad refers to a location toward the head or anterior section of the body, and caudal refers to a location toward the tail or distal end of the body.
- *Frontal/dorsal*—Frontal refers to a structure on the front of the body; whereas, dorsal refers to a structure on the back of the body (Figures 1-1 and 1-2).
- *Sagittal plane/coronal plane*—The sagittal plane passes from the frontal to the dorsal region and divides the body into right and left halves. The coronal plane passes from the left to the right side and divides the body into anterior (frontal) and posterior (dorsal) halves.
- *Abduction/adduction*—The motion of a segment away from the midline is referred to as abduction; the motion of a segment toward the midline is referred to as adduction (see Figures 1-1 and 1-2).

Koutures C, Wong V.
Pediatric Sports Medicine: Essentials for Office Evaluation (pp 2-8)

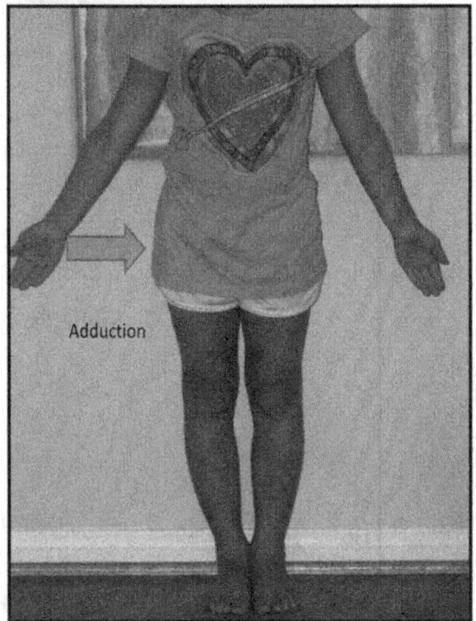

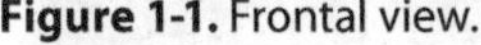

Figure 1-1. Frontal view.

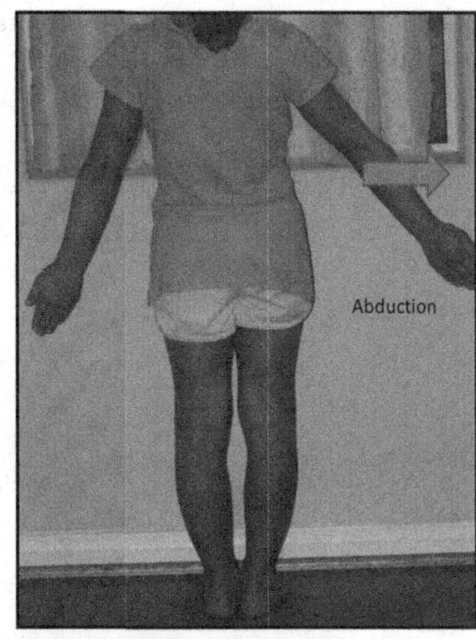

Figure 1-2. Dorsal view.

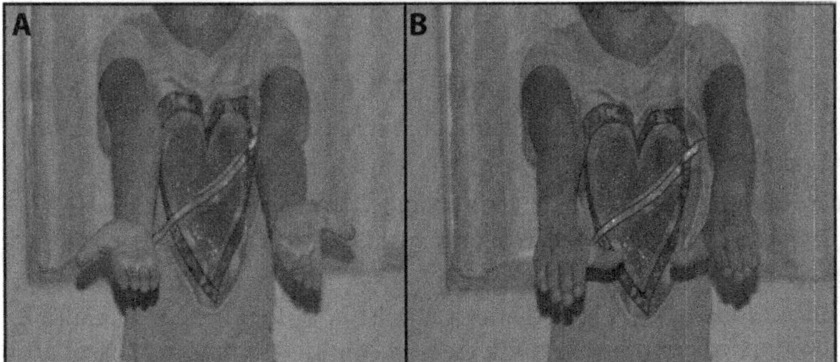

Figure 1-3. (A) Supination and (B) pronation.

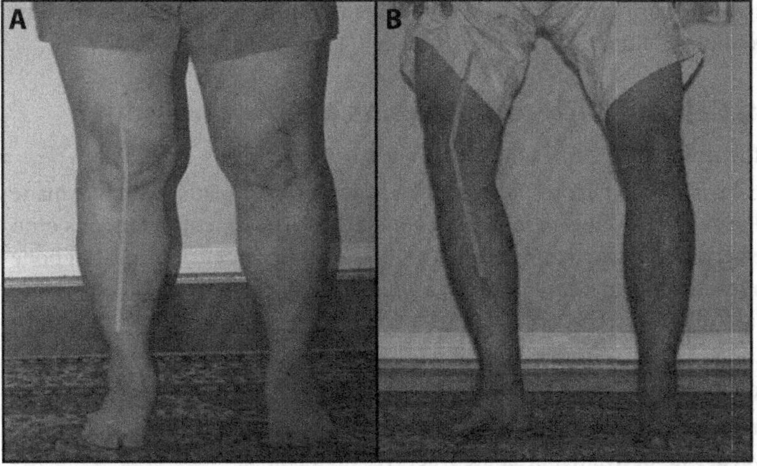

Figure 1-4. (A) Knee valgus and (B) knee varus.

- *Pronation/supination*—Pronation and supination refer to the position of the forearm or foot. Pronation means the hand is facing posteriorly and the foot is everted or flat. Supination means the hand is facing anteriorly and the foot is inverted or arched. (Figure 1-3).
- *Varus/valgus*—Valgus and varus refer to the position of the distal portion to the proximal portion. In the valgus position, the distal portion is lateral to the proximal portion. In the varus position, the distal portion is medial to the proximal portion (Figure 1-4).[1]
- *Dorsi-/plantarflexion*—The motion of a segment in the dorsal direction is dorsiflexion, and the motion of a segment in the plantar direction is plantarflexion.[2]

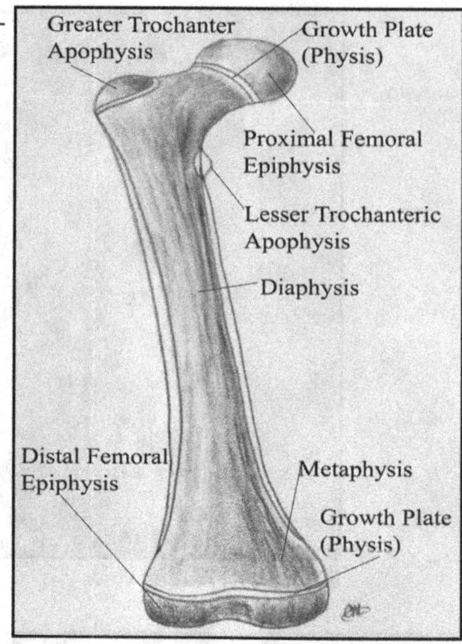

Figure 1-5. Regions of growing bone. (Graphite Pencil-Copyright © 2012 Cora Maglaya, PT, ATC, CSCS.)

- *Lordosis*—A curvature of the spine in the dorsal direction. There is normal lordosis in the cervical and lumbar spines. Loss of lordosis is common in the cervical spine with cervical muscle spasm after a patient sustains an injury.[3]
- *Kyphosis*—A curvature of the spine in the frontal direction. There is normal kyphosis in the thoracic and sacral spines. This rigid kyphosis is present in a patient with Scheuermann's disease of the spine (see Figure 33-1).[3]
- *Scoliosis*—A curvature in the sagittal plane that can consist of a single curve or multiple curves (see Figure 33-4). A curvature over 10 degrees is considered abnormal. Scoliosis also involves the rotation of the spine, which is often how it is discovered on a physical examination (during the Adam's forward bend test). There are multiple causes of scoliosis, ranging from congenital to idiopathic.[3]

2. What Do You Call the Different Regions of Growing Bone?

- Figure 1-5 depicts the different regions of growing bone.
- *Physis*—The primary ossification center (also known as the growth plate), which is made of cartilage and is located at the ends of long bones and at the attachment of tendons onto bone. The cartilage becomes ossified and is called an ossification center. This part of bone is often involved in fractures or overuse injuries, as it is made of cartilage and is therefore considered the "weak link in the chain."[4]
- *Epiphysis*—The secondary ossification center at the ends of long bones that is important for longitudinal growth of the skeleton.
- *Apophysis*—The tertiary ossification center located at the attachment of tendons. It is a common site for overuse (apophysitis) or acute fractures (avulsions).
- *Metaphysis*—The segment of bone that is being converted from cancellous bone (spongy) to cortical bone (diaphysis). It is located between the epiphysis and the diaphysis. This is a common site for buckle fractures.
- *Diaphysis*—The segment of bone in the shaft of long bones that has a thick outer cortex and hollow center (like a pipe). This is a common site for complete fractures.
- *Periosteum*—The membranous outer lining of the bone that is very vascular in children and allows for their faster healing time.
- *Cortex*—The hard outer shell of the shaft of bones.

3. What Are Some Key Soft Tissue Structures?

- *Ligament*—Connective tissue that connects two different bones that form a joint. Ligament injuries are called sprains and are graded as follows:
  - Grade 1 sprain = stretch[3]
  - Grade 2 sprain = partial tear[3]
  - Grade 3 sprain = complete tear[3]
- *Tendon*—Connective tissue that connects the muscle to the bone. Tendons are very well-organized parallel fibers that form a strong rope-like structure. Injury to a tendon can be acute (strain or tear) or chronic (tendinopathy).[3]
- *Meniscus*—Cartilage in the knee that is formed into two thin wafers. There is both a medial and lateral meniscus that are located between the tibia and the femur. Either meniscus can be torn in isolation or can commonly accompany a knee ligament tear. There is a similar structure in the wrist called the triangulofibrocartilage complex.[3]
- *Articular cartilage*—Cartilage attached to the end of a long bone that forms a joint (articulation) with the end of another long bone. It can be injured over time in degenerative arthritis or acutely with an articular cartilage defect.[3]
- *Muscle*—Soft tissue that is attached to a tendon that can elongate and contract, causing motion of joints. This tissue can be injured with a contusion, strain, or tear.[3] Muscle and tendon strains are graded as follows:
  - Grade 1: minor tear of muscle; mild pain, minimal loss of strength, no palpable muscle defect[3]
  - Grade 2: severe damage to muscle; moderate pain, moderate loss of strength, muscle defect occasionally palpable[3]
  - Grade 3: complete tear of muscle; severe pain, complete loss of strength, muscle defect palpable
- *Myotendinous junction*—Connection between the muscle and the tendon. It is a common site of weakness and tensile overuse in tendinosis and acute injuries.[3] Proximal myotendinous injuries have unique considerations due to the involvement of the bone attachment, while distal myotendinous injuries are treated more like muscle strains.[3]

4. What Pain Rating Scales Are Used in Children?

- *Visual analog scale*—A way of rating pain on a scale from 0 (no pain) through 10 (most severe pain).
- *Face scale*—The visual analog scale may be confusing for very young children, and therefore the face scale may be considered more appropriate. The faces can range from a big smile that represents no pain to a big frown that represents severe pain.

5. How Are Physeal Fractures Described Using the Salter Harris Classification?

Physeal fractures are a common fracture pattern in children, because the physis is made of cartilage and is therefore the weak link in the chain. Salter and Harris devised a well-known but poorly understood scheme for classifying these fractures (Figure 1-6). The most important features to recognize with physeal fractures are the amount of displacement and whether the joint is involved.[3]

- *Salter-Harris type I*—A fracture through the physis that does not involve the epiphysis or the metaphysis. It can be displaced or not, but is commonly nondisplaced and is therefore invisible on x-ray. If it is nondisplaced, this type of fracture can be treated conservatively in a cast.
- *Salter-Harris type II*—A common pattern that involves the physis and the metaphysis. Regardless of the amount of displacement, the metaphyseal fragment is usually easy to visualize. If it is nondisplaced, this type of fracture also can be treated conservatively. If it is displaced, it must be reduced.

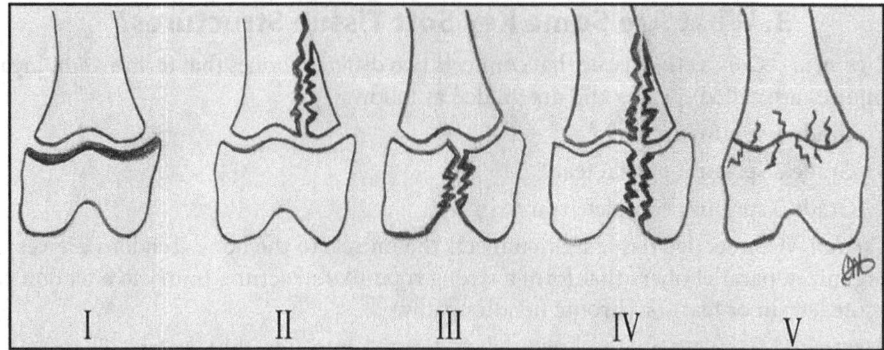

Figure 1-6. Salter-Harris types I to V fracture depictions. (Graphite Pencil-Copyright © 2012 Cora Maglaya, PT, ATC, CSCS.)

- *Salter-Harris type III*—A more unusual pattern that involves both the physis and the epiphysis, and therefore the joint. Even if it is nondisplaced, this fracture often requires open reduction and internal fixation. A patient presenting with this type of fracture should be referred to a specialist.
- *Salter-Harris type IV*—A fracture that is similar in frequency to the Salter-Harris type III fracture, but involves both the metaphysis and the epiphysis, and therefore the joint. Because of the joint involvement, treatment is the same as a type III fracture.
- *Salter-Harris type V*—The most unusual physeal fracture pattern. It involves a crush injury to the physis itself. The diagnosis is often made after the fracture is healed and a patient presents with abnormal growth.

6. What Are Key Terms to Describe Fractures?

- *Plastic deformity*—Bone that is bent without a fracture line.[3]
- *Buckle (torus) fracture*—Periosteum is folded upon itself (compression side).[3]
- *Greenstick fracture*—A fracture through a single cortex (tension side).[3]
- *Complete fracture*—A fracture through both cortices that may or may not be displaced.[3]
- *Simple fracture*—A single fracture with a proximal and distal fragment.[3]
- *Comminuted fracture*—A fracture that has multiple fragments.[3]
- *Avulsion fracture*—Fragment of bone is pulled off (tensile) by the tendon or ligament attachment (apophyseal fractures).[3]
- *Physeal fracture*—A fracture that involves the physis of the bone (see the Salter-Harris classification system describe previously).[3]
- *Displaced*—The distance that the distal fragment is moved from a proximal fragment; it is described using percentages (30%/50%/100% displaced).[3]
- *Angulated*—The angle that the distal fragment lies in relation to the axis of the proximal fragment; it is described using degrees (20 degrees of angulation).[3]
- *Open fracture*—When the skin over the fracture is lacerated, posing a higher risk for infection that could infiltrate the bone and cause osteomyelitis; prophylactic antibiotics are recommended for open fractures.[3]
- *Closed fracture*—When the skin over the fracture is intact.[3]

7. How Do Fractures Heal?

Most fractures heal in a short time with simple immobilization. The stages of healing are as follows:

- A clot forms.[5]

- Inflammation occurs above the fracture site.[5]
- Osteoclasts begin the process of bone removal.[5]
- Osteoblasts come in and begin laying down new bone.[5]
- The apex of the fracture is usually the last part to heal.[2,5]
- Callus or new bone formation begins very quickly in children and is often palpable (clavicle fractures). It is not usually visible on x-ray until the 3- to 4-week mark and initially appears as a faint white line that parallels the cortex of the bone. The periosteum in children is very vascular and allows for faster healing than in adults. Mature callus has a sharp border that is similar to the normal cortex.[3,5]
- Remodeling is important in the healing process in children. The extra callus that has been created is slowly removed until the bone takes on a more normal shape. Remodeling potential is based on the proximity to the physis, bone age, and plane of motion.[3,5]
- Timing of specialty referral after fractures—Closed (nonsurgical) reduction can be more readily done in the first week before significant callus formation that may require open (surgical) reduction; thus, ensure specialty evaluation of any concerning fractures in the first week.[5]

8. What Are Different Types of Muscle or Tendon Injury?

- *Tendinopathy*—Any disease of a tendon.[6]
- *Tendinitis*—Specific to inflammation of a tendon (only present early in the process).[6]
- *Tendinosis*—A process that involves degeneration of a tendon (most common).[6]
- *Strain*—A stretch injury of a muscle or tendon (think hamstring strain), usually at the myotendinous junction.[6]
- *Tear*—A complete rupture of a tendon or muscle.[6]

9. What Is the Spectrum of Stress Injuries?

- *Stress reaction*—Edema is present within the bone that is visible on magnetic resonance imaging, but no fracture line is present on x-ray.
- *Stress fracture*—The progression of a stress reaction where a fracture line is visible on one cortex.
- *Complete fracture*—The progression of a stress fracture where the fracture line crosses both cortices.[6]

10. What Are Recommendations for Splint Use, Casting and Cast Care, and Selection of Premade and Preformed Braces?

- *Splint*—After an acute fracture, a splint is generally preferred due to the initial swelling above the injury site. If a cast is applied and the swelling was to get worse, then the cast could constrict the extremity and cause more pain. Alternatively, if the swelling was to go down, then the cast could loosen and again cause more pain.[3]
    - Certain fractures do not swell significantly, so a cast could be applied initially in these cases (eg, buckle fracture of the wrist or a toddler's fracture of the tibia).
    - The application of a splint includes padding (cotton or synthetic) and the splint material (fiberglass or plaster).
    - In general, the splint should be form fitting and should include the joint above and below the fracture (eg, midshaft forearm fractures). For distal fractures, however, splinting only the joint below the fracture is usually sufficient (eg, distal radius buckle fractures).
- *Casting*—It is usually safe to apply a cast after the patient has been in a splint for 1 week.[3]

    - A cast consists of a single layer stockinette, several layers of padding (cotton or synthetic), and then finally the cast material itself (fiberglass or plaster). The advantage of synthetic padding is that it can be dried out if it gets wet. If a cast made with cotton padding gets wet, it needs to be removed and a new cast needs to be applied after the skin dries, otherwise skin irritation/sluffing can be significant. Fiberglass casting can get wet, but plaster comes apart in water.
- *Braces*—There are many different types of preformed off-the-shelf braces for various body parts, but ankle, knee, and wrist braces are the most common. They come in multiple sizes, including pediatric specific, and are usually more expensive than the splint or cast formed by the practitioner, but they can be more efficient and practical to use.[3]
    - Common braces should be stocked in the clinic (walking boot or wrist splint), and more uncommon ones (shoulder harness) can be ordered from the brace or durable medical equipment store.
    - Proper fitting is essential, so do not hesitate to refer patients to a professional who is familiar with braces for appropriate brace selection and fit.

References

1. Netter FH. *Atlas of Human Anatomy.* 5th ed. Philadelphia, PA: Saunders; 2010.
2. Anatomical terminology. SEER Training Modules. *National Cancer Institute.* http://training.seer.cancer.gov/anatomy/body/terminology.html. Accessed March 17, 2013.
3. Green NE, Swiontkowski MF, eds. *Skeletal Trauma in Children.* 3rd ed. Philadelphia, PA: Saunders; 2003.
4. LaBella CR. Overuse injuries unique to young athletes. Children's Hospital of Chicago Web site. http://www2.luriechildrens.org/ce/online/article.aspx?articleID=101. Accessed June 21, 2013.
5. Snider RK, ed. *Essentials of Musculoskeletal Care.* Rosemont, IL: American Academy of Orthopedic Surgeons, American Academy of Pediatrcs; 1997.
6. Bracker MD. *The 5-Minute Sports Medicine Consult.* 2nd ed. Philadelphia, PA: Wolters Kluwer Health/Lippincott Williams & Wilkins; 2011.

2 Sports Lingo Activities, Positions, and General Sports Terms

Valarie Wong, MD, FAAP

1. Cross Training—What Is It?

Cross-training is exercising in another sport or activity other than the athlete's main sport with the goal of improving overall performance and minimizing the risk of injury from overuse of muscle groups. Cross training can also develop an underutilized muscle group, leading to improved fitness. An example would be a long-distance runner running 3 days a week and adding 2 days of cross training with a bicycle, which may help with cadence training, or swimming, which will provide a cardiovascular workout minus the impact to the body.

2. What Is a Club or Travel Team?

Club or travel team—A team composed of above-average players for a sport. Playing on this type of team allows the athlete to hone his or her skills in a particular sport against highly skilled athletes in his or her same age group. Being a member of a club or travel team requires a significant commitment from the athlete and his or her families in terms of time and cost.

3. When Does an Athlete Have Overuse Syndrome or Suffer From Overtraining? What Is a Showcase or Tournament?

- *Overuse or overtraining*—Refer to Chapter 20, question 9 for definition and work-up.
- *Tournament or showcase*—See Chapter 4, questions 3.

4. What Are the Martial Arts?

The martial arts are ancient disciplines of combat practices. They are organized systems of defense and attack moves that may or may not include specialized equipment or protective gear. They are practiced for a variety of purposes, including self-defense, physical fitness, increased mental awareness, and spiritual development. There are over 1000 different types of martial arts. The following is a list of common types of martial arts[1,2]:

- *Aikido*—Originating in Japan, this style uses arm bars, holds, and takedowns to redirect and neutralize the energy of an opponent; few kicks are used; the martial artist moves with the attacker rather than against him or her.
- *Judo*—Japanese sport that uses mainly throws.
- *Jiu-jitsu*—Includes arm bars, holds, throws, joint locks, and takedowns. Law enforcement officers may use these techniques.
- *Karate*—Originating in Japan, this style uses kicks and punches for self-defense purposes.
- *Kickboxing*—Originating in America during the 1970s, this style utilizes kicking, punching, sparring, and kick blocks.

Koutures C, Wong V.
Pediatric Sports Medicine: Essentials for Office Evaluation (pp 9-13)

- *Kung fu*—Practiced by the Shaolin Monks in China, as well as by students all over the world, this style focuses on low stances and powerful blocks.
- *Muay Thai*—Also known as Thai boxing. Muay Thai uses punches, kicks, knee strikes, and elbow strikes.
- *Sumo*—Originating around 20 BC in Japan as a form of military combat, this style incorporates slapping, sweeps, and sacrifice throws.
- *Taekwondo*—A Korean sport that is 80% kicks and 20% hand techniques.
- *Mixed martial arts*—Incorporates both striking and grappling techniques. This style combines elements of the other styles of martial arts including Jiu-jitsu, wrestling, judo, karate, Muay Thai, and Taekwondo.

5. What Is the Proper Type of Helmet for a Particular Sport?

There are different types of helmets that are recommended for different sports. Motorcycle and bicycle helmets are governed by mandatory federal safety standards. Manufacturers who make helmets used in recreational sports other than cycling or motorcrossing may choose to follow recommended federal safety standards. A list of helmets and their safety standards can be found at www.cpsc.gov/PageFiles/117293/349.pdf.[3]

6. What Are the Different Positions Found in Cheerleading and the Skills That Are Required for Each?

There are 4 basic positions for a stunt: flyer, base, back spot, and front spot. Somtimes there is also a tumbler.

Cheerleading Positions and Skills[4]

- *Flyer* (also known as top, climber, floater, mounter)—The person who is thrown or pushed up into the air. A good flyer will have confidence, great body awareness and focus in space, good flexibility and strength, enjoys tumbling, and is aware of the surrounding environment. Also beneficial are a sense of timing and no fear of heights.
- *Base*—May include one or two people. Their main responsibility is getting the flyer into the air and then safely back down. Bases should have good upper-body and lower-body strength, and a good sense of timing.
- *Spotters* (also known as scoop, third base)—Should be fast thinkers and attentive to the flyer. They can be subdivided into back spot and front spot.
    - *Back spot*—Assists the base in getting the flyer into the air and helps with the safety of the flyer during the stunt. When the flyer comes out of a stunt, the back spot supports the flyer's back.
    - *Front spot*—Supports the wrists of the base or the ankles of the flyer at the beginning of a stunt. At the end of a stunt, the front spot is in charge of the flyer's legs and for the safety of the flyer when he or she is dismounting.
- *Tumbler*—Tumbles throughout the routine.

The major skills required in cheerleading are cheering and chanting (clearly and in a loud voice), jumps (eg, toe touch, spread eagle), and stunts (eg, back tuck, handstand, back handspring, cartwheel, splits, tumbling).

7. What Are the Most Popular Types of Dance in the United States?

- *Ballet*—Originated during the 15th century as a type of performance dance. Many dance types use ballet as a foundation for their style of dance. There are five basic ballet positions from which basic moves in ballet either start or end (Figures 2-1 through 2-5).

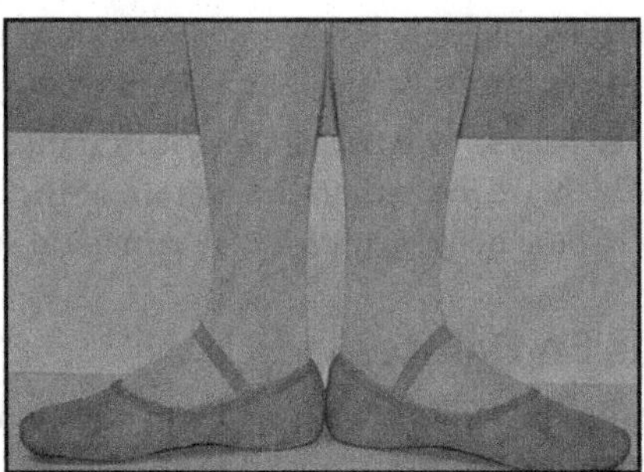

Figure 2-1. First position feet—heels pointed toward each other with hips externally rotated, feet should form a "V" close to 180 degrees.

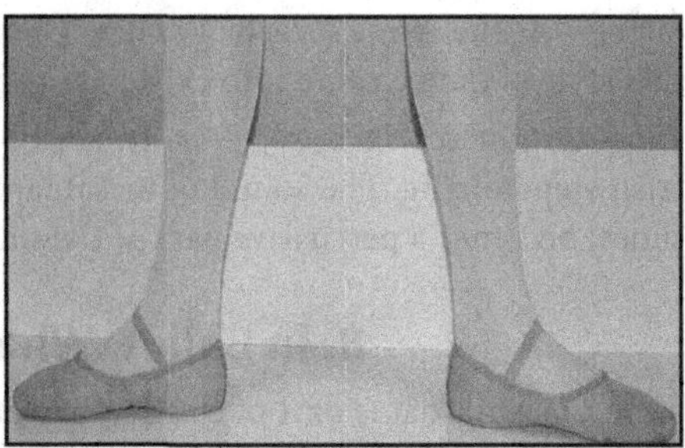

Figure 2-2. Second position feet—from position 1, slide heels apart about one and a half foot length.

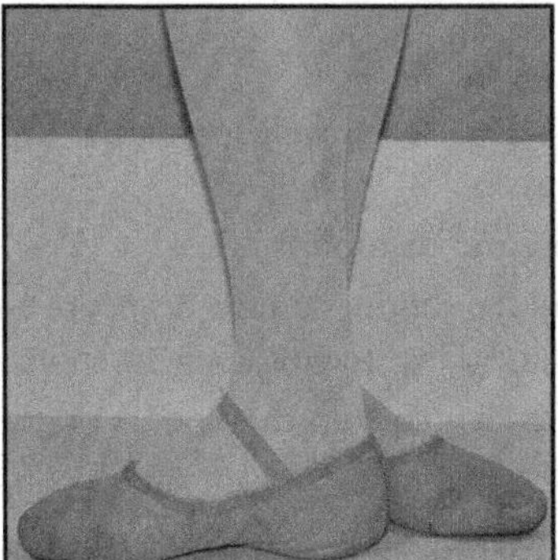

Figure 2-3. Third position feet—heel of one foot is in the arch of the other foot.

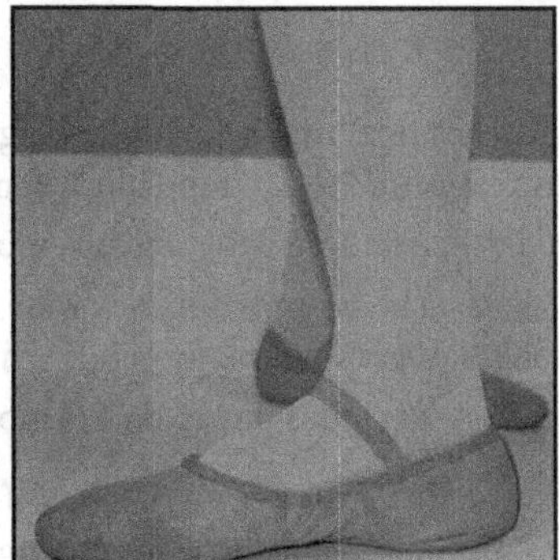

Figure 2-4. Fourth position feet—from position 3, slide front foot forward about 1 foot length.

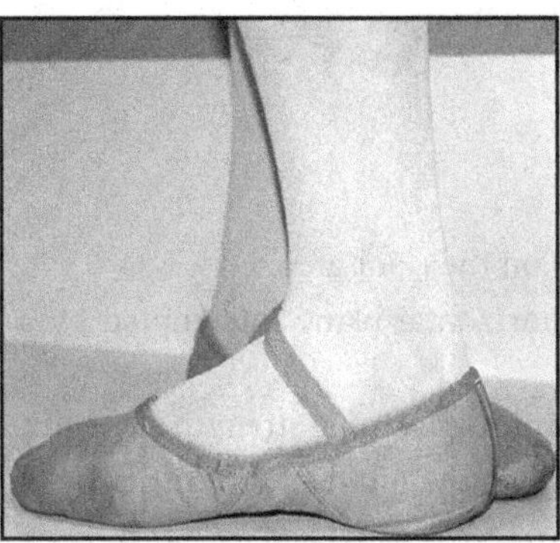

Figure 2-5. 5th position feet—heel of front foot is at the first metatarsal joint of back foot.

- *Ballroom*—A series of partner dances performed for social or competitive purposes. Origins can be traced back to the 16th century.
- *Hip hop*—A dance style that began in the 1970s in New York City. Incorporates various dance moves such as popping, locking, breaking, and krumping along with improvisation.
- *Jazz*—Developed in the early 1900s in New Orleans alongside jazz music; includes many different styles of dance, with an emphasis on improvisation, syncopated rhythm of the music, and isolation of body parts.
- *Modern*—Emerged in the early 20th century as a dance form that rejects the strictness of classical ballet. Highlights include a focus on expression of inner feeling, creativity, and choreography.

- *Swing*—As the swing style of jazz developed in the United States during the 1920s to 1940s, this style of dance came into existence and utilizes jumps, swing, and spin moves.
- *Tap*—Originated in mid-1800s. It can be traced back to African American dances and Irish stepdancing. The sound of metal taps, which are located on the bottom of the dance shoes, becomes a percussive part of the music. Some people consider tap a musical style.

8. In Ballet, What Is En Pointe?

En pointe is a skill that is part of classical ballet technique. Please see Chapter 4, question 6 for further discussion.

9. What Are the Different Gymnastic Disciplines and Skill Levels?

Female Gymnasts

Gymnastic Disciplines[5]

- *Vault*—Acceleration into the vault, height, distance traveled, number and difficulty of twists, and landing are all important elements.
- *Uneven bars*—Includes swing, release moves, and dismount.
- *Balance beam*—The beam is 4 inches wide and the routines on the beam are no more than 90 seconds long. The gymnast performs acrobatic and dance moves along the entire length of beam.
- *Floor exercise*—Includes dance and tumbling elements on the floor area.

Skill Levels 1 to 10 (Junior Olympic Program)[5]

- *Levels 1 to 4*—Starting at 4 to 6 years of age, learning of basic skills, considered recreational and noncompetitive (competition may begin at level 4).
- *Levels 5 to 6*—Starting at 7 years of age, compulsory levels, building on skills of the previous level.
- *Levels 7 to 10*—Starting at 7 to 9 years of age, competitive level. Level 10 is considered an elite level where a gymnast may attempt to qualify for the Olympics.

Male Gymnasts

Gymnastic Disciplines[5]

- *Floor exercise*—Tumbling passes and acrobatic elements on the floor area.
- *Pommel horse*—Continuous circling movements in a horizontal plane interrupted by a scissors element or handstand.
- *Still rings*—Requires stillness and proper body position while performing strength elements.
- *Vault*—Acceleration into the vault, height, distance traveled, the number and difficulty of twists, and landing are all important elements.
- *Parallel bars*—Includes swing and flight elements.
- *Horizontal/high bar*—Includes swings, release moves, and dismount.

Skill Levels 1 to 10 (Junior Olympic Program)[5]

- *Levels 1 to 3*—Starting at 5 years of age, Basic Skills Achievement Program, considered recreational and noncompetitive, focuses on learning basic skills.
- *Levels 4 to 6*—Competitive levels, progressing from basic to more complex movements.
- *Level 7*—Bridge between basic and advanced, includes the creation of the gymnast's own routines.
- *Levels 8 to 10*—Advanced competitive levels.

References

1. Mellion MB, Walsh WM, Madden C, Putukian M, Shelton GL. Martial Arts. In: Mellion MB, Walsh WM, Madden C, Putukian M, Shelton GL, eds. *The Team Physician's Handbook*. 3rd ed. Philadelphia, PA: Hanley & Belfus; 2002:732.
2. Types of Martial Arts. US Gyms Web site. http://www.usgyms.net/martial%20arts%20types.htm. Accessed August 1, 2012.
3. Which Helmet for Which Activity? U.S. Consumer Product Safety Commission brochure. www.cpsc.gov/PageFiles/117293/349.pdf. Accessed August 14, 2012.
4. Valasek AE, McCambridge TM. Cheerleading. In: Madden CC, Putukian M, Young CC, McCarty EC, eds. *Netter's Sports Medicine*. 1st ed. Philadelphia, PA: Saunders; 2010:693-694.
5. USA Gymnastics Web site. http://usagym.org/pages/index.html. Accessed June 23, 2013.

Preparticipation Physical Evaluation

3

Paul D. Brydon, DO; David Wang, MD; and Kenneth S. Taylor, MD

1. How Often Does a Young Athlete Need a Preparticipation Physical Evaluation, and When Is the Best Time to Perform It?

- High school—The American Heart Association recommends mandatory complete history and physical examination prior to any sports activities, and then every year thereafter. The National Federation of State High School Associations also recommends an annual preparticipation physical evaluation (PPE) as a precondition to participation.[1]
- College—Complete history and physical examination prior to any sports activities with a yearly interim history, heart and lung examinations, and blood pressure checkups.[2]
- Preparticipation Physical Evaluation Monograph Recommendations—The third edition of *Preparticipation Physical Evaluation* recommends a comprehensive PPE at entry into middle school and high school or upon transfer to a new school, and annual updates with a comprehensive history, vital signs, and problem-focused physical examination.[1]

It is recommended that the PPE be performed approximately 6 weeks prior to the start of the athlete's season to allow enough time to complete an appropriate work-up for abnormalities found, rehabilitate any injuries discovered, and condition athletes who might not be appropriately trained. Conversely, the PPE should not be completed too far in advance of the start of a season because this could allow new injuries or abnormalities to develop.

2. What Are the Pros and Cons of the Preparticipation Physical Evaluation at Mass Screenings Versus the Primary Care Office?

Some pros of the PPE at the primary care office are the continuity of care and easier management of chronic medical conditions, while some pros of the PPE at mass screenings for the individual include the fact that the sole emphasis is on the PPE and its low cost (Table 3-1).[3]

3. Is There a Recommended Form That Helps Me to Remember Everything That Should Be Covered on the Preparticipation Physical Evaluation?

The American Academy of Family Physicians, American Academy of Pediatrics, American College of Sports Medicine, American Medical Society for Sports Medicine, American Orthopaedic Society for Sports Medicine, and American Osteopathic Academy of Sports Medicine have developed a "Preparticipation Physical Evaluation" form that is available for free download at http://www2.aap.org/sections/sportsmedicine/PDFs/PPE-4-forms.pdf. The form includes pertinent personal and family history questions to screen for cardiovascular, pulmonary, musculoskeletal, dermatologic, and infectious disease, as well as central nervous system, women's health, and gastrointestinal/genitourinary issues. It also includes a complete physical examination form with reminders for specific pertinent positives that are most significant during a PPE.

Koutures C, Wong V.
Pediatric Sports Medicine: Essentials for Office Evaluation (pp 14-20)

Table 3-1. Pros and Cons of the Primary Care Office, Mass Screening (Stations), and Mass Screening (Individual)

	PRIMARY CARE OFFICE	*MASS SCREENING (STATIONS)*	*MASS SCREENING (INDIVIDUAL)*
Pros	• Continuity of care • Access to the patient's history and records • Easier management of chronic medical problems • Easier access to consultations • Offers privacy and a quiet setting • Often has better equipment and easier set-up • Able to see the athlete's entire story	• Efficient • Sole emphasis is on the PPE • Often little to no cost to the athlete • Studies have shown that multiple examiners find more abnormalities and recommend further evaluation[3] • Possibly can involve physicians with specific expertise/interest	• Sole emphasis is on the PPE • Often little to no cost to the athlete • Able to see the athlete's entire story • Efficient
Cons	• Often combined with annual health maintenance examination with less emphasis on PPE • Often less efficient • Requires that the patient or a parent schedules the appointment in correct time frame	• Less continuity of care • Often a louder, more chaotic setting • Only able to see one part of the patient's story • Less privacy	• Less continuity of care • Often a louder, more chaotic setting • Find fewer abnormalities[3] • Less privacy

There is no single form, however, that has been endorsed as a universal PPE form. It is important to ensure that whatever form is used includes the pertinent personal and family history questions as well as height, weight, vital signs, vision screening, and complete medical and musculoskeletal examination questions. The form must also require a parent or guardian signature for athletes who are minors. If the athlete does not supply a form from his or her state or school, many different organizations have forms available online.

4. What Are Key Questions That Should Be Asked About Personal and Family History of Potential Cardiovascular or Sudden Cardiac Death At-Risk Findings?

- Personal history—Clinicians should ask questions related to exertional chest pain, syncope, and cardiac murmur, among others (Table 3-2).[4]
- Family history
  - Sudden cardiac death (SCD) at an age < 50 years.
  - Unexplained fainting or seizures.[5]
    - More common causes of SCD: hypertrophic cardiomyopathy (HCM),[6] dilated cardiomyopathy, long QT syndrome, short QT syndrome, Brugada syndrome, catecholaminergic polymorphic ventricular tachycardia, arrhythmogenic right ventricular cardiomyopathy (ARVC), Marfan syndrome.

Table 3-2. Important Personal History Questions		
Exertional chest pain	Syncope	Palpitations
Dyspnea on exertion	History of cardiac murmur	History of cardiac work-up
Easy fatigue with exertion	Dizziness (estimated 10% with primary cardiovascular disease may present with dizziness)[4]	

5. What Are the Pros and Cons of Performing Routine Screening Electrocardiograms and Echocardiograms During the Annual Preparticipation Physical Evaluation?

- Pros
  - Multiple studies have shown increased sensitivity for identifying relevant underlying cardiac abnormalities when screening electrocardiograms (EKGs) added to the history and physical examination.[7,8]
  - When previous resting EKGs were available for review postmortem, studies have shown that 95% of SCD cases caused by HCM had EKG abnormalities, while 70% to 80% of SCD cases caused by ARVC also had EKG abnormalities.[7,8]
  - EKGs have a high negative predictive value (99.98%) for excluding HCM.[6]
  - EKGs can identify preexcitation, long/short QT interval, and Brugada syndrome.
- Cons
  - EKG does not detect all causes of SCD.
  - High false-positive rate given the high rate of EKG changes associated with normal physiologic adaptations to exertion (athlete's heart [Table 3-3]).
  - Potential for withholding an athlete from participation for benign EKG abnormalities.
  - The high cost of performing EKGs and any further work-up required. (The AHA estimated cost of $330,000 for each detected cardiac disease and $3.4 million for each death prevented.[8])
  - Liability for physicians performing an EKG with the potential for a missed diagnosis.
  - Large amount of resources required, including technicians and physician interpretation.

6. What Other Medical Conditions May Require Modified Clearance?

- Neurologic
  - *Well-controlled convulsive disorders in high-risk sports* (eg, skiing, gymnastics, high diving)—Neurologic consultation should be considered in these cases.
  - *Poorly controlled seizures*—Withhold from contact or collision and hazardous noncontact sports such as archery, riflery, swimming, sports involving heights, and weight lifting.[9]
- Pulmonary
  - *Asthma*—Only athletes with severe asthma may need to modify participation.
  - *Cystic fibrosis*—All sports are okay if oxygenation remains satisfactory; ensure acclimatization and good hydration.
- Skin
  - *Concerns*—Boils, herpes simplex virus, impetigo, scabies, and molluscum contagiosum.
  - *While contagious*—Mat sports, collision, contact, and limited contact sports not allowed.[2]

Table 3-3. Common and Uncommon Training-Related EKG Changes

Common and Training-Related EKG Changes	*Uncommon and Training-Unrelated EKG Changes*
• Sinus bradycardia • First-degree atrioventricular block • Incomplete right bundle branch block • Early repolarization • Isolated QRS voltage criteria for left ventricular hypertrophy	• Widespread T-wave inversion • Complete right bundle branch block/left bundle branch block • Brugada-like early repolarization • ST-segment depression • Pathological Q waves • Left atrial enlargement • Left axis deviation/left anterior hemiblock • Right axis deviation/left posterior hemiblock • Right ventricular hypertrophy • Ventricular pre-excitation • Long or short QT interval

- *Once cleared and no longer contagious*—Participation in all sports is allowed.
- Solitary organs
  - *Kidney*—Individual assessment for contact, collision, and limited-contact sports with understanding the risks to make an informed decision. No contact or collision sports are allowed if a single kidney is polycystic or abnormally located.[2]
  - *Testicle*—Higher risk of injury and loss of fertility in contact, collision, and limited-contact sports; use of a protective cup is recommended.[9]
  - *Ovaries*—Risk is possible but very slight, thus full participation is allowed.[2]
- Organomegaly
  - *Enlarged spleen*—Acute enlargement: avoid contact, collision, and limited-contact sports due to the risk of rupture. Participation is allowed after it is cleared by a physician. Chronic enlargement: individual assessment before contact, collision, or limited-contact sports.[2]

7. What Is a "Functional Single-Eyed" Patient and What Activity Restrictions or Protective Means May Be Needed?

- *"Functional single-eyed"*—Best-corrected visual acuity less than 20/40 in the patient's worst eye.
- If a "functional single-eyed" athlete were to lose function of his or her better eye, this would cause significant disability and have a significant effect on the athlete's lifestyle.
- The American Society for Testing and Materials has a list of approved eye guards that can allow participation in most sports; however, each situation is judged on an individual basis.
- If the sport is not conducive to wearing protective eye guards, this is a contraindication for a "functional single-eyed" athlete to participate.[10]

8. What Types of Functional Testing Can Be Performed as Part of Musculoskeletal Screening?

- *Neck*—Forward flexion, extension, rotation, and lateral flexion—range of motion (ROM).
- *Shoulder*—Resisted shoulder shrug (trapezius strength), resisted shoulder abduction (deltoid strength), internal and external rotation of the shoulder (glenohumeral ROM—degrees of internal rotation should roughly equal degrees of external rotation; limited internal rotation may be a risk factor for biceps tendon or shoulder labrum injuries).

- *Elbow*—Extension and flexion ROM, pronation and supination (ROM of elbow and wrist).
- *Hand*—Clenched fist and spread fingers (ROM of the hand).
- *Back*—Extension with knees straight (pain may indicate spondylolysis or spondylolisthesis); flexion with knees straight (ROM of the back and hamstring flexibility).
- *Duck walk*—4 steps (motion of the hip, knee, and ankle, as well as strength and balance; see Figure 37-3).
- *Single leg balancing test*—Reliable and valid test for predicting ankle sprains.[11]
- Standing on toes then standing on heels.
- *Single leg squat*—Hip, knee, and foot should be in straight line; knee going into valgus position with tibial internal rotation indicates poor hip and gluteal muscle control with potentially increased risk for anterior cruciate ligament damage and anterior knee pain.

9. How May Hearing Impairment Influence Sports Participation?

- Hearing impairment may impact acquisition of speech, social, and physical development.
- If related to vestibular apparatus damage, the athlete may have difficulties with balance.
- Most hearing-impaired individuals will have no physical disorders, unless the impairment is the result of a genetic or other disorder.[12]
- Deaf athletes can potentially participate in all sports with athletes who do not have hearing impairment; however, they may be at a slight disadvantage in team sports that require verbal directions from teammates and may require additional visual cues.
- National Collegiate Athletic Association: hearing-impaired athletes are eligible to compete "...if they qualify for a team without any lowering of standards for achievement...and do not put others at risk."[12]
- Hearing impairment >55 decibels qualifies an individual to participate in the USA Deaflympics.[13]

10. Many Athletes Must Make a Certain Weight to Participate in a Chosen Sport. What Are Guidelines To Determine Healthy Weights and Acceptable Weight Loss Goals/Practices?

- All physical examinations should include a history of weight, eating patterns, hydration practices, eating disorders, heat illness, and factors that influence weight control.
- No optimal values for body composition have been established for any sport. The body fat of "reference adolescents" ranges from 12.7% to 17.2% for male athletes and 21.5% to 25.4% for female athletes. "Low fat" is considered to be 10% to 13% for male athletes and 17% to 20% for female athletes. "Very low fat" is considered to be 7% to 10% for male athletes and 14% to 17% for female athletes.[14] Female athletes who are meeting their energy (caloric) needs will be eumenorrheic.
- Fluid or food deprivation should never be allowed. There is no substitute for a healthy diet consisting of a variety of foods from all food groups with enough energy (calories) to support growth, daily physical activities, and sports activities.
- A program for the purpose of gaining or losing weight should include the following:
  - Be started early to permit gradual weight gain/loss over a realistic time period.
  - Permit a change of 1.5% or less of one's body weight per week.
  - Permit the loss of weight to be fat loss and the gain of weight to be muscle mass.
  - Be coupled with an appropriate training program (both strength and conditioning).
  - Have a well-balanced diet with adequate calories, carbohydrates, protein, and fat.
  - Never be instituted before the 9th grade.

- Weight loss accomplished by overexercising; using rubber suits, steam baths, or saunas; prolonged fasting; fluid reduction; vomiting; or using anorexic drugs, laxatives, diuretics, diet pills, insulin, stimulants, nutritional supplements, or other legal or illegal drugs and/or nicotine should be prohibited at all ages.
- Weigh-ins for competition should be performed immediately before competition. Athletes should be permitted to compete in championship tournaments only at the weight class in which they have competed for most other athletic events that year.

Formulas and protocols have been established to help calculate minimal wrestling weight.[15]

11. An Inguinal Hernia Is Identified on a Preparticipation Physical Evaluation. How Does This Influence Clearance? Should There Be Any Modifications, and What Is the Urgency for Evaluation and Repair?

Athletes with an asymptomatic inguinal hernia can be cleared for participation in any sport. Participation should be limited based on symptoms and patient/parent/physician comfort. Close follow-up should be performed to monitor for pain or signs and symptoms of incarceration. If pain develops, withhold the athlete from participation until a repair can be performed. If signs or symptoms of incarceration develop, the athlete should be immediately referred for surgical repair. Asymptomatic athletes may be referred for repair during the off season.[16]

12. Are There Any Routine Tests That I Should Order During an Athletic Preparticipation Physical Evaluation?

- There are no routine screening tests that are recommended during a PPE. However, certain findings may prompt further testing:
  - *Complete blood count*—Consider in cases with fatigue, pallor, performance decline, heavy menstrual bleeding, low-calorie intake,[2] sore throat, lymphadenopathy, or mononucleosis exposure.
  - Lipid panel if a family history of premature atherosclerosis or dyslipidemia is present.[2]
  - Urinalysis if dysuria, hematuria, or a family history of kidney disease is reported.[2]
  - Mandatory HIV or hepatitis testing is not recommended and should be encouraged based on risk factors.[2]
  - *Sickle cell trait*—See Chapter 13, questions 7 and 8, for further detail.

References

1. American Academy of Family Physicians, American Academy of Pediatrics, American College of Sports Medicine, American Medical Society for Sports Medicine, American Orthopaedic Society for Sports Medicine, American Osteopathic Academy of Sports Medicine. *Preparticipation Physical Evaluation*. 3rd ed. Minneapolis, MN: McGraw-Hill; 2005.
2. Maron BJ, Thompson PD, Ackerman MJ, et al. Recommendations and considerations related to preparticipation screening for cardiovascular abnormalities in competitive athletes: 2007 update. *Circulation*. 2007;115:1643–1655.
3. DuRant RH, Seymore C, Linder C, Jay S. The preparticipation examination of athletes: comparison of single and multiple examiners. *Am J Dis Child*. 1985;139(7):657–661.
4. Newman-Toker DE, Dy FJ, Stanton VA, Zee DS, Calkins H, Robinson K. How often is dizziness from primary cardiovascular disease true vertigo? A systematic review. *J Gen Intern Med*. 2008;23(12):2087–2094.
5. Campbell RM, Berger S, Drezner J. Sudden cardiac arrest in children and young athletes: the importance of a detailed personal and family history in the pre-participation evaluation. *Br J Sports Med*. 2009;43(5):336–341.
6. Basavarajaian S, Wilson M, Whyte G, et al. Prevalence of hypertrophic cardiomyopathy in high trained athletes: relevance to pre-participation screening. *J Am Coll Cardiol*. 2008;51(10):1033–1039.
7. Borjesson M, Dellborg M. Is there evidence for mandating electrocardiogram as part of the pre-participation examination? *Clin J Sport Med*. 2011;21(1):13–17.
8. Drezner J, Corrado D. Is there evidence for recommending electrocardiogram as part of the pre-participation examination? *Clin J Sport Med*. 2011;21(1):18–24.

9. Kurowski K, Chandran S. The preparticipation athletic evaluation. *Am Fam Physician.* 2000;61(9):2683–2690.
10. American Academy of Pediatrics Council on Sports Medicine and Fitness. Protective eyewear for young athletes. *Pediatrics.* 2004;113(3 Pt 1);619–622.
11. Trojian TH, McKeag DB. Single leg balance test to identify risk of ankle sprains. *Br J Sports Med.* 2006;40(7):610–613.
12. McKeag DB, Moeller JL. *ACSM's Primary Care Sports Medicine.* Philadelphia, PA: Lippincott Williams & Wilkins; 2007.
13. Patel D, Greydanus DE, Baker R. *Pediatric Practice Sports Medicine.* New York, NY: McGraw Hill; 2009.
14. Haschke F. Body composition during adolescence. In: Klish WJ, Kretchmer N, eds. *Body Composition Measurements in Infants and Children: Report of the 98th Ross Conference on Pediatric Research.* Columbus, OH: Ross Laboratories; 1989:76–83.
15. American Academy of Pediatrics Council on Sports Medicine and Fitness. Promotion of healthy weight-control practices in young athletes (published correction appears in Pediatrics. 2006;117[4]:1467). *Pediatrics.* 116(6);1557–1564.
16. Ouellette LR, Dexter WW. Inguinal hernias: value of preparticipation examination, activity restriction decisions, and timing of surgery. *Curr Sports Med Rep.* 2006;5(2):89–92.

4 Injury Prevention Guidelines

Emanuel Elias, MD and David Kruse, MD

1. What Sports Are Appropriate for Each Age Group?

To predict a child's sport readiness and to determine his or her ability to engage in a certain sport, one must evaluate the child's cognitive, social, and motor development. Appropriate sporting activities can also be selected based on the developmental skills and limitations of the child's specific age group.

Early Childhood (Aged 2 to 5 Years)

Growth is rapid, with a decrease in fat percentage. During this time, children experience improvement in gait due to straightening of the legs and longer stride, but their balance is still limited because of their inefficiency at integrating visual, vestibular, and proprioceptive cues. Also, attention span is still limited. At this age, emphasis should be placed on the development of fundamental skills through play and experimentation rather than competition. Suggested activities include running, tumbling, throwing, catching, and tricycle riding.[1]

Middle Childhood (Aged 6 to 9 Years)

Children will begin to learn transitional skills, which are combinations or variations of fundamental skills. Growth during this period is slower; however, there is increased aerobic and anaerobic exercise capacity. Posture, balance, and visual tracking improve, while attention span, memory, and rapid decision-making skills are still limited. Emphasis for this age group should be placed on fundamental and transitional skill development. Suggested activities and entry-level sports include soccer, baseball, swimming, running, gymnastics, skating, dancing, racquet sports, bicycle riding, and noncontact martial arts.[1]

Late Childhood (Aged 10 to 12 Years)

Due to an earlier onset of puberty, girls are temporarily taller and heavier than boys during this age, and both are able to compete equally. Children can perform complex motor skills, and transitional skills improve. Attention span expands but remains selective, and children at this age are ready to learn strategy and increasingly complex play combinations. Children attain more adult patterns of vision. Emphasis should be placed on development of skills, strategy, and tactics. Suggested entry-level sports include football, basketball, and ice hockey.[1]

Early Adolescence (Aged 13 to 15 Years)

Children at this age experience the greatest increase in muscle mass, strength, and cardiopulmonary endurance. Compared with boys, girls experience a lesser increase in muscle strength and accumulate fat mass at a greater rate with puberty. Attention span and memory are improved, and adult-patterned vision is attained. However, there is a decrease in flexibility, coordination, and balance. Early maturing boys become taller with more strength and muscle mass, while late-maturing

Koutures C, Wong V.
Pediatric Sports Medicine: Essentials for Office Evaluation (pp 21-27)

Table 4-1. Risks of Early Specialization		
Social isolation	Overdependence on others	Manipulation and exploitation
Overuse injuries	Stunted growth and maturation	Burnout

Table 4-2. Symptoms of Burnout		
Changes in cognition and mood	Fatigue	Disturbances in sleep
Chronic muscle or joint pain	Impaired athletic performance	Impaired academic performance

girls have narrower shoulders and hips. Emphasis at this age should be placed on individual strengths. Suggested sports include the following:

- Early-maturing boys—Track and field, basketball, and ice hockey.
- Late-maturing girls—Gymnastics and skating.[1]

Late Adolescence (Aged 16 to 18 Years)

Girls continue to accumulate fat mass, and boys continue to increase in strength, size, and speed, although at a slower rate compared with early adolescence. Late maturers will catch up by this age but will tend to be lighter and not as strong as those who matured at an earlier time. Muscular strength and aerobic capacity will increase into adulthood. All sports are appropriate at this age and may help develop independence, identity, and social interaction.[1]

2. What Are the Pros and Cons of Early Sports Specialization and Playing on Multiple Teams at the Same Time? What About the Risks of Psychological and Physical Burnout, and How Can "Free Play" Be Encouraged to Prevent Burnout?

Early sports specialization is the systematic training in a single sport at a relatively young age with the goal of attaining elite status, often including year-round training and simultaneous participation on multiple teams. Young athletes may also begin specialized sport training to gain an advantage in pursuing scholarships and professional contracts, and for the opportunity to be labeled as gifted or talented. However, the chance that a young athlete will make it to the elite level or a professional status in sports remains small. This approach of early specialization poses many potential risks for the adolescent athlete (Table 4-1).

One potential risk is burnout. Burnout develops over time and is associated with the athletes' perception that they cannot meet the physical or psychologic demands placed upon them. Three primary factors involved in burnout include negative performance evaluations, mixed messages, and overtraining. Burnout can manifest clinically in many ways (Table 4-2).

Young athletes can avoid burnout by being encouraged to explore different activities and develop their own skills and interests. Hence, the American Academy of Pediatrics (AAP) recommends that sport specialization be avoided before adolescence.

3. Do Multiday Tournaments or Showcases Increase the Risk of Injuries in Children?

- With more opportunities for competition, increased playing time, and the need to maximize the use of sports facilities, youth athletes are now routinely expected to compete in multiday tournament play. This is of particular concern, since the duration and frequency of exercise, as determined by the scheduling of practices and games, are important risk factors for both acute and overuse injury. Although an increased injury rate during multiday tournaments

Table 4-3. Resistance Training Injury Prevention	
Ensure supervision and instruction from qualified professionals	Modify the training program according to the individual athlete's needs
Have the emotional maturity to accept and follow coaching instructions	Utilize appropriate equipment

Table 4-4. Benefits of Resistance Training			
Increased strength, power, and endurance	Enhanced skill and performance	Increased bone density	Improved body composition
Improved insulin sensitivity	Improved lipid profile	Reduced risk of sports injury	Promotes interest in lifetime physical activity

may result from higher intensity and level of play, overscheduling may also contribute to injury due to inadequate hydration, nutrition, and excessive fatigue between games.

- To prevent injury during multiday tournaments, a schedule should be in place that allows for adequate rest and nutrient recovery. Such a schedule depends on the type, intensity, and duration of physical activity; environmental conditions; nutritional challenges; and psychosocial factors. General recommendations include the following:
    - At least 2 hours of recovery time between games for games of moderate-to-vigorous intensity lasting more than 1 hour. More time should be allotted in warmer environments.
    - At least 7 hours of sleep between tournament days.
    - Limited volume and intensity of practice sessions within a 48-hour time period prior to tournament play.
- Showcases are programs designed to market and display athletic abilities to scouts and potential coaches. These have the potential to add unneeded physical and mental stress due to the increased effort exerted by the athletes to impress their observers. Additionally, showcases often occur in the off season, placing the athlete at an increased risk of acute and overuse injury due to suboptimal physical conditioning and decreased recovery time between seasons. As such, athletes are recommended to avoid participation in showcases. Should the athlete continue to participate in showcases, close monitoring for injury is warranted.

4. Is There Any Benefit for Young Athletes to Lift Weights? Is There a "Safe" Way to Lift?

Resistance training (also known as "weight training" by the general public) in young athletes was once considered harmful to a developing musculoskeletal system. However, resistance training has not been found to cause more injury than any other sports or recreational activities in which children and adolescents regularly participate. Most injuries that occur during resistance training are a result of inadequate professional supervision, poor exercise techniques, and inappropriate training loads. Multiple steps can be taken to prevent injury (Table 4-3).

If appropriately managed, there are many potential benefits of resistance training for young athletes, including increased bone density and improved body composition (Table 4-4).

Increasing strength in a young child can be achieved with exercises incorporating his or her body weight, such as push-ups and sit-ups. When a child is mature enough to follow directions for proper form and technique and has good body awareness and balance (usually around 7 to 8 years of age), then a more formal strength-training program can be initiated. Children with health issues should have a medical examination prior to starting a strength-training program.

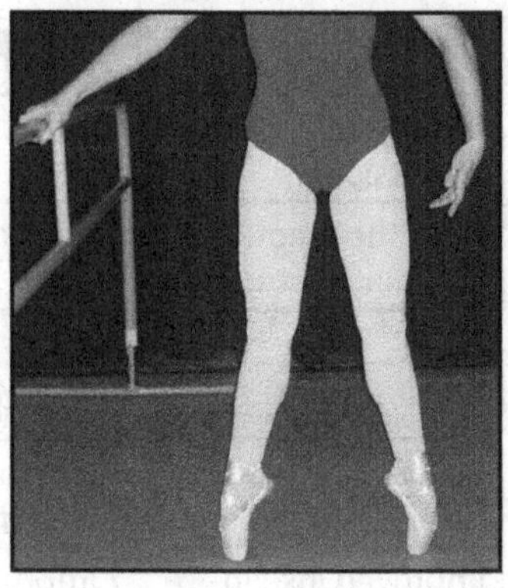

Figure 4-1. First position pointe. (Reprinted with permission of Dr. Jeffrey A. Russell.)

The explosive and rapid lifting of weights during routine strength training is not recommended by the AAP.[2]

5. What Are Performance-Enhancement Classes, and in What Circumstances May These Classes Be Beneficial for Young Athletes? When Is It "Too Much?"

In the United States, there has been a rapid increase in classes and programs designed to enhance sports performance and athleticism. These include the use of resistance training, dynamic stability, plyometric exercise, or a combination of the previous. These training programs can improve running and jumping capabilities in children. They can also reduce the rates of acute and overuse injury, likely by addressing the risk factors associated with certain youth sports, such as low fitness level, muscle imbalances, and errors in training. However, such programs may contribute to chronic and repetitive stress placed on the developing musculoskeletal systems of young athletes. Therefore, it is important that such classes structure their programs with periodization, in which the volume and intensity of training periodically changes throughout the year, such that the athletes have sufficient time to recover.

6. What Are the Latest Recommendations on When a Young Girl Can "Safely" Go En Pointe?

- In classical ballet, dancing "en pointe" means dancing "on the tips of the toes" with the use of specially designed pointe shoes (Figure 4-1).
- The following factors need consideration when determining dancer readiness for en pointe: age, technique, flexibility, strength, proprioception, placement, and training.[3]

Age

Traditionally in the United States, dancers are not allowed to progress to pointe work until the age of 11 or 12 years due to potential negative effects on the growth plates and the need for further technical development. However, it is more important that the dancer demonstrate adequate mental and physical capability for en pointe transition, in addition to age recommendations.

Technique

In ballet, adequate turnout is important. Turnout is the pointing of the feet outward (Figure 4-2). This turnout should be accomplished evenly across all involved joints. However, dancers may cheat to achieve turnout by overpronating the feet, increasing lumbar lordosis, or using excess external tibial torsion—all of which may increase the risk of injury, especially during pointe work. Dancers should be evaluated in various stances (first, second, and fifth positions—see Chapter 2)

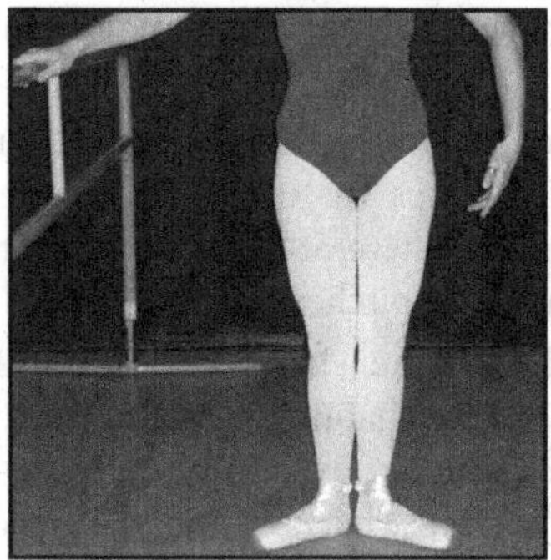

Figure 4-2. First position. (Reprinted with permission of Dr. Jeffrey A. Russell.)

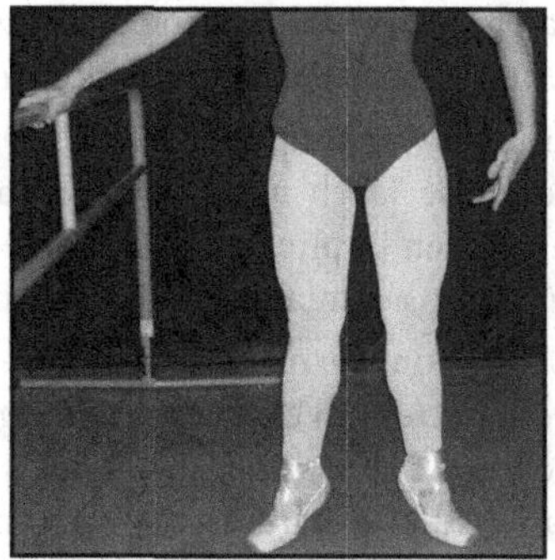

Figure 4-3. First position demi-pointe. (Reprinted with permission of Dr. Jeffrey A. Russell.)

to evaluate for such compensatory malalignments. Mastery of precursor positions is also required to ensure that the dancer has an adequate level of ability to transition to pointe work (Figure 4-3).

Flexibility

The ability to properly relevé (to rise from any position on one or both feet with the heels off of the floor) is a precursor to pointe work. During relevé, the foot should be aligned with the tibia in a straight line. This requires a minimum of 90 degrees plantar flexion, achieved at the ankle and midfoot, and 80 to 90 degrees of dorsiflexion at the metatarsophalangeal joints.

Strength, Proprioception, and Placement

These qualities may be assessed with the "Airplane," "Sauté," and "Topple" tests.

- *"Airplane" test* will test the dancer's trunk and lower-extremity strength and alignment.
- *"Sauté" test* will test the dancer's pelvic and trunk stability, as well as lower-extremity alignment.
- *"Topple" test* will test the dancer's pelvic, trunk, and lower-extremity strength, as well as proprioceptive control.

Training

No universal standard of training prior to en pointe exists. Typical schools have several levels of ballet classes. Transition to pointe work should emphasize the previous factors as opposed to years and quantity of training.

7. What Is a Little League Pitch Count, How Did It Originate, and How Does It Relate to Injury Prevention in Young Pitchers?

The Little League pitch count is a regulation for all levels of Little League Baseball that limits the number of pitches a pitcher may throw based on age, with a goal of preventing upper-extremity injury. In the mid-1990s, an increase in serious arm injuries in adolescent pitchers was documented. The pitch count originated in 2007 after studies found that the number of pitches thrown was the most significant contributor to arm injury.

Regular season pitch counts and rest requirements can be found at www.littleleague.org/Assets/forms_pubs/media/PitchingRegulationChanges_BB_11-13-09.pdf

8. What Is the Best Warm-Up Routine for Throwers/Pitches to Prevent Injuries?

- Although ineffective warm-up technique is considered a risk factor for injury, it is unclear in the current literature whether warm-ups actually prevent injury. Regardless, a warm-up prior to a physically demanding activity is widely accepted, and an adequate warm-up is recommended for youth baseball pitchers.

- The traditional warm-up includes aerobic exercise followed by stretching and then sport-specific exercise (such as arm circles and push-ups for overhead throwers). Warm-up pitches have been implicated as a source of injury; therefore, young throwers and pitchers should warm up adequately prior to throwing these pitches.
- Another common warm-up routine for pitchers is the Thrower's Ten routine, which was developed for strength and conditioning as well as rehabilitation after injury for the overhead thrower. This routine, through 10 specific upper-extremity exercises using weights or resistance tubing, targets the rotator cuff, biceps, triceps, and the flexors, extensors, pronators, and supinators of the wrist.[4]
- The AAP 2012 revised policy statement on baseball and softball states that "Young pitchers should avoid pitching on multiple teams with overlapping seasons."[5]

9. What Is the Best Warm-Up Routine for Runners to Prevent Injuries?

The traditional warm-up includes aerobic exercise followed by stretching and then sport-specific exercise. However, to date, there is lack of high-quality evidence to support the stance that a warm-up or stretching prior to running prevents running injuries.[6] Despite this, the majority of sports practitioners still strongly favor stretching, with the belief that it decreases the risk of injury.

Ballistic stretching, which is a rapid, bouncing, stretch-shortening cycle, should generally be avoided due to suspected increased muscle stress and stress-induced injury. The following are four generally accepted techniques for stretching:

1. *Passive stretching with a partner*—Stretching of muscles beyond the limit of what can be done alone.
2. *Contract-relax/agonist-antagonist/muscle energy*—Stretching with the use of the muscle's physiologic contraction and reciprocal relaxation cycle.
3. *Static stretching*—Lengthening the muscle and holding the position for 30 to 60 seconds with slow buildup; the most common form of stretching.
4. *Dynamic stretching*—Controlled movement through the active range of motion of each joint. Static dynamic stretching is performed while stationary, whereas active dynamic stretching is performed while walking or jogging (Table 4-5).[7]

10. What Are Good Recommendations for Proper Helmet Selection and Fit?

- In regards to helmet selection, it is important that the helmet is standards certified or standards approved. There are multiple organizations that maintain standards for devices such as helmets to ensure that they are safe and reliable and that they consistently perform as they are intended to. These organizations include the American National Standards Institute, the American Society for Testing and Materials (ASTM), the National Operating Committee on Safety in Athletic Equipment, and the Canadian Standard Association.
- For assessing fit, see Chapter 11, question 3, for details.
- For football, there are specific parameters for proper fit that should be followed (Table 4-6).

11. What Are the Good Recommendations for Proper Eye Protection Materials and Fit?

- The appropriate use of eye protection, usually in the form of goggles or helmet-mounted face guards, is recommended to reduce the risk of considerable sport-related eye injury by approximately 90%. About 30% of ocular injuries in children younger than 16 years of age are attributed to sports, with baseball being the most common cause of sport-related

Table 4-5. Dynamic Stretching Techniques
• Bringing the knee to the chest while walking stretches the gluteal muscles. • Walking while actively swinging the forward leg into hip flexion, keeping the knee extended and foot in plantar flexion stretches the hamstrings. • While walking or jogging forward, the trailing leg is raised and the hip is placed in flexion in an abducted and internally rotated position with the knee flexed at 90 degrees (as if the athlete were stepping over a waist-high obstacle) stretches the hip adductors. • Kicking the heels up and toward the buttocks while walking or jogging stretches the quadriceps.
Adapted from Turki O, Chaouachi A, Behm DG, et al. The effect of warm-ups incorporating different volumes of dynamic stretching on 10- and 20-m sprint performance in highly trained male athletes. *J Strength Cond Res*. 2012;26(1):63–72.

Table 4-6. Proper Football Helmet Fit			
One-inch clearance above the eyebrows	Minimal anterior/ posterior movement with pressure	Two-inch clearance from the nose to the facemask	Cheek pads snug to the face
Adequate coverage of the posterior cranium	Centered chinstrap	Ear hole alignment	

ocular injury in children younger than 15 years of age.[8] For a list of low-, moderate-, and high-risk sports in terms of eye injury, please visit www.nei.nih.gov/sports/risk.asp

- The AAP and the American Academy of Ophthalmology (AAO) strongly recommend the use of protective eyewear for sports with increased risk for ocular injury, such as baseball. Furthermore, all sport-related eyewear should meet the standards set by the ASTM. A list of the protective eyewear that is recommended for a particular sport can be found at www.aao.org/about/policy/upload/Protective-Eyewear-for-Young-Athletes.pdf
  - Lenses should be made of polycarbonate or similar material, which provides 20 times more protection than typical eyeglass lenses and can withstand a projectile traveling at up to 90 miles per hour. Polycarbonate lenses are also thinner and lighter than glass and block most ultraviolet radiation; however, the material scratches easily and may have optical distortions. Contact lenses, fashion sunglasses, regular eyeglasses, and industrial safety glasses do not offer adequate eye protection during sports, according to the AAO.
  - When assessing fit, it is important to follow the manufacturer's fitting guidelines provided with the eyewear or faceguard. In general, eye protection should fit firmly but comfortably.
  - All athletes with one functioning eye require eye protection at all times. Sports such as boxing, wrestling, and full-contact mixed marital arts are not recommended for these patients.

References

1. Purcell L. Sport readiness in children and youth. *Paediatr Child Health*. 2005;10(6):
2. Council on Sports Medicine and Fitness. Revised Policy Statement, Strength Training by Children and Adolescents. *Pediatrics*. 2008;121(4):836–837.
3. Shah, S. Determining a young dancer's readiness for dancing on pointe. *Curr Sports Med Rep*. 2009;8(6):295–299.
4. Huang J, Pietrosimone B, Ingersoll C, Weltman A, Saliba S. Sling exercise and traditional warm-up have similar effects on the velocity and accuracy of throwing. *J Strength Cond Res*. 2011;25(6):1673–1679.
5. American Academy of Pediatrics Council. Sports Medicine and Fitness Policy Statement Baseball and Softball. *Pediatrics*. 2012;129(3):e842–e856.
6. Yeung S, Yeung E, Gillespie L. Interventions for preventing lower limb soft-tissue running injuries. *Cochrane Database of Systematic Reviews*. 2011;7:CD001256.
7. Turki O, Chaouachi A, Behm DG ,et al. The effect of warm-ups incorporating different volumes of dynamic stretching on 10- and 20-m sprint performance in highly trained male athletes. *J Strength Cond Res*. 2012;26(1):63–72.
8. Goldstein M, Wee D. Sports injuries: an ounce of prevention and a pound of cure. *Eye Contact Lens*. 2011;37:160–163.

5 Sports Nutrition and Hydration

Kyle B. Nagle, MD, MPH and David T. Bernhardt, MD

1. What Are the Recommendations for Types and Amounts of Fluids During Exercise?

Athletes should drink fluids during exercise to avoid excessive dehydration (> 2% of bodyweight loss) and electrolyte imbalances. The amount, rate, and composition of fluid replacement should be individualized depending on many factors, including sweat rate and exercise duration. Sweat rates and electrolyte concentrations are influenced by multiple factors, including bodyweight, degree of acclimatization, genetics, metabolic efficiency, activity, environmental conditions, and equipment being used. Generally, rates of sweating vary between 0.5 and 2 L/h. As periods of exercise get longer, more care should be taken to replace fluids and electrolytes lost as any mismatch becomes greater.[1]

The best method for determining replacement fluids is to monitor pre- and postexercise weights, adjusting for fluids ingested during the activity. After monitoring these rates over multiple events in similar environmental conditions, a sense of the individual's general sweat rate can be assessed. An appropriate amount of fluid can then be ingested during the activity to replace the sweat losses.

For short-duration activities, plain water may be sufficient.[1] For activity lasting longer than 1 hour, carbohydrates (30 to 60 g/h) can be beneficial to maintain blood glucose and exercise performance; the best absorption occurs with a mixture of sugars (eg, glucose, sucrose, fructose, maltodextrin). Carbohydrate concentrations greater than 8% can cause delayed gastric emptying and symptoms of nausea, bloating, and vomiting. Consuming electrolytes can help prevent excessive imbalances such as exertional hyponatremia that result from excessive hypotonic fluid intake and sweat electrolyte losses. Electrolyte composition typically recommended includes 20 to 30 mEq/L of sodium and 2 to 5 mEq/L of potassium.[1]

Fluids with electrolytes and carbohydrates may be ingested in forms such as sports drinks or as plain water combined with nonfluid sources of electrolytes and carbohydrates. Water can generally be absorbed quicker if it is accompanied by some electrolytes and carbohydrates.

2. Are Sports Drinks Better Than Water?

Sports drinks may be better than plain water for certain reasons, such as the following[1]:

- They are often more palatable than water and can encourage more fluid intake.
- The addition of carbohydrates may be beneficial for exercise lasting longer than 1 hour.
- The carbohydrates and electrolytes in sports drinks can also aid fluid absorption from the gut and prevent excessive electrolyte loss.
- Drinking 0.5 to 1 L/h of a sports drink with 6% to 8% carbohydrates provides 30 to 80 g/h of carbohydrates and sufficient fluid to avoid dehydration.

Koutures C, Wong V.
Pediatric Sports Medicine: Essentials for Office Evaluation (pp 28-33)

3. Is There a Role for Chocolate Milk After Exercise?

Chocolate milk may be an effective postexercise recovery drink. Suggested recommendations of postexercise recovery intake are 1 to 1.5 g/kg of carbohydrate with some protein (0.2 to 0.4 g/kg) and approximately 16 to 24 oz of fluid for every pound of bodyweight loss (or 1 to 1.5 L/kg).[2] Generally, a carbohydrate-to-protein ratio of 3 to 1 to 5 to 1 has shown some benefit in rehydration,[2] as well as in providing substrates for glycogen replenishment and muscle and tissue repair. A recent review summarizing a number of studies found that chocolate milk provided better recovery after exercise than water or sports drinks.[3] Chocolate milk contains about 26 g of carbohydrate and 8 g of protein in an 8-oz serving for a carbohydrate to protein ratio of roughly 3.5 to 1, along with about 150 mg sodium (6.6 mEq) and 425 mg of potassium (10.8 mEq) per serving.[4] It is also delicious and inexpensive!

4. What Are the Potential Signs of Inadequate Hydration During Exercise?

- Thirst, dry mouth, fatigue, decreased performance, irritability, and headache.
- As dehydration worsens, athletes may experience cramps, dizziness, and even nausea and vomiting.
- Decreased and more concentrated urine output.

5. Is There a Risk of Too Much Fluid Intake, and What Are High-Risk Sports/Activities?

In endurance events lasting over 4 hours, too much fluid intake increases the risk of exertional hyponatremia due to hypotonic fluid consumption exceeding sweat losses. Occasionally, in extremely long events, it may be the result of excessive sodium losses through sweating. Risk factors for hyponatremia include small athlete size, overdrinking, slow speed (increased time to complete event), and lack of experience in endurance events.[1] Female gender and the use of nonsteroidal anti-inflammatory drugs are also associated risk factors.[5] Symptomatic hyponatremia occurs when serum sodium drops to 130 mEq/L or below. Signs and symptoms include confusion, headache, vomiting, extremity swelling and edema, pulmonary edema, and eventually encephalopathy, seizures, and death.[1] Any amount of weight gain during endurance events is inappropriate and should be a red flag. The keys to avoiding significant illness and death are preventing excessive fluid intake (ie, not encouraging fluid intake on a schedule or at every aid station) and providing access to salt sources (eg, pretzels, chicken soup) in endurance events.

6. Is There an Easy Way to Guide How Many Calories Young Athletes Should Consume in a Given Day?

There is no easy way to determine how many calories any specific individual needs. Resting metabolic rate, energy expenditure during exercise, and nonexercise energy expenditure vary significantly between individuals, even those engaged in the same sport. If an athlete has stopped growing and is interested in maintaining a stable weight, enough calories must be ingested to offset daily energy expenditure. If a young athlete is still growing, enough calories are needed to offset daily needs while also providing for normal growth and development requirements.[6]

7. How Much Caloric Intake Should Be in the Form of Carbohydrate, Protein, and Fat, and What Are Some Sources?

Generally the recommendations for an athlete's diet mirror those of any individual in the general population—calories composed of 50% to 60% carbohydrates, 15% to 30% protein, and 20% to 35% fat. As the overall intake of athletes increases due to the increased demand of their training, a greater percentage of their diet needs to be carbohydrates, resulting in a mixture approaching 60% to 75% carbohydrates, 10% to 20% protein, and 20% to 35% fat.

- **Carbohydrates** are the primary fuel source for working muscle. Generally, athletes will require 6 to 10gm/kg per day of carbohydrates.[7] Endurance athletes need quantities on the higher end of this range.[6] Some good choices for healthy carbohydrates include pasta, rice, whole grain breads and cereals, potatoes, fruits, and vegetables. Athletes should attempt to eat more whole foods while avoiding processed foods when possible as these contain higher fat, lower fiber, and decreased micronutrients.[6]
- **Protein** is required as a substrate for tissue synthesis and multiple systems in the body. The amount of protein required for adult athletes is generally 1.2 to 1.7gm/kg per day, with resistance trained athletes requiring 1.2 to 1.7gm/kg and endurance trained athletes 1.2 to 1.4gm/kg.[7] Sedentary adults need 0.8gm/kg of protein per day, compared to 0.85gm/kg for 14 to 18 year olds and 0.95gm/kg for 4 to 13 year olds. Adult athletes have higher protein requirements than their sedentary counterparts and younger athletes likely do as well.[2] Diets with higher than 2gm/kg of protein have shown no additional benefit, as people have no reservoir for storing excess protein.[2] Some good food options for protein include lean meats, eggs, fish, poultry, nuts, beans, whole grain breads and cereals, and low-fat dairy products.[6]
- **Fat** is an important part of the diet as we need it for protection of organs, energy, insulation, and vitamin source and transport. Athletes can use it as a fuel source, particularly in low-intensity activities. The diet should include 20% of 35% fat, or 1 to 1.2gm/kg.[6,7] It is important to try to ingest these fats as heart healthy fats, such as omega-3 fatty acids and unsaturated fats. Some good sources for healthy fats include fatty fish, nuts, and olive and canola oils.[6]

8. What Is Carboloading, How Is It Done, and Is There Any Evidence for Its Use?

For several days before a competition, athletes will decrease their level of physical activity while increasing carbohydrate intake to maximize the level of glycogen in muscles and the liver and to improve athletic performance. Techniques range from 6 days to as low as 1 day of high carbohydrate intake (10 g/kg/day) coupled with inactivity, while some methods suggest a hard, glycogen-depleting workout prior to initiating a high-carbohydrate diet. Some studies, however, have not found a glycogen-depleting workout to be necessary.[8] Studies have shown that this technique can increase the level of glycogen stored in the muscles, but results have been inconsistent regarding performance improvement following carboloading and when compared with a general athletic diet.[2,8] If carboloading is effective, it is most likely to work for activities exceeding 90 minutes.[8]

9. What Are Some Good Food Choices for Before, During, and After Exercise?

- Variation in palates, tolerance, and experience make specific activity-related food recommendations difficult, so some general guidelines are provided.
- Encourage athletes to experiment with different food choices to determine what works best for them. This experimentation is best done prior to practices or less-important competitions to reduce the possibility of experiencing a poor outcome on the day of an important competition.

Pre-Exercise

If possible, an athlete should consume a pre-activity meal with approximately 4 g/kg of carbohydrates 3 to 4 hours before the exercise.[2,7,9] If an athlete has trouble tolerating solid foods, liquid meals such as smoothies can be an alternative.

- *Example*—Pasta with sauce, a dinner roll, and fruit. Or, if earlier in the day, oatmeal, granola, or whole-wheat pancakes, along with 1 or 2 eggs, yogurt, and fruit.
- *1 to 2 hours before exercise*—A snack of 0.5 to 1 g/kg of carbohydrates, which can be as simple as a banana or an energy bar.[2,9]

During Exercise

Carbohydrates (30 to 60 g/h), particularly if exercise lasts over 1 hour, can be broken down to 0.7 g/kg/h divided every 15 to 20 minutes.[2,7,9]

- If the athlete is having trouble tolerating pre-exercise meals, start replacement earlier during the activity.

The carbohydrates can be ingested as liquids in the form of sports drinks. Other choices include energy gels or bars accompanied by water and, depending on the type of exercise and the athlete's tolerance, more solid foods such as fig bars, dried fruit, or squares of jelly sandwiches.

Postexercise

It is important to provide nutrients and substrates to start replenishing losses.

- Carbohydrates (1 to 1.5 g/kg), particularly in the first 30 minutes after exercise, can help restore muscle glycogen stores.[7] Some experts suggest that adding a small amount of protein (0.2 to 0.4 g/kg) may also help with recovery.[2,6,7]
- One should ingest approximately 16 to 24 oz of fluid per pound of bodyweight lost.[7]
- Options include chocolate milk, a sports drink, or water accompanied by salty foods such as pretzels. String cheese, an egg, or yogurt (particularly protein-rich Greek yogurt) are all good sources of the small amount of protein that is needed.

10. What Are Some Good Nutritional Recommendations for Young Athletes Playing on Travel Teams or Participating in All-Day Tournaments?

- Following the guidelines previously mentioned can help with making good decisions.
- Avoiding fast food will likely result in better nutrition and performance.
- Easy-to-make, cold breakfast foods while travelling include peanut butter and jelly sandwiches, as well as granola or oatmeal, nuts, and fruit.
- Athletes, coaches, and parents should work together to ensure that the athlete is obtaining enough calories to meet his or her energy and fluid needs, particularly if there is little time between workouts or competitions.

During an all-day tournament, the general guidelines regarding fluids and nutrition replenishment during exercise should be followed.

- It is important to remember to replenish fluids and nutrients throughout the day.
- Sometimes during extended bouts of exercise, it is difficult on the palate to continue fueling on sports drinks. In this case, ingesting a combination of plain water and some solid carbohydrates such as bagels or breads, or some salty snacks such as pretzels, can help encourage fluid and nutrient intake.
- If there is enough time between games, athletes may want to approach refueling between games as postexercise recovery. Peanut butter and jelly sandwiches are a great option, as they have a good amount of carbohydrates mixed with some protein to aid recovery.
- If there are 3 to 4 hours or more before the next game, a full pre-exercise meal may be warranted to help with recovery before the next event.

11. Are There Any Particular Nutritional Concerns for Teenage Female Athletes?

- Young female athletes do have some particular nutritional concerns, although some of these concerns are relevant to male athletes as well. Calcium is a necessary mineral for bone growth and muscle function. Many male and female youth in the United States who are older than 6 years of age do not get the daily recommended amounts of calcium in their diets, which is 1300 mg per day for adolescents aged 9 to 18 years. Peak bone mass is attained during adolescence for both genders, and low calcium intake may be related to lower bone mass and issues with bone density later in life.[9]

- Iron requirements in athletes do not appear to be greater than those for the general population, despite some increased losses from the gut during exercise and through exercise-related hemolysis. Female athletes are at a greater risk of having low levels of iron, primarily due to iron losses from menstruation. Iron deficiency anemia is related to poor athletic performance. Controversy remains over the effect of nonanemic iron deficiency on athletic performance. Adolescent females should be encouraged to eat 4 servings of iron-rich foods each day compared with 3 servings for male athletes.[9] If it is determined that a need for iron supplementation is required, oral supplementation 3 times a day is usually sufficient, should be accompanied with vitamin C supplementation between meals, and should not be taken at the same time as calcium supplementation.
- Many female athletes have a negative energy balance in general. This can be particularly true in aesthetic sports, running, and weight-dependent sports, where a leaner body can promote an athletic advantage. This negative energy balance may put female athletes at risk for energy-availability issues, menstrual dysfunction, and low bone density (known as the "Female Athlete Triad"). Correcting that energy imbalance is the key to addressing the triad.[10] It can often be helpful to frame discussions regarding diet and adequate caloric intake with female teenage athletes around the importance of adequate energy balance to maintain health and athletic performance.
- Athletes who adopt a vegetarian or vegan diet may be at risk of insufficient iron and protein intake and are strongly recommended to work with a dietician to ensure that they ingest adequate amounts of nonmeat or nonanimal product sources of iron and protein.

12. Many Young People Are Drinking "Energy Drinks." Are These the Same as Sports Drinks, and What Are the Possible Risks?

Energy drinks are not the same as sports drinks, although adolescents and parents may not be aware of the differences.

- Sports drinks are flavored fluids, usually consisting of 6% to 8% carbohydrates, and often with electrolytes, designed for fluid, nutrient, and electrolyte replacement
- Energy drinks are commercial beverages marketed as providing energy. Often, they do contain carbohydrates; however, they also usually contain stimulants such as caffeine and guarana (a plant extract) as the primary sources of energy. They may also contain other supplements such as amino acids.

Carbohydrates in energy drinks often can be in greater concentrations than recommended for optimal athletic performance. This can lead to delayed gastric emptying and gastrointestinal distress. The levels of caffeine and stimulants can also be dangerously high. In fact, some energy drinks can have over 500 mg of caffeine per bottle, which is equivalent to over 14 cans of common soft drinks. Guarana contains 40 mg caffeine/g, further increasing the amount of caffeine. Effects of caffeine include increased heart rate, elevated blood pressure, increased attention, diuresis, and disturbances in sleep and mood. Anxiety can be worsened by caffeine, and caffeine can also trigger arrhythmias. Caffeine use can lead to physical and psychological dependence, with withdrawal symptoms including headache, fatigue, drowsiness, irritability, difficulty concentrating, depressed moods, and muscle pain. Further, the effects of amino acid supplements in energy drinks also have not been supported in clinical trials. Energy drinks are strongly discouraged in youth in general and in athletes of any age.[11]

References

1. Sawka MN, Burke LM, Eichner ER, et al. Exercise and fluid replacement. American College of Sports Medicine position stand. *Med Sci Sports Exerc.* 2007;39(2):377–390.
2. Kleinman RE, ed. Sports nutrition. In: *Pediatric Nutrition Handbook*. Elk Grove Village, IL: American Academy of Pediatrics; 2009:225–247.
3. Spaccarotella KJ, Andzel WD. Building a beverage for recovery from endurance activity: a review. *J Strength Cond Res.* 2011;25(5):1210–1224.
4. Low-fat chocolate milk (1%). CalorieKing Web site. www.calorieking.com/foods/calories-in-milk-flavored-milk-chocolate-low-fat-1_f-ZmlkPTExNjc0MA.html. Accessed June 10, 2013.
5. Divine J, Takagashi J. Exercise in the heat and heat illness. In: Madden CC, Putukian M, Young CC, McCarty EC, eds. *Netter's Sports Medicine.* Philadelphia, PA: Saunders Elsevier; 2010:139–148.
6. Gruner, M. Sports nutrition. In: Madden CC, Putukian M, Young CC, McCarty EC, eds. *Netter's Sports Medicine.* Philadelphia, PA: Saunders Elsevier; 2010:31–37.
7. Rodriguez NR, DiMarco NM, Langley S. Nutrition and athletic performance. American College of Sports Medicine position stand. *Med Sci Sports Exerc.* 2009;41(3):709–731.
8. Sedlock DA. The latest on carbohydrate loading: a practical approach. *Curr Sports Med Rep.* 2008;7(4):209–213.
9. LaBotz M. Sports nutrition. In: Harris SS, Anderson SJ. *Care of the Young Athlete.* 2nd ed. Elk Grove Village, IL: American Academy of Pediatrics; 2010:71–80.
10. Frankovich RJ. The female athlete. In: Madden CC, Putukian M, Young CC, McCarty EC, eds. *Netter's Sports Medicine.* Philadelphia, PA: Saunders Elsevier; 2010:72–85.
11. American Academy of Pediatrics Committee on Nutrition and Council on Sports Medicine and Fitness. Sports drinks and energy drinks for children and adolescents: are they appropriate? *Pediatrics.* 2011;127(6):1182–1189.

6 Supplements and Performance-Enhancing Agents

David V. Smith, MD, FAAP and Joel S. Brenner, MD, MPH, FAAP

1. What Is the History of the Federal Laws Governing Supplements?

- Federal laws governing food, drugs, and supplements have evolved over time and have been driven by the competing interests of consumer safety through regulation and freedom of business and commerce. Historically, advancements in consumer protection and patient safety have been made following adverse public events that spur the development of more federal regulation.[1]
- Prior to 1906 there was only one food and drug safety law in the United States. The Food and Drugs Act was passed by congress in 1906 and criminalized the misbranding or adulteration of foods, drinks, and drugs. Before the Food and Drugs Act, patent medications or medicinal elixirs were largely unregulated and often contained opiates or cocaine. There were no legal restrictions governing their sale or labeling accuracy.
- The Federal Food, Drug, and Cosmetic Act of 1938 (FFDCA) was passed after more than 100 patients died secondary to toxicity from a solvent similar to antifreeze that was used to prepare a liquid antibiotic.[2] The solvent was known to be toxic and was banned from foods, but it still caused a rash of deaths because prior to 1938, there was no requirement to test patent medications for their safety. The FFDCA mandated that manufacturers premarket drug test their products for safety. Further amendments strengthened the FFDCA and mandated premarket testing of drug effectiveness following the tragic effects of thalidomide in Europe and, to a lesser extent, in the United States. These laws did not apply to a relatively new class of products: dietary supplements.
- The Dietary Supplement Health and Education Act of 1994 (DSHEA) created the modern regulatory framework for dietary supplements. Dietary supplements are defined by the US Food and Drug Administration (FDA) as one or any combination of a vitamin, a mineral, an herb or other botanical, an amino acid, a dietary substance for use by man to supplement the diet by increasing the total dietary intake (eg, enzymes or tissues from organs or glands), or a concentrate, metabolite, constituent, or extract.[3] Dietary supplements that were sold in the United States before 1994 may be marketed without any evidence of efficacy or safety.[4] Ingredients introduced since 1994 must provide the FDA with evidence supporting a "reasonable expectation of safety"[4]; however, this aspect of the DSHEA has not been enforced. Since the introduction of the DSHEA, the number of available dietary supplements has increased from approximately 4000 to 55,000.[4] Under the DSHEA, there are no premarket requirement for safety or efficacy testing of supplements as there is for drugs, so a supplement can reach the marketplace without FDA approval. In addition, manufacturer claims do not need to be proven before being put on labels as long as they

Koutures C, Wong V.
Pediatric Sports Medicine: Essentials for Office Evaluation (pp 34-39)

do not claim to treat a specific disease, and they have a disclaimer that "the health benefit claims have not been evaluated by the FDA."[3] Currently, the FDA has the burden of proof in establishing that claims are actually false.[5] Under the DSHEA, the FDA has little oversight and regulatory control of supplements and faces great difficulty in getting a supplement removed from the marketplace.

2. Do the List of Ingredients on the Supplement Labels Accurately Reflect What Is in That Supplement? Are Athletes Responsible for What Is in an Ingested Supplement if They Are Drug Tested Even Though It May Not Have Been Mentioned on the Label?

- To be compliant with the DSHEA, manufacturers are required to list the ingredients in their supplement and the strength of the ingredients, and the product is supposed to contain what is represented on the label.[5] The manufacturer is responsible for ensuring that the "Supplement Facts" label and ingredients are accurate, that the dietary ingredients are safe, and that the contents match the amount declared on the label.[6]
- There have been numerous studies documenting ingredients in supplements being dramatically different than what is indicated on their labels. These studies have also detailed the contamination and/or adulteration of products with ingredients not listed on the label. A study from 2001 documented that when 12 different supplement brands were tested with liquid gas chromatograph, only one of the 12 met the labeling requirements set forth in the DSHEA. Eleven of the supplements had less than the stated dose, one had nearly twice the stated dose with 177% of the reported dose, and one was found to contain testosterone.[5,7]
- Rules governing the use of performance-enhancing substances in sports vary depending on the governing body for each sport. Often, the athletes are responsible for whatever substance enters their body whether or not they knew they were consuming it.

3. Are There Any Supplements That Cause a Gain in Muscle Mass?

- Protein and amino acid supplements can assist in building muscle when taken along with resistance training. However, these supplements are no more or less effective than food sources when energy is adequate for gaining lean body mass. If an athlete consumes an appropriate amount of energy and protein in his or her diet, additional supplementation with proteins or amino acids will not increase muscle mass.[8]
- Creatine is the most widely used ergogenic aid in athletes seeking to build muscle and enhance recovery. It is effective in assisting in repeated bouts of high-intensity exercise and can help gain muscle through hypertrophy of muscle.[8]
- Athletes take supplements containing precursors to testosterone in the hopes that they will achieve the androgenic effects of testosterone. While testosterone use can cause an increase in muscle mass, studies of prohormones such as androstenedione (Andro), dehydroepiandrosterone (DHEA), and androstenediol have not shown similar increases.[9] While prohormone supplements have not been shown to be beneficial to athletes, they have the same risks and side effects that are associated with anabolic steroids.[10]

4. How Can Protein Supplements Help Athletes? What Are the Concerns When Using Protein Supplements? Is It Banned in Athletic Competition?

- The American College of Sports Medicine and the American Dietetic Association recommend a higher intake of protein for endurance and strength training in adult athletes. However, it is recommended that these increased protein intakes be reached through diet alone, rather than through supplementation. While protein or amino acids consumed near the time of strength

TABLE 6-1. DIETARY PROTEIN REFERENCE		
AGE (Y)	*PROTEIN, MALE (G/DAY)*	*PROTEIN, FEMALE (G/DAY)*
1 to 3	13	13
4 to 8	19	19
9 to 13	34	34
14 to 18	52	46
19 to 30	56	46
31 to 50	56	46
Adapted from Institute of Medicine. *Dietary Reference Intakes for Energy, Carbohydrate, Fiber, Fat, Fatty Acids, Cholesterol, Protein, and Amino Acids.* Washington, DC: The National Academies Press; 2005.		

or conditioning can enhance maintenance of or gain in skeletal muscle, protein or amino acid supplementation has not been shown to increase athletic performance.[8]

- In adults, the current recommended dietary amount (RDA) of protein is 0.8 g/kg of body weight. In adult endurance athletes, it is recommended that they increase their protein intake to 1.2 to 1.4 g/kg. In adult strength athletes, it is recommended that they increase their protein intake to 1.2 to 1.7 g/kg (Table 6-1).[8]
- Very little data are available on the protein requirements for young athletes, although it is generally recommended that children and adolescents obtain a similar proportion of their diet in protein as compared with adults. Some limited data have suggested that adolescent athletes may require higher protein intake than adolescent nonathletes.[11] Adequate intake of total energy should be emphasized to children and adolescents, as inadequate intake of energy with prolonged exercise can lead to muscular protein being used as a substrate for energy. In most cases, young athletes will spontaneously increase their food intake for energy needs and will naturally meet their protein needs.[12]
- The safe way for an athlete to increase his or her protein intake is through increasing his or her dietary intake of protein and not through supplements.
- Protein supplements are not banned in competition, but under most governing bodies of sport, the athletes are responsible for whatever substance enters their body whether or not they knew they were consuming it.

5. How Can Creatine Supplementation Help Athletes? What Is the Evidence Behind the Use of Creatine? What Are the Concerns When Using Creatine Supplementation? Is It Banned in Athletic Competition?

- Creatine acts as a readily available source of energy in muscle tissue. It acts as a phosphate donor for adenosine diphosphate in muscle and is responsible for a substantial fraction of adenosine triphosphate synthesis during short-duration, high-intensity exercise. During the initial 10 seconds of high-intensity anaerobic activity, creatine phosphate serves as the primary source of energy for muscle.[13] Supplementation with creatine can increase muscle phosphocreatine stores by up to 20%, and has been shown to increase strength and performance in short-duration events reliant upon short-duration anaerobic output.[10]
- Common side effects of creatine include gastrointestinal discomfort, diarrhea, weight gain, and muscle cramping. There are some concerns regarding potential renal effects of creatine: at least two published case studies of patients developed renal compromise while taking creatine. The first case was a previously healthy 20-year-old man who developed

a transient nephritis after starting creatine and the second was a person with a history of focal segmental glomerulosclerosis who had a transient loss of 50% of glomerular filtration rate while on creatine.[14,15]

- The American College of Sports Medicine currently recommends against creatine supplementation in patients less than 18 years of age.[16] Like all supplement products, creatine is regulated under the DSHEA, and therefore there is no premarket requirement for safety or efficacy testing and no mandated testing to confirm that there is no contamination or adulteration of the product. Creatine typically is not banned in competition, but under most governing bodies of sport, the athletes are responsible for whatever substance enters their body, whether or not they knew they were consuming it.

6. How Can Caffeine Intake Help Athletes? What Are Issues to Watch Out for When Using Caffeine as a Performance-Enhancing Substance? Is It Banned in Athletic Competition?

- Caffeine's beneficial effects are on alertness and neurocognitive performance, particularly during periods of sleep deprivation. There have been studies conducted on the effects that caffeine has on exercise and athletic performance, especially on endurance sports such as distance running and cycling. Generally, in endurance sports, caffeine has been found to improve or sustain exercise performance.[17] Some of these studies have attributed caffeine's performance-enhancing effect to a delay in the time to fatigue. There are a number of proposed mechanisms of how caffeine may act to enhance performance and exercise, although little data to support specific mechanisms exist.[18]
- Adverse effects can occur with moderate to high doses of caffeine. Moderate doses have been associated with agitation, tachycardia, diuresis, insomnia, irritability, and increased anxiety. Severe toxicity has been linked to seizures and arrhythmias.[17] Recently, energy drinks have become increasingly popular with adolescent and pediatric patients. Energy drinks oftentimes combine caffeine with other ingredients and supplements, such as Taurine, Glucuronolactone, Guarana, Ginseng, and Ginkgo Biloba.[19] Side effects resulting from high doses of caffeine combined with these other ingredients have potential to be more significant than caffeine alone and less predictable. Adverse effects with their consumption have been reported including cardiac arrest.[20]

7. How Do Steroids and Precursors to Steroids (Prohormones) Help Athletic Performance? What Are the Potential Side Effects From Steroid Use? Is It Banned in Athletic Competition?

- Anabolic steroids taken at supraphysiologic dosing have demonstrated gains in muscle, fat-free mass, and strength.[21] Precursors to testosterone, also known as prohormones, are often marketed in supplements as having similar anabolic effects of testosterone. The most commonly marketed prohormones include androstenedione (Andro), DHEA, and androstenediol. Controlled studies have repeatedly shown that acute and long-term use of oral androstenedione, DHEA, and androstenediol do not effectively increase serum testosterone levels and do not produce any significant changes in lean body mass, muscle strength, or performance compared with placebo.[9]
- Athletes who use testosterone prohormones place themselves at risk of the same side effects as those associated with anabolic steroid use. These include, but are not limited to, hepatic damage, lipid abnormalities, mood changes, increased cancer risk, gynecomastia, and androgenization in females.[13] Testosterone precursors are banned by most

major sports-governing bodies, including the World Anti-Doping Agency (WADA), the International Olympic Committee, and the National Collegiate Athletic Association.

8. What Is Nitric Oxide, and How Does It Help Athletic Performance? Are There any Side Effects From Nitric Oxide Use? Is It Banned in Athletic Competition?

- Nitric oxide (NO) has been a focus of research over the past two decades. NO has been found to have an important role in the regulation of vasodilation, blood flow, platelet function, and immune function.[22,23] Early studies examined the therapeutic use of NO as a vasodilator in individuals with vascular compromise.[22] A number of studies have shown improvements with the use of arginine, a precursor of NO, through beneficial hemodynamic effects in patients with congestive heart disease and improved exercise capacity in patients with stable angina.[22] NO and arginine supplementation have been areas of interest for enhancing athletic performance.
- Supplements containing L-arginine are the supplements most commonly used that are purported to affect NO production. L-arginine is a semi-essential amino acid and is the only substrate for synthesis of NO. The supposed acute effects of L-arginine supplementation are the promotion of vasodilation through increased NO synthesis in muscle during exercise. Claims have been made that L-arginine supplementation can lead to increased blood flow to exercising muscle, increased nutrient delivery to muscle, and increased removal of byproducts of exercise such as lactate and ammonia.[24] While there have been well-designed studies showing that arginine supplementation has benefits to patients with cardiac compromise or endothelial dysfunction, the evidence for an ergogenic effect with exercise in the general population is lacking.[22]
- At higher doses, L-arginine has been reported to cause tachycardia, hypotension, and diarrhea. Allergic reaction and anaphylaxis have been documented. NO and L-arginine are not typically banned substances in sport. However, it is of note that supplements that contain L-arginine often contain other substances that are banned by governing bodies. In addition, as with all supplements regulated by the DSHEA, supplements containing L-arginine could be contaminated or adulterated with banned substances not listed as ingredients.

9. Growth Hormone and Erythropoietin Have Been Used by Athletes as Performance-Enhancing Agents. Is There Any Scientific Basis for Their Use in Enhancing Athletic Performance? If an Athlete Has a Medical Condition That Requires the Administration of Growth Hormone or Erythropoietin, Is It Possible to Get a "Therapeutic Use Exemption" When Competing?

- Erythropoietin (EPO) stimulates the growth of red blood cells, thereby increasing the number of circulating erythrocytes and increasing muscle oxygenation. There is a recombinant version (rEPO). EPO is used illegally in endurance sports such as cycling, cross-country skiing, and triathlons. EPO and rEPO were added in 1990 to the WADA Prohibited List of Substances that cannot be used in athletic competition.[25]
- Growth hormone (GH) has effects on many organ systems in the body. Athletes use this substance and peptide secretagogues, which cause the pituitary gland to release more GH because of its proposed anabolic effects. The scientific evidence for the performance-enhancing effects of GH is weak.[26] It is also listed on the WADA Prohibited List of Substances.
- Athletes may have a medical condition that requires them to take a medication that is on the WADA Prohibited List of Substances. The athlete may then apply for a Therapeutic Use

Exemption (TUE), which may allow him or her to use the medication during competition. GH deficiency may qualify an athlete for the use of GH through a TUE.[27]

References

1. Phillips GC. Medicolegal issues and ergogenic aids: trade, tragedy, and public safety, the example of ephedra and the Dietary Supplement Health and Education Act. *Curr Sports Med Rep.* 2004;3(4):224–228.
2. US Food and Drug Administration. The history of drug regulation in the United States. www.fda.gov/AboutFDA/WhatWeDo/History/FOrgsHistory/CDER/CenterforDrugEvaluationandResearchBrochureandChronology/ucm114470.htm. Accessed April 1, 2012.
3. US Food and Drug Administration. Overview of dietary supplements. www.fda.gov/Food/DietarySupplements/ConsumerInformation/ucm110417.htm#what. Accessed April 1, 2012.
4. Cohen PA. Assessing supplement safety—the FDA's controversial proposal. *N Engl J Med.* 2012;366(5):389–391.
5. Calfee R, Fadale P. Popular ergogenic drugs and supplements in young athletes. *Pediatrics.* 2006;117(3);e577–e589.
6. US Food and Drug Administration, Overview of dietary supplements. www.fda.gov/Food/DietarySupplements/ConsumerInformation/ucm110417.htm#safe Accessed April 1 2012.
7. Green GA, Catlin DH, Starcevic B. Analysis of over-the-counter dietary supplements. *Clin J Sport Med.* 2001;11(4):254–259.
8. American Dietetic Association; Dietitians of Canada; American College of Sports Medicine, Rodriguez NR, Di Marco NM, Langley S. American College of Sports Medicine position stand. Nutrition and athletic performance. *Med Sci Sports Exerc.* 2009;41(3):709–731.
9. Smurawa TM, Congeni JA. Testosterone precursors: use and abuse in pediatric athletes. *Pediatr Clin North Am.* 2007;54(4):787–796.
10. Smith DV, McCambridge TM. Performance enhancing substances in teens. *Contemporary Pediatrics.* 2009;26(2):36–46.
11. Boisseau N, Vermorel M, Rance M, Duché P, Patureau-Mirand P. Protein requirements in male adolescent soccer players. *Eur J Appl Physiol.* 2007;100(1):27–33.
12. Petrie HJ, Stover EA, Horswill CA. Nutritional concerns for the child and adolescent competitor. *Nutrition.* 2004;20(7-8):620–631.
13. Terjung RL, Clarkson P, Eichner ER, et al. American College of Sports Medicine roundtable. The physiological and health effects of oral creatine supplementation. *Med Sci Sports Exerc.* 2000;32(3):706–717.
14. Millman RB, Ross EJ. Steroid and nutritional supplement use in professional athletes. *Am J Addict.* 2003;12 Suppl 2:48–54.
15. Koshy KM, Griswold E, Schneeberger EE. Interstitial nephritis in a patient taking creatine. *N Enl J Med.* 1999;340(10):814–815.
16. Smith, J, Dahm DL. Creatine use among a select population of high school athletes. *Mayo Clini Proc.* 2000;75(12):1257–1263.
17. Keisler BD, Armsey TD 2nd. Caffeine as an ergogenic aid. *Curr Sports Med Rep.* 2006;5(4):215–219.
18. Rogers NL, Dinges DF. Caffeine: implications for alertness in athletes. *Clin Sports Med.* 2005;24(2):e1-13, x–xi.
19. Higgins JP, Tuttle TD, Higgins CL. Energy beverages: content and safety. *Mayo Clin Proc.* 2010;85(11):1033–1041.
20. Berger AJ, Alford K. Cardiac arrest in a young man following excess consumption of caffeinated "energy drinks." *Med J Aust.* 2009;190(1):41–43.
21. Bhasin S, Storer TW, Berman N, et al. The effects of supraphysiologic doses of testosterone on muscle size and strength in normal men. *N Engl J Med.* 1996335(1):1–7.
22. Hauk JM, Hosey RG. Nitric oxide therapy: fact or fiction? *Curr Sports Med Rep.* 2006;5(4):199–202.
23. Bescós R, Sureda A, Tur JA, Pons A. The effect of nitric-oxide-related supplements on human performance. *Sports Med.* 2012;42(2):99–117.
24. Álvares TS, Meirelles CM, Bhambhani YN, Paschoalin VM, Gomes PS. L-arginine as a potential ergogenic aid in healthy subjects. *Sports Med.* 2011;41(3):233–248.
25. Reichel C, Gmeiner G. Erythropoietin and analogs. *Handb Exp Pharmacol.* 2010;(195):251–294.
26. Baumann GP. Growth hormone doping in sports: a critical review of use and detection strategies. *Endocr Rev.* 2012;33(2):155–186.
27. World Anti-Doping Agency. *Therapeutic Use Exemptions.* www.wada-ama.org/en/Science-Medicine/TUE/. Updated December 2011. Accessed on January 6, 2013.

Section II

Medical Issues

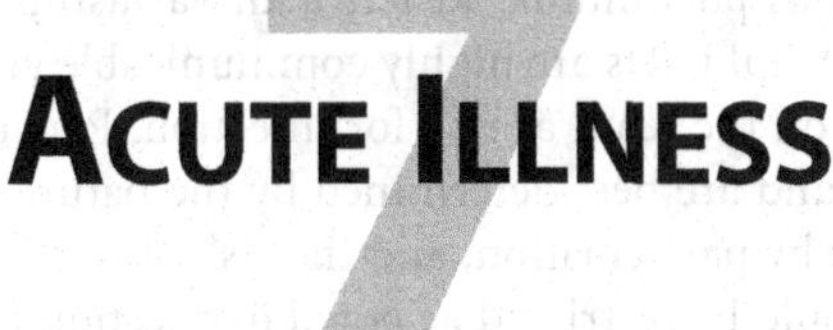

7 Acute Illness

Megan Groh Miller, MD and Rob Monaco, MD

1. What Effects Does an Elevated Temperature Have on Exercise? What Are Some Sensible Recommendations for Exercising With a Fever?

Fever is the temporary increase in body temperature in response to an illness or disease. A significant fever is an oral temperature above 100.4°F or 38°C. Fever is most often caused by the body's response to an infection, but it can be caused by other matters such as heat illness or chronic diseases (eg, cancer, autoimmune processes). The physiological effects of fever and illness on exercise include the following[1]:

- *Respiratory*—Increased airway resistance/respiratory rate, and decreased diffusion capacity.
- *Cardiovascular*—Increased heart rate and oxygen consumption, decreased blood pressure and peripheral resistance, and decreased maximal cardiac output/workload.
- *Musculoskeletal*—Decreased muscle strength and premature fatigue.
- *Temperature regulation*—Increased temperature set point in the hypothalamus, increased risk of dehydration and heat-related illness, and increased fluid requirements.
- *Athletic performance*—Decreased endurance, strength, aerobic power, and coordination/concentration/cognition.
- Fever can place significant strain on the thermoregulatory system of the body, increasing the risk of dehydration and heat-related illness. Therefore, more aggressive fluid replacement may need to be initiated.

It is essential to try to determine the underlying cause of the fever to help better determine individual decisions regarding return to play (RTP). Fever above 100.4°F suggests that a systemic reaction is ongoing and that exercise should be avoided. Strenuous exercise has been shown to temporarily impair immune function, and therefore may increase the time period for recovery or potentiate the severity of the illness. This effect generally lasts 3 to 24 hours after exercise and is most pronounced when exercise is continuous, prolonged (> 1.5 h), has a 55% to 75% maximum oxygen uptake, and is performed without food intake.[2]

The effects of fever in those who continue to exercise may lead to an increased injury rate and potentially worsening of illness. Therefore, exercise should be restricted when fever is present.

2. A Patient Has Upper Respiratory Symptoms and Wants to Exercise. What Issues Should Be Considered?

Upper respiratory infections (URIs) are the most common acute illness found in the general population. URIs can have a wide range of presentations, pathogenic causes, and treatment options. They are generally self-limiting in nature, typically lasting 5 to 14 days. Occasionally,

Koutures C, Wong V.
Pediatric Sports Medicine: Essentials for Office Evaluation (pp 41-46)

URIs can be complicated by other matters, such as sinusitis, Streptococcal *pharyngitis*, or lower respiratory tract disease such as pneumonia. Reactive airway/asthmatic exacerbations are often triggered by these infections. Viral URIs are highly communicable via direct contact and aerosols and may place other athletes on the team at risk for infection. Participation decisions should be made on an individual basis and are best determined by the nature of the type of infection, the demand placed on the athlete by participation, and the risk of transmission to other team members. Athletes with a fever should be restricted as noted in question #1.

In general, the sports medicine provider can follow the "neck check" as a general guide. In the absence of fever, myalgias, severe cough, or systemic symptoms (below-the-neck symptoms), the athlete with isolated upper respiratory tract symptoms can try to train at half of his or her usual intensity for 10 minutes. If symptoms do not worsen, then the workout can continue as tolerated. If the symptoms worsen in the initial 10-minute period, the workout should end and training should not resume until symptoms improve. Exercise should be delayed until all symptoms below the neck have resolved.[1,3]

When resuming training after recovery from an illness, the athlete should start at a moderate pace and gradually increase his or her training intensity to the pre-illness level over 1 to 2 days for every training day missed.

3. Do Common Over-the-Counter Medications Have Any Adverse Influences on Exercise?

Many common over-the-counter (OTC) medications can have mild effects on athletic performance. Individuals and sports medicine providers need to weigh the risks versus the benefits with all medications.

Antipyretics such as acetaminophen and ibuprofen are common in many OTC cold products and as stand-alone therapy. In general, they have no significant effect on athletic performance. Sports providers should monitor the dosing of these agents, as they are often overused and may cause liver toxicity and excessive renal load, particularly in the face of significant dehydration. Athlete education in this area should be considered.

Oral decongestants such as pseudoephedrine and phenylpropanolamine are effective in reducing nasal congestion but can cause insomnia, loss of appetite, and excessive nervousness. While some early studies have shown some mild to modest ergogenic benefits with these agents, the predominance of the literature supports that these substances do not have any significant benefits to performance. These common decongestants are not prohibited by most sports medicine organizing bodies. Some individuals may have hypersensitivity to these products (heart racing/palpitations), and therefore caution should be considered when using these products.

Antihistamines are common OTC medications used in the treatment of allergic disorders such as allergic rhinitis. Antihistamines, the most common of which is diphenhydramine, are also commonly used in combination cold products. There are two primary types of antihistamines: older first generation and newer second generation. The older first-generation antihistamines (eg, diphenhydramine, chlorpheniramine) can cause significant sedation and anticholinergic adverse effects, which may compromise important psychomotor skills (eg, reaction time, visual discrimination), and therefore should be avoided. The newer second-generation antihistamines (eg, loratadine, certirizine) are preferred because of their longer duration of action and minimal, if any, central nervous system adverse effects.

Antitussive medications such as dextromethorphan act centrally to help control cough. These agents can be taken individually, but are also frequently found in combination OTC cold-relief medications. In some individuals, these drugs may cause sedation, fatigue, and nausea, which can affect athletic performance. Athletes with a significant cough requiring medications should be restricted from participation, as discussed in the "neck check" section in question #2. Other medications such as beta 2 agonists may be considered for short-term use for those not tolerating or responding to typical antitussive drugs.

4. An Athlete Has Streptococcal Pharyngitis. How Long Before He or She Can Return to Play?

Group A *Streptococcus* accounts for about 10% of adult cases, but it is seen more frequently in children. Patients present with the classic symptoms of sore throat, fever, enlarged exudative tonsils, and tender anterior cervical lymphadenopathy. In younger patients, a sandpaper rash may appear on the trunk. These athletes are also at risk for dehydration due to poor oral intake secondary to pain. Diagnosis can be either by rapid streptococcal testing or culture. Studies show a sensitivity of 80% to 90% and a specificity of 90% to 100% for rapid testing.[4]

The risk of complications from *Group A Streptococcus* can be significant and may include rheumatic fever, acute glomerulonephritis, and peritonsillar abscess. Early diagnosis and treatment may be able to shorten the disease course and minimize the potential for complications. Treatment is usually with a penicillin-based antibiotic or erythromycin in those allergic to penicillin.

Individuals are considered contagious until they have been on 24 hours of antibiotic treatment. Athletes should take particular care to reduce the chance of exposure to teammates and others by following careful hygiene guidelines, such as washing hands, using hand sanitizers, covering their mouths when coughing or sneezing, and not sharing water containers or other common items. In general, it is not recommended that they participate in sports until they have been on 24 hours of antibiotic treatment to minimize the transmission to other teammates. However, RTP needs to be evaluated on a case-by-case basis, as other factors may affect the decision.

5. What Are Return-to-Play Suggestions for Water Sport Athletes With Otitis Externa, and What Are Some Sensible Prevention Tips?

Otitis externa is common in water sport athletes secondary to the prolonged exposure to moisture in the ear canal. Common infectious causative organisms include *Pseudomonas aeruginosa* (50%) followed by *Staphylococcus aureus*. Fungi such as *Candida* and *Aspergillus* can also be implicated in more chronic cases.[5] Athletes with otitis externa present with a tender, swollen external auditory canal, sometimes with exudate. Systemic symptoms such as fever and vertigo are generally absent. Treatment starts with the removal of any débris and the use of topical antibacterial drops containing neomycin, polymyxin B, aminoglycosides, or quinolones. Ototopical therapy usually should continue for 5 to 10 days, depending on disease severity, or for 3 days after the resolution of symptoms. The addition of hydrocortisone may initially help decrease inflammation. Oral antibiotics should be reserved for severe or chronic disease. Fungal infections (< 10%) are treated with antifungal medications. Chronic otitis externa is more likely associated with underlying dermatologic, allergic, or other medical issues.

For patients with frequent bouts of otitis externa, a discussion of preventive strategies is warranted, which includes drying the ear canals after swimming, using prophylactic acidifying drops (isopropyl alcohol/acetic acid mixtures), and avoiding cotton swabs to clean the ear canals (decreased cerumen predisposes to infection). In chronic recurrent cases, one should also avoid sensitizing agents around the ear, such as metal earrings or chemical shampoos. The use of a hair dryer on the lowest setting with or without a head tilt to aid fluid clearance after swimming may help accelerate drying. The use of hypoallergenic ear canal molds (hearing aid or water exclusion varieties) with or without tight swim caps to diminish recurrent infections is controversial.

RTP is handled on a case-by-case basis. In general, competitive water athletes can usually return in 2 to 3 days to their sport after the onset of treatment for mild disease. Abstaining from sports for 7 to 10 days or until the infection is eliminated is reasonable in recreational athletes.

6. What Kind of Signs or Symptoms Can Lead to a Diagnosis of Infectious Mononucleosis in a Young Athlete, and What Laboratory Tests Might Assist in Making the Diagnosis?

The classic triad for infectious mononucleosis (IM) is fever, pharyngitis, and lymphadenopathy. Many patients have a prodrome of malaise and headache. Pharyngitis occurs in 80%, with exudative

Table 7-1. Interpretation of Specific Antibody Tests for Infectious Mononucleosis			
	VCA-IgM	*VCA-IgG*	*EBNA*
Susceptible	–	–	–
Acute infection	+	+/ –	–
Chronic/reactivated	+/ –	+	+
Past infection	–	+	+
EBNA, Epstein-Barr nuclear antigen; IgG, immunoglobulin G; IgM, immunoglobulin M; VCA, viral capsid antigen.			

pharyngitis in greater than 50% of patients.[6] Exudative pharyngitis and tonsillar enlargement can cause airway compromise. The characteristic lymph nodes involved in IM are the posterior cervical chain more than the anterior chain. Lymphadenopathy may also include the axillary and inguinal regions in IM, which helps to distinguish it from other etiologies of pharyngitis. Nodes are typically large and moderately tender, subsiding over a 2- to 3-week period. Other important signs include fatigue, splenomegaly (50% to 100%), palatal petechiae (25%), and rash (10% to 40%).[6] Unfortunately, the clinical reliability of determining splenomegaly by physical examination is poor; studies show sensitivities ranging from 20% to 70% and specificity ranging from 69% to 100%.[6] A maculopapular, urticarial, or petechial rash may be found on the trunk and upper arms. A rash is more common with concomitant administration of ampicillin/amoxicillin and does not represent an allergy to these antibiotics. Rash has also been described with the use of azithromycin, levofloxacin, and cephalexin. It should be noted that among youth, symptoms of Epstein-Barr virus (EBV) infection are frequently less severe than in older adults. Symptoms usually resolve in 4 to 8 weeks, although in some individuals a more protracted time course occurs.[6]

To establish a diagnosis of IM, one should look for the presence of fever, pharyngitis, and adenopathy, in addition to typical laboratory data. One could consider ordering a complete blood count (CBC), liver function panel, heterophile antibody, and specific EBV antibody tests. The CBC will demonstrate at least 50% lymphocytes and at least 10% atypical lymphocytes.[6] Hepatic transaminase levels are usually mildly elevated in IM, occurring in approximately 50% of cases.[6] For the interpretation of specific antibody tests, see Table 7-1.

7. A Patient Has Been Diagnosed With Infectious Mononucleosis. How Long Before He or She Can Return to Play, and What Criteria Should Be Used to Make That Return-to-Play Decision?

RTP decisions have traditionally focused on clinical resolution of symptoms and the absence of splenomegaly.[6] Exertion of any kind can cause splenic rupture, which is highest in the first 3 weeks and can last longer than 7 weeks.

- For the first 3 weeks of the illness, rest without exertion is recommended.
- The current consensus from the literature is that light, noncontact activities may commence 3 weeks from symptom onset,[6] providing at this time the athlete is afebrile, well hydrated, asymptomatic, has good energy levels, and has achieved an appropriate level of physical fitness. Progression of noncontact activity should then be gradually individualized, as determined by the athlete's clinical progress.

Returning to contact activity is more controversial, and generally is not advised before 4 weeks from symptom onset. The risk of rupture may be increased in contact sports and in those activities associated with an increased abdominal pressure or Valsalva, such as weightlifting or rowing. A more cautious timing of return to activity may be recommended in these situations.[6]

It should be kept in mind that it may take several months for a highly trained athlete who has IM to return to a high fitness level. Returning an athlete too quickly to sports participation risks splenic injury and also raises the possibility of prolonging the time necessary for a full recovery.

8. Can Serial Laboratory Testing Help Determine Return to Play in Patients With Infectious Mononucleosis?

There is no firm evidence to advocate for or against the use of serial laboratory testing to help determine RTP guidelines in patients with IM. While it may be prudent to ensure normalization of any abnormalities found in laboratory screening, it is likely more reasonable to rely on the patient's clinical presentation and symptoms as the sign that infection is improving over time when making RTP decisions.

9. Is There a Role of Serial Ultrasonography Examinations to Look for Enlargement of the Spleen in Making a Return-to-Play Decision in a Patient With Infectious Mononucleosis?

The potential for splenic rupture during IM is a concern. Splenomegaly in IM is nearly universal, but splenic rupture is rare. While difficult to determine the true incidence, splenic rupture is cited to occur in 0.1% to 0.2% in most reviews.[6] Given the concern for splenic rupture, along with the poor ability of the physical examination to detect splenic enlargement, serial ultrasonography examinations have been advocated in the evaluation of the athlete with IM.[6]

In general, ultrasonography is not needed in typical IM cases, but it can be considered in certain instances, such as when there is concerning abdominal pain or controversies surrounding the timing of RTP. There is controversy surrounding ultrasonography use to assess spleen size because of both the variation in "normal" spleen size and the fact that ultrasonography does not accurately predict risk of rupture. Determining the presence or absence of splenomegaly is controversial because there are no large natural history studies of splenomegaly or ruptures in athletes. Many experts advocate that the spleen size should be "normal" prior to RTP. The quoted "normal" spleen size is 11 cm, but 2006 data describing normative spleen size in a population of 631 collegiate athletes demonstrated considerable variability of normal splenic size among the athletes.[5] One-time imaging of the spleen for assessment of splenomegaly at the time of illness is not recommended because of the wide variability encountered in normal values. One could, however, consider serial ultrasonography measurements even if there is no baseline available. The assumption is that the spleen will generally enlarge with the onset of IM and that the risk for rupture is greatest as the spleen is enlarging. However, these results would need to be interpreted with caution because the relationship between splenomegaly and the risk of splenic rupture remains controversial and unclear; the spleen, even if not enlarged, may be more susceptible to injury as a result of fragility due to the infectious disease process of EBV itself. Therefore, finding a "normal" spleen size, or a decreasing spleen size, may provide a false sense of security of decreased rupture risk in a spleen still at risk for rupture, thereby adding further controversy to the use of serial ultrasonography.

10. What Precautions Should Be Taken in a Patient With Diarrhea Before Allowing Him or Her to Return-to-Play Activity?

RTP decisions in an athlete with diarrhea will need to be made on a case-by-case basis, depending on the severity of the illness, including the frequency of the loose stools and other factors such as hydration status and infectivity of the illness. If an athlete is believed to be dehydrated, he or she likely should be held from play until his or her fluid status can be improved. To assess the degree of hydration, one should look for the return of fully hydrated bodyweight, as well as normal urine output and blood pressure. Hydration status is particularly important when exercising in the heat. In addition, if there is a concern about an infectious process leading to the diarrhea, one may consider keeping the ill athlete away from other team members to prevent an outbreak. RTP may be limited further by reconditioning if the athlete has been held out for a significant period of time.

References

1. Metz JP. Upper respiratory track infections: who plays, who sits. *Curr Sports Med Rep.* 2003;2:84–90.
2. Natarajan B. Gastrointestinal problems. In: Madden CC, Putukian M, Young CC, McCarty EC, eds. *Netter's Sports Medicine.* Philadelphia, PA: Sauders Elsevier; 2010:203–207.
3. Eichner R. Infection, immunity and exercise: what to tell your patients. *Phys Sports Med.* 1993;21:125.
4. Page CL, Diehl JJ. Upper respiratory tract infections in athletes. *Clin Sports Med.* 2007;26:345–359.
5. Osguthorpe JD, Nielsen DR. Otitis externa: review and clinical update. *Am Fam Physician.* 2006;74(9):1510–1516.
6. Putukian M, O'Connor FG, Stricker P, et al. AMSSM Consensus Statement: mononucleosis and athletic participation: evidence-based subject review. *Clin J Sports Med.* 2008;18(4):309–315.

8 Respiratory and Chest Issues

Byron Patterson, MD and Valarie Wong, MD, FAAP

1. Can Children With Asthma Play Sports? Which Sports Might Present Unique Challenges to the Asthmatic Athlete?

Children with inadequate or poorly controlled asthma may experience extreme difficulty participating in sports and might be prevented from any participation all together. However, when asthma is controlled, these children can go on to be highly competitive, successful athletes. In fact, there are well-known athletes with asthma who are Olympic champions. The ability to participate will always be based on symptoms that the athlete may be experiencing, such as shortness of breath, chest pain, and being easily fatigued. With that said, there are some sports in which environmental factors may pose potential triggers for asthma attacks. The following is a list of such triggers:

- Cold weather is a known trigger for potential asthma attacks. Therefore, winter sports such as skiing or snowboarding can pose potential challenges for these athletes. Participation in winter sports may be restricted when medical management fails.
- An outdoor environment may include exposure to pollen and grass, which can easily trigger asthma attacks. These can often be the only triggers for some asthmatics. Knowledge of these triggers can allow the athlete to properly prepare for participation in sports by using the appropriate medication prior to exposure or to switch to indoor training, if possible. Minimizing exposure to possible triggers can be especially advantageous during high-pollen count periods.
- Indoor swimming pools and ice rinks contain triggers that are by-products of the decontamination of swimming pools (chlorine derivatives) or the combustion end products from ice resurfacing machines (carbon monoxide, carbon dioxide, and nitrogen dioxide). These triggers can lead to increased airway reactivity and possible asthma attacks. For example, elite athletes who spend hours of training in these environments are at higher risk. Some factors that can help to lower the concentration of the by-products in these buildings are having proper ventilation systems and controlling the amount of chlorine or decontamination product that is used. For indoor swimming, the literature is unclear as to what level exposure of the by-product is needed to cause increased airway reaction.[1]

2. What Is Exercise-Induced Bronchospasm? For Athletes Being Drug Tested for Participation in Sports, What Medications Can Be Used?

- Exercise-induced bronchospasm (EIB) occurs as a result of airway constriction triggered by exercise. This phenomenon occurs mainly in asthmatics as well as a small percentage of nonasthmatics.[2] The symptoms (cough, shortness of breath, wheezing, and chest tightness) may occur during or following exercise.[2] Pollution, cold weather, and dry air can act as triggers for EIB. The exact mechanism of EIB is not well understood. One of the main

Koutures C, Wong V.
Pediatric Sports Medicine: Essentials for Office Evaluation (pp 47-52)

accepted theories for EIB is based on an increase in airway osmolarity.[2] There is heat loss from the respiratory mucosa when large amounts of dry, cold air move in and out of the lungs during exercise. This heat loss causes an osmolarity change within the mucosa, leading to an inflammatory reaction causing subsequent edema.

- The pharmacologic treatment for EIB in recreational athletes (exercises < 3 times per week) is the use of a short-acting beta 2-agonist (SAβ2), such as albuterol, 15 to 20 minutes prior to exercise. If the EIB is not controlled with an SAβ2, then a leukotriene receptor antagonist or inhaled corticosteroids may be used (see next).[3]
- Elite athletes (exercises > 3 times per week) may want to include the use of a leukotriene receptor antagonist such as montelukast.[3] This newer class of medications appears to be effective in preventing or controlling EIB. Inhaled corticosteroids are known to be effective for the long-term control of EIB and can be used by the elite athlete.[3] For acute attacks, an SAβ2 may be used as back-up medication if necessary; however beta-agonists should not be used frequently because they become less effective in preventing EIB over time.[3]
- There are many tests that are used to diagnose EIB, including the test most familiar to primary care physicians: pulmonary function testing. Currently, the International Olympic Medical Committee does not require testing to formally diagnose asthma.[4] Oral steroids are prohibited unless the athlete has a therapeutic use exemption (TUE) and a formal diagnosis of EIB.[4]
- In addition, athletes may try nonpharmacologic treatments such as warming up (see question 4), nose breathing in cold climates to warm the air before it reaches the lungs, and training indoors when outdoor factors (eg, pollen) cause symptoms.[2]

3. How Can a Peak Flow Meter Be Used to Help Develop Adequate Preactivity Management and to Help Monitor Asthma Control During Activity?

- Pre- and postexertion peak flow measurements in athletes can help to monitor the usefulness of treatments. A pre-exertion measurement is done at rest. The patient should then exercise to the point of causing shortness of breath or when he or she reaches 80% of his or her maximum heart rate. Then, a postexertion measurement is performed. If there is a > 15% drop from the pre- to postexertion measurements, then this indicates that the current treatment is inadequate.
- If the athlete's pre-exertion peak flow measurement is below his or her normal or expected level, then the athlete should consider taking an SAβ2 prior to exercise or avoiding exercising until he or she can meet with his or her physician to consider possible triggers and/or changes to his or her medications.

4. What Is the "Asthma Refractory Period," and How Can the Combination of Preactivity, Short-Acting Beta-Agonist Use, and a Proper Warm-Up Use This Concept to Reduce the Risk of Asthma Exacerbation During Exercise?

- For individuals with EIB, it is postulated that there is a refractory period for the onset of EIB-associated symptoms following a warm-up period. A 15- to 20-minute period of warming up at a heart rate of around 50% of the maximum heart rate will give a 1- to 2-hour window when the symptoms are abated, allowing the athlete to exercise symptom free. Along with the use of an SAβ2 when needed, most athletes should be able to perform their exercise without the onset of EIB.[5]

5. Can Asthmatics Participate in Scuba Diving? Are There Any Activities That Should Be Limited in Asthmatics?

- Scuba diving is not contraindicated for the mild or well-controlled asthmatic if the person has normal peak flow measurements prior to diving as well as not having EIB to cold temperature or emotional triggers.[6-8]

6. What Is Vocal Cord Dysfunction, and How Can It Mimic Exercise-Induced Bronchospasm?

- Vocal cord dysfunction (VCD), simply put, is the inability of the vocal cords to separate during inspiration (inappropriate adduction), a condition that can be misdiagnosed as asthma. The exact cause of VCD is unknown and probably multifactorial, as psychopathologic origins (stress) and environmental exposures (gastroesophageal or laryngopharyngeal reflex and/or sinusitis) have been postulated. Exercise-induced VCD occurs mainly in elite athletes.
- The presence of VCD may be suspected if there is an abrupt onset of symptoms that mimic asthma (wheezing, coughing, dyspnea) that do not worsen but may last from a few hours to days, or the presence of inspiratory stridor (sometimes mistaken as wheezing, with or without labored breathing).
- Often, VCD can be considered when patients are undergoing pulmonary function testing, with the flow volume loops showing a decrease in inspiratory flow, causing the classic flattening of the inspiratory loop. However, the diagnosis is made with direct visualization of the cord dysfunction during laryngoscopy.
- Treatment of VCD includes treating the reflux or sinusitis, with the mainstay of treatment being speech therapy and counseling, which can result in a high rate of resolution of symptoms over time.[9]

7. Can Children With Cystic Fibrosis Participate in Sports? What Are the Risks and Benefits? What Are the Recommendations for Safe Sport Participation?

- Currently, participation in sports and recreational activities are recommended for all patients with cystic fibrosis (CF) as a modality of treatment. Patients who are asymptomatic or with mild to moderate disease can often follow the same exercise guidelines that individuals without CF follow, which is up to 1 hour of exercise per day. However, patients with moderate to severe CF need to be closely monitored with an individualized exercise program and should have an exercise challenge test at least every 6 to 12 months.
- There are many postulated benefits of exercise in patients with CF to improve survival rates (Table 8-1).
- Patients with CF are at risk for hyponatremic dehydration as a result of high sweat-related salt loss, especially in hot or humid weather. This condition can be treated with appropriate ingestion of sports drinks that contain sodium chloride (500 mg/L). Gatorade (PepsiCo Inc) contains 450 mg of sodium per liter.
- The most significant risk for patients with CF is the decrease in lung function, which presents as a drop in oxygenation during exercise. This is mainly seen in patients with moderate to severe CF (patients with abnormal lung function), and is the reason to closely follow, test, and develop an individualized program for these patients. Scuba diving should be avoided in such patients.[10,11]

TABLE 8-1. BENEFITS OF EXERCISE IN PATIENTS WITH CYSTIC FIBROSIS	
Improves sputum clearance	Improves ion transport
Lowers the rate of lung function decline	Improves bone density
Possibly improves CF-related diabetes	Improves cardiac function

8. An Athlete Develops Pneumonia. What Are the Criteria for Return to Play?

- There is a lack of solid evidence in the literature concerning when an athlete may return to play (RTP). Many sports practitioners use the "neck check" guidelines developed by Eichner:
  - If the symptoms are present are "above the neck" (rhinorrhea, congestion, sore throat) then it is ok to participate in sports.
  - If the symptoms are "below the neck" (malaise, fever, gastrointestinal symptoms, significant cough, myalgias) then the athlete should refrain from sports participation.
  - Thus, an athlete with pneumonia should not participate in sports until symptoms have resolved.[12]
- If the pneumonia has a bacterial source, then the athlete should be on antibiotics for at least 24 hours and also have no fever before returning to sports participation. Full RTP may take weeks after having pneumonia.
- When returning to sports, a brief trial of activity can be undertaken to see if there is a reoccurrence or worsening of symptoms. If symptoms worsen, activity should postponed.

9. What Are the Signs and Symptoms of a Pneumothorax? How Does an Athlete Get a Pneumothorax? What Is the Work-Up and Management for a Pneumothorax, and When Can the Athlete Safely Return to His or Her Sport?

- A pneumothorax is air or gas in the pleural space of the chest usually causing varying degrees of lung collapse. A tension pneumothorax is when the air is under pressure and forces a collapse of one or both lungs, with a possible shift of mediastinal structures and decreased cardiac output. It may be life-threatening.
- The most common cause of a pneumothorax is blunt trauma to the chest.[13] A spontaneous pneumothorax may occur in teenagers and young adults who are tall, thin males that engage in strenuous physical activities.[13] The peak age of incidence of spontaneous pneumothoraces is the early 20s but they can occur well into the 40 year old age group.[14] More than half of these patients were found to have blebs and bullae in their lungs even though there was no history of pulmonary disease.[14]
- A pneumothorax in the majority of patients causes sudden dyspnea and chest pain that is located on the involved side of the chest. The pain may be referred to the tip of the shoulder on the involved side.
- On physical exam, there may be decreased breath sounds on one side of the chest, retractions, and hyperresonance to percussion. A chest x-ray may be helpful in making the diagnosis. Treatment options depend on the degree of the collapse and should be individualized. A small to moderate pneumothorax in a person with minimal respiratory symptoms can spontaneously resolve without specific treatment in 1 to 2 weeks. For a pneumothorax that may be causing respiratory distress or affecting cardiac function, interventions can include supplemental oxygen, needle aspiration, thoracostomy with chest tube, use of a

sclerosing agent, or open thoracotomy. The goal is to re-expand the collapsed lung. Of note is that the option of a sclerosing agent may cause issues with long-term pulmonary function in an athlete.

- After resolution of the pneumothorax there is always a chance that it may reoccur, usually within the first year of the initial incident.
- For an athlete, the process to RTP is not well described. A gradual RTP is prudent. It is recommended that the athlete not participate in any vigorous activity for 2 to 3 weeks after chest tube removal (if a chest tube was needed as part of the management plan).[13] The team physician, certified athletic trainer, and parent should monitor the athlete for chest pain or dyspnea, especially the first year after the initial episode due to the chance of recurrence.

10. What Is the Differential Diagnosis for Chest Wall Pain? What Is the Work-Up and Management for Each of These Entities, and When Can the Athlete Safely Return to His or Her Sport?

See Table 8-2 for information on common causes of noncardiac and cardiac chest wall pain in an athlete, his or her work-up, and when the athlete can RTP.

References

1. Weisel CP, Richardson SD, Nemery B, et al. Childhood asthma and environmental exposures at swimming pools: state of the science and research recommendations. *Environ Health Perspect.* 2009;117(4):500-507.
2. Weder MM, Truwit JD. Pulmonary disorders in athletes. *Clin Sports Med.* 2011;30(3):525-536.
3. Fitch KD, Sue-Chu M, Anderson SD, et al. Asthma and the elite athlete: summary of the International Olympic Committee's consensus conference, Lausanne, Switzerland, January 22-24, 2008. *J Allergy Clin Immunol.* 2008;122(2):254-260.
4. Couto M, Horta L, Delgado L, Capão-Filipe M, Moreira A. Impact of changes in anti-doping regulations (WADA Guidelines) on asthma care in athletes. *Clin J Sport Med.* 2013 Jan;23(1):74-76.
5. Stickland MK, Rowe BH, Spooner CH, Vandermeer B, Dryden DM. Effect of warm-up exercise on exercise-induced bronchoconstriction. *Med Sci Sports Exerc.* 2012;44(3):383-391.
6. Davies MJ, Fisher LH, Chegini S, Craig TJ. Asthma and the diver. *Clin Rev Allergy Immunol.* 2005;29(2):131-138.
7. Olson S, Moore LA. Persons with special needs and disabilities. In: Auerbach PS, ed. *Wilderness Medicine.* 6th ed. Philadelphia, PA: Mosby; 2012:2021-2059.
8. de Lisle Dear G. Asthma & Diving. Divers Alert Network Web site. http://www.diversalertnetwork.org/medical/articles/Asthma_Diving. Accessed June 30, 2013.
9. Morris MJ, Christopher KL. Diagnostic criteria for the classification of vocal cord dysfunction. *Chest.* 2010;138;1213-1223.
10. Philpott J, Houghton K, Luke A. Physical activity recommendations for children with specific chronic health conditions: Juvenile idiopathic arthritis, hemophilia, asthma and cystic fibrosis. *Paediatr Child Health.* 2010;15(4):213–218.
11. Rand S, Prasad SA. Exercise as part of a cystic fibrosis therapeutic routine. *Expert Rev Respir Med.* 2012;6(3):341–352.
12. Eichner ER. Infection, immunity, and exercise: what to tell patients? *Phys Sportsmed.* 1993;21:125-135.
13. Mellion MB, Walsh WM, Madden C, Putukian M, Shelton GL. Athletic injuries of the thorax and abdomen. In: *Team Physician's Handbook.* 3rd ed. Philadelphia, PA: Hanley & Belfus; 2011:448.
14. Davis PF. Primary spontaneous pneumothorax in a track athlete. *Clin J Sport Med.* 2002;12(5):318-319.
15. Maron BJ, Zipes DP. 36th Bethesda conference: eligibility recommendations for competitive athletes with cardiovascular abnormalities. *J Am Coll Cardiol.* 2005;45(8):1312-1375.

TABLE 8-2. DIFFERENTIAL DIAGNOSIS OF NONCARDIAC AND CARDIAC CHEST WALL PAIN, WORK-UP, AND RETURN TO PLAY	
NONCARDIAC	*WORK-UP AND RETURN TO PLAY*
Asthma	Spirometry testing pre- and postexercise Decrease in forced expiratory volume (FEV_1) RTP when symptoms are controlled during exercise
Costochondritis	Diagnosis is by history and examination "Pain" is reproduced by palpation over affected rib Return to play after a short break from activity; may treat with nonsteroidal anti-inflammatory drugs (NSAIDs)
Intercostal muscle strain	Diagnosis is by history and examination Dull or sharp pain with breathing Return to play after a short break from activity; may treat with NSAIDs
Rib contusion or fracture	X-ray, may need computed tomography scan, magnetic resonance imaging, or bone scan Gradually resume training when symptoms resolve
Gastroesophageal reflux	Trial of H2 blockers 4 hours prior to exercise, alteration of eating habits (timing of food and beverages in relation to exercise); work-up by standard gastrointestinal methodology (eg, ambulatory pH monitoring, endoscopy) Temporary decrease in training; return to full play when symptoms are controlled
Spontaneous pneumothorax	See text (question 9)
Infection (eg, myocarditis, pericarditis)	Diagnosis by history, electrocardiogram, echocardiogram, possible blood cultures Stop participation in all competitive sports during acute phase; see Bethesda Conference recommendations for RTP guidelines[15]
CARDIAC (EXERTIONAL CHEST PAIN, IMPROVES WITH REST)	*MINIMUM WORK-UP INCLUDES ELECTROCARDIOGRAM, ECHOGRAM, POSSIBLE EXERCISE STRESS TEST, AND USUALLY CONSULTATION WITH A CARDIOLOGIST*
Hypertrophic cardiomyopathy	See Chapter 9, question 7[15]
Marfan syndrome	See Chapter 9, question 9; See Bethesda Conference recommendations for RTP guidelines[15]
Myocardial ischemia (eg, coronary artery anomaly, aortic stenosis)	See Bethesda Conference recommendations for RTP guidelines[15]
Mitral valve prolapse	See Bethesda Conference recommendations for RTP guidelines[15]

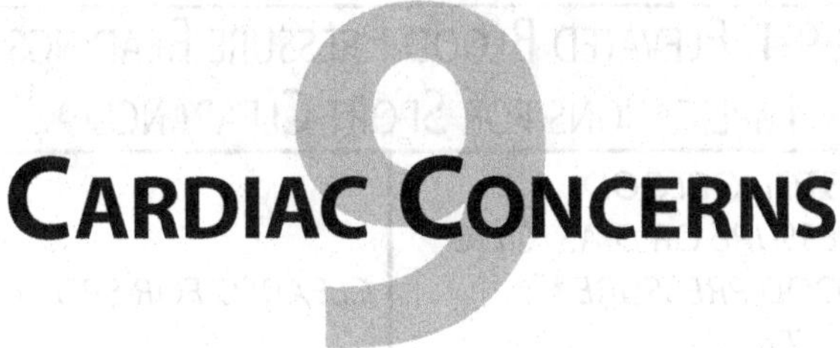

Cardiac Concerns

Kirk Mulgrew, MD and Chris Koutures, MD, FAAP

1. What Are the Criteria for Staging Elevated Blood Pressure in Children and Adolescents, and What Are the Implications for Sports and Exercise Clearance?

Blood pressure in children is graded by percentiles based on gender, age, and height. For blood pressure levels in children, please refer to: www.nhlbi.nih.gov/guidelines/hypertension/child_tbl.pdf. Table 9-1 reviews sport-specific clearance and follow-up for elevated blood pressure findings.[1-3]

2. Which Blood Pressure Medications Might Have Adverse Consequences on Exercise, and Which Ones Might Be More Favorable for Exercise?

Table 9-2 lists more preferable and less preferable blood pressure medications for use in athletes based on general side effects, adverse consequences to athletic performance, and potential as banned substances for certain sports or activities.[1,3,4]

3. What Common Arrhythmias May Cause Collapse or Sudden Cardiac Death?

Table 9-3 outlines cardiac syndromes that may cause exercise-related collapse or sudden death due to arrhythmias, and also lists key historical characteristics along with pertinent EKG/work-up findings and management recommendations.[1,5,6]

4. What Findings on History or Examination Require Urgent Versus Routine Specialist Evaluation and Temporary Removal From Exercise or Sport Participation?

- Urgent specialist evaluation
  - Syncope or near-syncope (especially if exercise related)
  - Auditory-induced syncope (even if unrelated to exercise)
  - Exercise-related frequent and/or persistent palpitations
  - Exercise-related dyspnea
  - Angina pectoris
  - Signs of myocarditis or congestive heart failure
  - Confirmed Stage 2 hypertension, and those with prehypertension or Stage 1 hypertension that have symptoms or target organ abnormalities.

Koutures C, Wong V.
Pediatric Sports Medicine: Essentials for Office Evaluation (pp 53-59)

Table 9-1. Elevated Blood Pressure Readings and Implications for Sport Clearance[1-3]

BLOOD PRESSURE STAGE	*SYSTOLIC BLOOD PRESSURE OR DIASTOLIC BLOOD PRESSURE PERCENTILE*	*CLEARED FOR SPORTS?*
Normal	< 90th	Yes
Prehypertension	90th to < 95th or if blood pressure > 120/80 mm Hg (if both values are below the 95th percentile)	Yes, if no target organ abnormalities.* Check blood pressure every 1 to 3 months
Stage 1 hypertension	95th to 99th + 5 mm Hg	Yes, if no target organ abnormalities.* Recheck blood pressure in 1 to 2 weeks or sooner if symptomatic; if 3 or more blood pressures elevated, refer within 1 month
Stage 2 hypertension	> 99th + 5 mm Hg	No competitive sports/static exercise. Cardiovascular conditioning may be okay. Evaluate/refer within 1 week (immediate if symptoms)

*If hypertension established, obtain echocardiogram for presence of left ventricular hypertrophy.

Table 9-2. Adverse Effects of Blood Pressure Medications on Athletes[1,3,4]

MORE PREFERRED AGENTS	*IMPORTANT SIDE EFFECTS FOR ATHLETES*	*PROHIBITED?*
ACE inhibitors/ARBs	Hyperkalemia and azotemia (recommend periodic monitoring of serum potassium and creatinine)	No
Calcium channel blockers	Headache, flushing, and local ankle edema	No
LESS PREFERRED		
Beta-blockers	Lower heart rate and myocardial contractility, inhibit muscle and hepatic glycogenolysis, inhibit lipolysis, hyperkalemia and muscle fatigue, and hypoglycemia	Yes (shooting, golf, archery, and ski jump)
Noncardioselective beta-blocker	Same effects as beta-blockers above, plus contraindicated in asthmatics (including EIA)	Yes (same as beta-blockers)
Alpha/beta blocker	Same effects as beta-blockers above	Yes (same as beta-blockers)
Diuretics	Affect hydration status and electrolytes and worsen total body sodium deficit after prolonged and/or repeated exercise	Yes (may be masking agent)
Alpha-agonist	Sedation and dry mouth	No
Vasodilators	Flushing, headache, tachycardia, and palpitations	No

ACE, angiotensin-converting enzyme; ARBs, angiotensin receptor blockers; EIA, exercise-induced asthma.

TABLE 9-3. COMMON ARRHYTHMIAS THAT MAY CAUSE SUDDEN DEATH OR COLLAPSE[1,5,6]		
SYNDROME/HISTORY	EKG/WORK-UP FINDINGS	TREATMENT
Arrhythmogenic right ventricular dysplasia/ cardiomyopathy • Exercise-induced arrhythmias or syncope, SCD • Fibro-fatty replacement of myocytes causing ventricular enlargement (MRI or endocardial biopsy)	• EKG: 1 or more left bundle branch QRS tachycardias, small deflection at terminal QRS, "epsilon" wave (pathognomonic —can be absent in 90%[1]) • Echocardiogram: RV enlargement	• Antiarrhythmic therapy, catheter ablation, or surgery (but unclear if these reduce SCD risk) • ICD may be appropriate • Athletes with ICDs should avoid contact sports due to risk of damage to ICD
Wolf-Parkinson-White syndrome/ventricular pre-excitation • Incidence: 1:1500 • Often asymptomatic • May have palpitations, syncope • SCD is rare (1/1000) • Higher risk often associated with accessory pathways with short refractory periods, syncope, structural heart disease, or family history of Wolf-Parkinson-White syndrome	• EKG: delta wave, evident after conversion to sinus rhythm	• EKG, exercise test, echocardiogram • Consider 24-hour EKG during activity • EPS if impaired consciousness, prolonged palpitations, ablation for rapid rates • If asymptomatic and no structural disease ◦ ~20 y/o or older: all sports OK ◦ <20 y/o may need EPS before sports • If successful ablation and no structural heart disease, (–) F/U EPS ◦ Sports maybe in several days
Long QT syndrome • Syncope • Polymorphic VT • Familial SCD • May be acquired from electrolyte abnormalities, hypothermia, CNS injury, liquid protein diets, starvation, antiarrhythmic medications, nonsedating antihistamines, and macrolides	• "Priori-Schwartz" score of 4 or more* • EKG: QTc 470 ms or more (males), 480 ms or more (females) • Genetic testing • Long QT syndrome 1: physical activity (particularly swimming) • Long QT syndrome 2: auditory or emotional triggers • Long QT syndrome 3: rest/inactivity	• Often require beta-blocker and/ or ICD • If out-of-hospital cardiac arrest or suspected long QT syndrome syncope: restrict all sports except lowest intensity • If QTc >470 (males) or >480 (females) without symptoms: restrict all sports except class lowest intensity (if long QT syndrome 3, then may liberalize sports) • If long QT syndrome mutation but asymptomatic and normal EKG, may participate in sports (long QT syndrome 1: avoid competitive swimming) • If has ICD, avoid contact sports

(continued)

TABLE 9-3 (CONTINUED). COMMON ARRHYTHMIAS THAT MAY CAUSE SUDDEN DEATH OR COLLAPSE[1,5,6]		
SYNDROME/HISTORY	*EKG/WORK-UP FINDINGS*	*TREATMENT*
Short QT syndrome • Atrial fibrillation • SCD	• EKG: QTc less than 300 ms (may only be seen when heart rate <80 bpm)	• Restrict all sports except possibly lowest intensity
Catecholaminergic polymorphic ventricular tachycardia • Syncope • Exercise-induced polymorphic VT • SCD	• EKG: includes bidirectional VT, polymorphic VT, and VF • 50% have mutation in RyR2-encoded[5] ryanodine receptor	• If symptomatic, ICD and restriction from sports except possibly lowest intensity • Restrict from swimming • If asymptomatic but with exercise or isoproterenol-induced VT, restrict all sports except possibly lowest intensity • If asymptomatic with no inducible VT, may liberalize sports
Brugada syndrome • Syncope • SCD • Spontaneous ST-segment elevation in leads V1 to V3 and syncope suggests greater risk of arrhythmia	• EKG: accentuated J-wave (V1 to V3) with ST elevation, often followed by (−)T-wave + R′. • Hyperthermia can cause polymorphic VT	• Antiarrhythmics have been ineffective • May need ICD if symptomatic or if inducible VT/VF during programmed electrical stimulation • Restrict all sports except class IA • If has ICD, no contact sports

* "Priori-Schwartz" score incorporates EKG findings including QTc durations, Torsades de pointes, T-wave alternans, Notched T wave in three leads, low heart rate, and history of syncope, congenital deafness or a immediate family history of LQTS or unexplained SCD. Points are given for each condition described above.

SCD, sudden cardiac death; MRI, magnetic resonance imaging; EKG, electrocardiogram; RV, right ventricular; ICD, implantable defibrillator; EPS, electrophysiologic study; VT, ventricular tachycardia; CNS, central nervous system; VF, ventricular fibrillation.

- Routine specialist evaluation (if asymptomatic)[1,4,5]
  - Examination suggestive of valvular disease, hypertrophic cardiomyopathy (HCM), or connective tissue disorders
  - Occasional palpitations not during physical activity
  - Stage 1 hypertension without symptoms or target-organ abnormalities

5. What Findings in Family or Personal History Might Indicate an Arrhythmia Risk?

- Personal medical history[1,4,5]
  - Metabolic—Thyroid issues, hypo-/hyperkalemia, hypomagnesemia
  - History of structural heart disease or cardiac surgery
  - Medications—Cardiac medications, caffeine, amphetamines, cocaine, ephedra (ma huang), phenothiazines, antidepressants

   - Infection—Viral myocarditis, Lyme disease, Chagas disease, diphtheria, typhoid, valvular endocarditis
   - Inflammatory—Rheumatoid or reactive arthritis (formerly Reiter syndrome), Guillain-Barré syndrome
- Family history[1,4,5]
   - Genetic arrhythmia syndromes (see question 3)
   - Premature sudden cardiac death or heart disease in relatives < 50 years old
   - Unrecognized arrhythmias—Unexplained seizures, drowning, or automobile accidents
   - Marfan syndrome (see question 9)

6. Why Is It Recommended That Cardiac Auscultation for Preparticipation Screenings Be Performed in Both the Upright and the Supine Positions?

The only murmur heard more in upright position is that of HCM. Not all cases of HCM will have an audible murmur. In those cases where a murmur is heard, it will be a crescendo-decrescendo murmur found more in the upright position or with increased intrathoracic pressure (Valsalva) due to decreased venous return. This transiently reduces stroke volume and left ventricular (LV) size, bringing together the hypertrophied septum and mitral valve anterior leaflet, obstructing outward flow and increasing the murmur. Lying down or squatting increases venous return and reduces murmur intensity.

7. Hypertrophic Cardiomyopathy Is One of the More Common Conditions Found in Sudden Cardiac Death. What Is It, How Common Is It, and How Is It Diagnosed and Managed?

- *Hypertrophic cardiomyopathy* is hypertrophy of the LV septum and free wall in the absence of LV dilation.
- Patients with HCM have an increased risk of spontaneous ventricular fibrillation.
- It occurs in approximately 0.2% of population, and most are asymptomatic.[5]
- Symptoms of HCM include dyspnea, fatigue, orthopnea, syncope/near syncope, palpitations, and chest pain.
- The electrocardiogram (EKG) may be abnormal in approximately 90% to 95% of probands (positive genetic test).[1]
   - *Abnormalities*—LV hypertrophy, significant inferior or lateral precordial T-wave inversion, left atrial enlargement, abnormal deep and narrow Q waves, and diminished R waves in lateral precordial leads.
   - *Diagnosis*—2-dimensional echocardiography or cardiac magnetic resonance (CMR) imaging with maximal LV wall end-diastolic thickness 2 standard deviations or more from mean relative to body surface area.
   - *Genetic studies*: over 400 mutations—A rapid genetic test is available.
- Treatment for symptomatic children—Beta-blockers and/or calcium channel blockers and surgical septal myectomy for severe cases; consider implantable defibrillator placement.
- Asymptomatic positive genotype, negative phenotype—Follow every 12 to 18 months with regular echo (less frequently, CMR), EKG, Holter monitoring, and stress testing. If all are negative, sports participation is acceptable.
- Probable/unequivocal HCM: restrict from participation in sports, except possibly those of the lowest intensity.[1,5]

TABLE 9-4. HYPERTROPHIC CARDIOMYOPATHY VERSUS ATHLETE'S HEART	
HCM	*ATHLETE'S HEART*
Family history of HCM or genetic testing indicating HCM mutation	Regression of LV wall thickness after 4 to 8 weeks of deconditioning
Doppler showing altered LV relaxation and filling LV end-diastolic cavity < 45 mm	LV end-diastolic cavity > 55 mm
HCM, hypertrophic cardiomyopathy; LV, left ventricular.	

TABLE 9-5. PHYSICAL FINDINGS SUGGESTING MARFAN SYNDROME, BY SYSTEM	
SYSTEM	*PHYSICAL FINDINGS*
Cardiac	Murmur and/or mid-systolic click
Skeletal	Pectus excavatum, scoliosis, wrist and thumb signs* Decreased upper-segment to lower-segment ratio Arm span > 1.05 times height, joint hypermobility, thoracic lordosis
Ophthalmologic	Ectopia lentis, myopia
*Wrist sign = the distal phalanges of thumb and 5th digit overlap when grasping opposite wrist. Thumb sign = thumb projects beyond ulnar border of palm when hand is clenched.	

8. What Is "Athlete's Heart," and How Is It Differentiated From Pathologic Issues?

Athlete's heart is a nonpathological enlargement of the heart along with resting bradycardia that is commonly confused with pathologic conditions such as HCM. High dynamic endurance and high static demand power sports can cause increased cardiac mass and structural remodeling with normal function (enlargement and increased volume of right ventricular and LV chambers, occasionally increased thickness of LV wall, and increased size of left atrium) that may be difficult to distinguish from HCM. Some criteria to help one distinguish between HCM and athlete's heart are listed in Table 9-4.

9. What Physical Findings or Observations May Suggest Marfan Syndrome, and What Further Evaluation Should Occur if Suspected?

Table 9-5 lists the physical findings that suggest Marfan syndrome.

If Marfan syndrome is suspected, then cardiovascular evaluation (echocardiography including aortic arch) is mandatory prior to starting or continuing sports activity.

- *Major criteria*—Dilatation of ascending aorta +/– aortic regurgitation, dissection of ascending aorta.
- *Minor criteria*—Mitral valve prolapse +/– mitral valve regurgitation, dilatation of main pulmonary artery, calcification of mitral annulus, dilatation or dissection of descending thoracic or abdominal aorta.

10. What Is the Differential Diagnosis of Syncope During Exercise, and Is There a Difference Between Syncope During Exercise Versus After Exercise?

In general, syncope *during* exercise has a higher likelihood of an association with cardiac abnormalities such as arrhythmias or cardiac outflow obstructions. Initial evaluation of syncope during exercise often includes EKG, echocardiography, Holter monitoring, and treadmill/bike exercise tolerance stress testing with electrophysiologic studies indicated if there are abnormalities found on initial testing or cardiac outflow obstructions. In addition to cardiac evaluation, hypoglycemia, hyperventilation, seizure, and cerebrovascular occlusion must be considered in syncope during exercise.

Syncope *after* exercise is commonly due to neurocardiogenic causes from decreased peripheral muscle contraction, reducing venous return while the heart continues to contract forcefully. The decreased volume stimulates vagal reflexes, causing vasodilation, bradycardia, and hypotension. This phenomenon has also been called orthostatic intolerance or postexercise hypotension. At a minimum, many recommend an EKG in any athlete with syncope. Prevention includes having athletes continue to walk after they finish exercising and possibly increasing their fluid and salt intake if orthostasis is found.[1,4]

11. A Patient Has Been Diagnosed With a Cardiac Condition. What Resources Can Help to Determine Some Appropriate Exercise Recommendations?

The 36th Bethesda Conference Eligibility Recommendations for Competitive Athletes With Cardiovascular Abnormalities[5] provides guidance regarding exercise/sports participation in athletes with cardiac abnormalities.

References

1. Allen HD, Shaddy RE, Driscoll DJ, Feltes TF. *Moss and Adams' Heart Disease in Infants, Children, and Adolescents.* Philadelphia, PA: Lippincott Williams & Wilkins; 2008.
2. Demorest RA, Washington RL, AAP Council on Sports Medicine and Fitness. Athletic participation by children and adolescents who have systemic hypertension. *Pediatrics.* 2010;125;1287–1294.
3. Falkner B, Daniels SR. Summary of the fourth report on the diagnosis, evaluation, and treatment of high blood pressure in children and adolescents. *Hypertension.* 2004;44(4):387–388.
4. Park MK. *Pediatric Cardiology for Practitioners.* Philadelphia, PA: Mosby, Inc; 2008.
5. Maron BJ, Zipes DP. 36th Bethesda Conference: eligibility recommendations for competitive athletes with cardiovascular abnormalities. *J Am Coll Cardiol.* 2005;45(8):1317–1375.
6. Priori SG, Schwartz PJ, Napolitano C, et al. Risk stratification in the long-QT syndrome. *N Engl J Med.* 2003;348:1866–1874.
7. Lilly, LS. *Pathophysiology of Heart Disease.* Philadelphia, PA: Lippincott Williams and Wilkins; 2007.
8. Maron BJ, Peliccia A, Spirito P. Cardiac disease in young trained athletes. Insights into methods for distinguishing athlete's heart from structural heart disease, with particular emphasis on hypertrophic cardiomyopathy. *Circulation.* 1995;91:1596–1601.
9. Loeys BL, Dietz HC, Braverman AC, et al. The revised Ghent nosology for the Marfan syndrome. *J Med Genet.* 2010;47(7):476–485.
10. Birrer RB, Griesemer BA, Cataletto MB. *Pediatric Sports Medicine for Primary Care.* Philadelphia, PA: Lippincott Williams & Wilkins; 2002.

Environmental Factors
Heat, Cold, Altitude, Humidity, and Anaphylaxis

Nate Waibel, MD and William O. Roberts, MD, MS, FACSM

1. What Are the Three Main Types of Heat-Related Illnesses, and How Can They Be Differentiated?

- The three main types of exertional heat-related illnesses are outlined in Table 10-1.
- The following are a few additional key points that are worth emphasizing:
  - Altered mental status or a change in physical ability on the field may indicate severe heat illness.
  - The diagnosis of hyperthermia can only be reliably established with a rectal temperature measurement.
  - Children are not at an increased risk of developing exertional heat-related illnesses when compared with adults.

2. How Can an Athlete Prevent Heat-Related Illness and Promote Proper Acclimatization?

- Proper preparation through education and activity modification in high-stress conditions is fundamental to preventing heat-related illness. Those who should be educated about heat-related illness include the athletes, coaches, parents, and game officials. Children should be properly acclimatized to hot conditions during training by gradually increasing intensity and duration of activity, limiting the use of protective equipment (eg, football pads), and including frequent rest breaks for water. Children should acclimatize to the heat with graduated exposure to game-day conditions over a minimum of 10 to 14 days.[1]
- Participation in physical activity should be adjusted based on the Wet Bulb Globe Temperature or dew point, which includes ambient temperature and relative humidity. In general, decreasing the length and/or intensity of the activity, increasing access to water and frequency of rest breaks, and removing helmets and pads will reduce the risk of heat-related illness.
- Children should be able to identify the signs and symptoms of heat-related illness in themselves and their teammates. Children need to feel safe to report their symptoms. Between practices or games, children should understand the importance of rehydrating, staying out of the sun and heat, and going into an air-conditioned space to recover prior to participating in the next activity.

Koutures C, Wong V.
Pediatric Sports Medicine: Essentials for Office Evaluation (pp 60-65)

Table 10-1. Types of Heat-Related Illness			
TYPE	*SYMPTOMS*	*SIGNS*	*INITIAL TREATMENT*
Exercise-associated muscle (heat) cramps	Muscle fatigue, spasm, and pain typically in the legs, arms, or abdomen	Normal to elevated core temperature up to 104°F, normal mentation, muscle spasm(s) in affected area, sometimes profuse sweating	Rest, neuroinhibition stretches to affected muscle group, hydration with sodium/glucose-containing fluids Diffuse or severe spasms may require intravenous normal saline Serum sodium should be checked
Exertional hyperthermia (heat exhaustion)	Severe fatigue, thirst, nausea, vomiting, diarrhea, headache, incoordination, dizziness, syncope, weakness	Core temperature normal to 104°F, normal mentation and clear sensorium, profuse sweating, goose flesh, pallor, tachycardia, hypotension	Move to cool location; cool with alternating cool towels applied to arms, legs, trunk, neck, groin, and axillae; hydrate with sodium-containing fluids; monitor rectal temperature; transfer to emergency facility if not improving or unable to tolerate fluids
Heat stroke	Diffuse encephalopathy with nausea, vomiting, confusion, delirium, headache, dizziness, hallucination, syncope, collapse	Core temperature ≥104°F, altered mental status, pale, sweaty, sometimes hot, sometimes flushed, sometimes dry skin, hypotension, tachycardia, seizure, coma	Begin immediate rapid cooling with immersion in cold or ice-water bath, O_2 supplementation, intravenous hydration (if possible), transfer for advanced medical care after body cooling

3. In Cases of Suspected Heat Stroke, What Are the Important Initial Management Steps?

It is essential to stop the activity and reduce the core body temperature rapidly, preferably by immersing the athlete in an ice water bath (see Table 10-1).

4. What Are Hypothermia, Frostnip, and Frostbite, and How Can They Be Prevented?

Hypothermia

- *Accidental hypothermia* is defined as the unintended cooling of core body temperature below 35°C (95°F). It can occur in both cool and wet conditions. Children are more susceptible than adults due to decreased insulation by fat and large surface-to-mass ratio. At first, the child might shiver and report feeling cold, but later becomes withdrawn and apathetic, exhibits poor judgment, or develops ataxia. Hypothermia can progress to muscle rigidity, dilated pupils, waning consciousness, extreme bradycardia, and ultimately lead to death.
- Accidental hypothermia management
  - Treatment of accidental hypothermia begins by recognizing its presence and documenting the child's rectal temperature measurement.

  - First, remove the child from the environment that caused the loss of body heat and remove all wet clothing. For mild hypothermia, it is suggested to insulate with warm, dry blankets and to encourage the ingestion of warm liquids. The next steps can include the use of forced air rewarming blankets, warmed blankets (using the microwave or oven) or warm packs, warm (38°C to 40°C) intravenous fluids, and heated (40°C to 44°C) humidified oxygen. More severe cases will require hospital-based treatment modalities, a discussion of which is beyond the scope of this text.
- Accidental hypothermia prevention
  - Adequate preparation, proper clothing, and nutrition should occur prior to the scheduled cold weather event.
  - Environmental risk assessment on the day of the event is essential and should include the current/anticipated air temperature, wind speed, rain potential, and altitude.
  - The child should be dressed in layers. Being overdressed will increase sweating.
  - Metabolic rates increase in the cold and sweat rates can be high with exertion so a child should have access to snacks and fluids to maintain energy stores and hydration.

Frostnip and Frostbite

- *Frostnip* is defined as superficial tissue "near-freezing"; is associated with intense vasoconstriction; and is characterized by discomfort, itching, or mild pain of the involved part(s). Symptoms usually resolve spontaneously within 30 minutes; neither frozen extracellular water nor progressive tissue loss is routinely demonstrated.[2] *Frostbite* is the actual freezing of tissue and can be very destructive depending on the depth and length of the freeze injury. Table 10-2 discusses the classification of frostbite injuries.
- Frostnip and frostbite management
  - The freeze-thaw-freeze cycle will lead to worse tissue damage, so rewarming should not be attempted until there is no risk of refreezing.
  - Warming by applying friction or massage to frostbite tissue should be avoided, as mechanical movement of the ice crystals will cause more damage.
  - Rapid rewarming by immersion in a hot-water bath between 40°C and 42°C (104°F to 108°F) will preserve the tissue. A mild antiseptic such as chlorhexidine added to the water will reduce the risk of infection.
  - Ibuprofen helps control pain and has selective antiprostaglandin activity that may reduce endothelial cell damage. Topical aloe gel also improves outcomes.
  - Consider giving a tetanus toxoid booster.
  - A child who has suffered from frostbite may require hospitalization for pain and surgical management (see Table 10-2).
- Frostnip and frostbite prevention
  - Risk assessment should take place prior to cold weather activities. When the wind chill temperature falls below –27°C (–18°F), frostbite in exposed skin occurs in ≤30 minutes.[3]
  - Frostbite prevention also relies on adequate training, hydration, and nutrition combined with layering clothes; keeping clothing layer next to the skin dry; and utilizing gloves/mittens, socks, and hats.

5. What Are Some Different Types of Altitude-Induced Illnesses, and How Can They Be Prevented?

There are three main types of altitude-induced illness described in children: (1) acute mountain sickness (AMS); (2) high-altitude pulmonary edema (HAPE); and (3) high-altitude cerebral edema (HACE). All types typically develop as a result of rapid ascent to an altitude >2500 m. AMS and HACE may share a common pathophysiology.

Table 10-2. Classification of Frostbite Injuries				
MILD (SUPERFICIAL) FROSTBITE INJURY			*SEVERE (DEEP) FROSTBITE INJURY*	
	First Degree	*Second Degree*	*Third Degree*	*Fourth Degree*
Clinical Appearance				
Depth of tissue freezing	Partial-thickness skin freezing	Full thickness skin freezing, soft subcutaneous tissue	Freezing of the skin and subcutaneous tissue; mobile	Freezing of the skin, subcutaneous tissue, muscle, and tendon to bone; immobile
Color of tissues after thawing	Erythematous or hyperemic	Erythematous	Blue or black	Initially deep red and mottled; eventually black and mummified
Blistering or necrosis	None	Blisters containing clear fluid	Hemorrhagic blisters and some tissue necrosis	Profound necrosis
Edema	Minor	Substantial	Substantial	Little or none
Severity				
Typically requires 4 to 8 weeks to see full extent of initial injury	No loss of tissue, no long-term sequelae	Skin loss and injury, fingernail sequelae	Tissue loss, functional sequelae	Amputation of bone, ± systemic illness, functional sequelae

Children with AMS manifest the following symptoms: fussiness, lack of playfulness, anorexia, nausea, vomiting, and disordered sleep.[4] The Lake Louise Scale (LLS) is applied to adults to assess for evidence of AMS. Children who are 4 to 11 years of age, even those with adequate verbal skills to answer the questions on the LLS, may underestimate their symptoms.[5] There is a modified scale for children called the Children's Lake Louise Score that can assist in recognizing AMS.

Although it is easy to attribute changes in a child's behavior to travel alone, most parents will likely be able to discern the difference between traveling issues and altitude illness. While it may be possible to miss the signs and symptoms of AMS, HAPE, and HACE are much easier to recognize. Children developing HACE will often have exhibited signs of AMS in addition to the following: ataxic gait; severe lassitude; headache; nausea and vomiting; behavioral changes, confusion, impaired mentation, drowsiness, stupor, and coma.[4,6] There have been reports of hallucinations, cranial nerve palsy, hemiparesis, hemiplegia, seizures, and focal neurologic signs. Children with HACE will have an elevated intracranial pressure and white matter edema on either computed tomography scan or magnetic resonance imaging. Children with HAPE present with hypoxemia, dyspnea at rest, reduced exercise tolerance, cough and hemoptysis, tachycardia, cyanosis, fever, rales, and positive chest radiograph.[4,6] It is imperative that these conditions be recognized and treated as early as possible, as HACE and HAPE can be fatal.

The single best way to prevent the altitude-induced illnesses in children is a slow ascent. A graded ascent of 300 m/day above 2500 m and a rest day for every 1000 m is typically recommended in adults and has been extrapolated to also work for children.[4] There is a subset of children for whom it may be reasonable and safe to give acetazolamide as prophylaxis, although this is purely based on expert opinion and again extrapolated from research in adults. This subset of children are those either at moderate or high risk of developing AMS and/or HACE.[6] Those at moderate risk would be the following:

- Individuals who have a history of AMS and are ascending to 2500 to 2800 m in 1 day
- No history of AMS and ascending to >2800 m in 1 day
- All individuals ascending >500 m/day (increase in sleeping elevation) at altitudes above 3000 m but with an extra day for acclimatization every 1000 m

Those at high risk would be the following:

- Individuals who have a history of AMS and are ascending to >2800 m in 1 day
- All individuals with a history of HACE
- All individuals ascending to >3500 m in 1 day
- All individuals ascending >500 m/day (increase in sleeping elevation) above >3000 m without extra days for acclimatization, very rapid ascents (eg, <7-day ascents of Mount Kilimanjaro)

Acetazolamide is contraindicated in patients who are allergic to sulfonamide-containing products. The most common adverse reactions are paresthesias, taste alteration, rash, tyramine reaction, and dehydration. Nifedipine is the mainstay of pharmacologic prophylaxis against the development of HAPE in adults. Nifedipine is used in the treatment of HAPE in children, but there are no studies involving nifedipine in children for HAPE prophylaxis.

6. What Is Exercise-Induced Urticaria, and Can It Be Prevented?

Exercise-induced urticaria (EIU) falls under a more broadly termed illness called *cholinergic urticaria*. It presents as small, 1 to 3 mm, punctate urticaria that usually begin on the upper thorax and neck and spread distally. It is caused by a rise in core body temperature by 1°C. EIU can occur not only during exercise, but also in response to stress, anxiety, hot baths or showers, or spicy or hot foods. Regardless of the inciting factor, EIU is prevented and treated in the same manner. Advising the child to not bathe in hot water or perform strenuous exercise during hot weather will reduce the risk of EIU. Second-generation antihistamines are the mainstay of pharmacologic prevention and treatment, as the sedation of first-generation antihistamines is not typically tolerated. EIU will often require twice the recommended dose of a second-generation antihistamine to control symptoms well. If second-generation antihistamines do not control symptoms adequately, then the first-generation antihistamine hydroxyzine can be tried.

7. What Is Exercise-Induced Anaphylaxis, and Can It Be Prevented?

Exercise-induced anaphylaxis (EIAn) is a rare but well-recognized condition that, unlike EIU, only develops in response to exercise. EIAn is thought to result from mast cell activation and the subsequent release of vasoactive mediators. The exact etiology that triggers mast cell activation is not known. Ingestion of certain medications such as nonsteroidal anti-inflammatory drugs (NSAIDs), including aspirin, prior to exercise may predispose an athlete to EIAn. Early signs and symptoms of EIAn are as follows: (1) generalized pruitus; (2) warmth and flushing; (3) sudden fatigue; and (4) urticaria. The urticaria is usually large (10 to 15 mm in diameter).

With continued exercise, signs and symptoms may progress to the following:

- Gastrointestinal symptoms such as nausea, abdominal cramping, and diarrhea
- Headache
- Angioedema of the face and/or extremities
- Wheezing from laryngeal edema
- Hypotension and/or collapse

It is important to differentiate EIAn from food-dependent exercise-induced anaphylaxis (FDEIAn). Patients with FDEIAn only have the reaction if they have eaten one or two specific foods within 1 to 3 hours prior to or after exercising.

Both EIAn and FDEIAn are managed like any anaphylactic reaction. Affected athletes should carry an epinephrine auto-injector device and inform coaches and teammates of their condition and subsequent care protocol. Once EIAn is recognized, stop all physical activity immediately; this will typically lead to a full resolution of the symptoms. If EIAn symptoms progress after stopping activity, then epinephrine from an auto-injector should be administered. The injection can be repeated one time in 5 to 15 minutes if symptoms do not improve. The child should have follow-up medical attention for further management and observance.

Reducing EIAn and FDEIAn incidents is focused on trigger avoidance. If the ingestion of NSAIDs preceded an attack of EIAn, then the athlete should be advised to not take NSAIDs for at least 24 hours prior to exercising. If it is not clear that the problem is purely EIAn versus FDEIAn, then the athlete should be advised to not eat for 4 to 6 hours prior to exercising. Athletes can try taking nonsedating antihistamines, but pharmacologic pretreatment does not appear to be an effective strategy and should not be relied upon as a means for preventing future attacks. A child who has experienced one attack already should gradually return to exercise over a span of weeks to months; should always have injectable epinephrine immediately available; and should exercise with a companion who is aware of the signs, symptoms, and treatment of EIAn.

8. What Is Venom-Induced Anaphylaxis, and Can It Be Prevented?

Venom-induced anaphylaxis (VIA) is typically caused by envenomation by the *Hymenoptera* order of insects, which includes bees, wasps, hornets, yellow jackets, and ants. Most people when stung by one of these insects will develop local pain, erythema, edema, and pruritus at the site. A much smaller percentage of people will go on to develop a systemic anaphylactic reaction. This reaction will develop quickly (often within 10 to 15 minutes of the sting) and progress to death if not recognized and treated appropriately. Common signs and symptoms include the following:

- Gastrointestinal tract—Metallic taste, nausea, vomiting, diarrhea, or abdominal cramping
- Genitourinary—Incontinence
- Nervous system—Lightheadedness or dizziness
- Cardiopulmonary—Dyspnea, stridor, bronchospasm, hypotension, or arrhythmias

Children may not complain of the sense of impending doom that adults often experience. Instead, children may have a sudden change in behavior, be more irritable, or just stop playing.

VIA is managed much like any anaphylactic reaction as outlined above for EIAn. Many VIA deaths occur because of a delay in the administration of epinephrine.

The prevention of VIA is achieved by avoiding exposure to these insects when possible. Patients with VIA should seek counsel from an allergist regarding allergen testing and venom immunotherapy after they are envenomated.

References

1. Armstrong LE, Casa DJ, Millard-Staffor M, et al. Exertional heat illness during training and competition. *Med Sci Sports Exerc.* 2007;39(3):556-572.
2. Freer L, Imray CHE. Frostbite. In: Auerbach PS. *Wilderness Medicine.* Philadelphia, PA: Elsevier Mosby; 2011:181-201.
3. Castellani JW, Young AJ, Ducharme MB, et al. American College of Sports Medicine position stand: prevention of cold injuries during exercise. *Med Sci Sports Exerc.* 2006;38(11):2012-2029.
4. Pollard AJ, Niermeyer S, Barry P, et al. Children at high altitude: an international consensus statement by an ad hoc committee of the International Society for Mountain Medicine, March 12, 2011. *High Alt Med Biol.* 2001;2(3):389-403.
5. Southard A, Niermeyer S, Yaron M. Language used in Lake Louise Scoring System underestimates symptoms of acute mountain sickness in 4- to 11-year-old children. *High Alt Med Biol.* 2007;8:124-130.
6. Hackett PH, Roach RC. High-altitude medicine and physiology. In: Auerbach PS. *Wilderness Medicine.* Philadelphia, PA: Elsevier Mosby; 2011:2–33.

11 Headache and Migraine Issues

Terra Blatnik, MD, FAAP and Susannah Briskin, MD, FAAP

1. What Are Some Common Headache Presentations Associated With Exercise, and How Can They Be Differentiated by History?

It is estimated that the incidence of exercise-associated headache is 35%.[1] Runners and weight lifters are the most commonly affected, but headaches can happen in any type of athlete.

Benign Exertional Headache

- A benign exertional headache (BEH) is associated with straining or Valsalva maneuver. It is most common in wrestlers and weight lifters and is believed to be associated with vascular spasm.
- A BEH is usually bilateral, severe, throbbing, and has a relatively rapid onset that fades to a dull ache over several hours.
- The location of the pain can be variable from athlete to athlete, but it is always in the same location for an individual.[1]

Effort-Associated Migraine

- An effort-associated migraine can often be difficult to distinguish from a BEH; however, it is commonly not triggered by the Valsalva maneuver or straining, but rather by aerobic exercise or reaching maximal aerobic threshold.
- Warm weather increases the risk of occurrence.[1]
- Pain in individuals with effort-associated migraines is unilateral, throbbing, and may be mild or intense, and typically lasts for several hours.
- Patients with effort-associated migraines may describe a history of migraines.
- It is believed to be related to vascular changes in the brain.

Cervicogenic Headache or "Weight Lifters Headache"

- A cervicogenic headache (also known as "weight lifters headache") is a unilateral headache that typically manifests as pain in the occipital or parietal regions that may radiate to the anterior part of the head.
- It may originate from various structures of the neck, including ligaments, joints, disks, muscles, or nerve roots. The patient may report that movement of his or her neck exacerbates the symptoms.
- Pain is constant and may last for days to weeks.

Koutures C, Wong V.
Pediatric Sports Medicine: Essentials for Office Evaluation (pp 66-70)

Tension Headache

- A tension headache can present with symptoms very similar to a cervicogenic headache with pain in the back of the neck/occipital region that may last hours to days.
- It can also present as a frontal headache and may occur during activities of daily living, not just exercise.

Postconcussive Headache

- Headache tends to be a very prominent symptom after a concussion.
- Diffuse constant or intermittent headache in association with recent head injury that may be exacerbated by physical and/or mental activity.
- Other symptoms include nausea, dizziness, balance issues, feeling foggy or tired, sleep problems, visual changes, and difficulty concentrating.[2]
- A postconcussive headache can last for days to months.

Headache Caused by Ill-Fitting Sports Equipment

- Supraorbital neuralgia, or "swimmer's headache," has been described in the literature as pain in the forehead/scalp area that occurs when an athlete's goggles do not fit appropriately or have a poor seal.[3]
- Hockey and football helmets can also cause diffuse headaches if not fitted appropriately.

When taking a history from an athlete with a headache, it is important to document headache onset and duration, quality of pain, and exacerbating and alleviating factors. By taking a thorough history, you may be able to discover warning signs that a more concerning headache is occurring. Concerning red flags include severe/sudden onset; stiff neck/meningeal signs; systemic symptoms such as fever, amnesia, headache waking the patient from sleep; recurrent or early morning emesis; changes in mental status; and/or loss of consciousness. The presence of these symptoms may indicate a tumor, subarachnoid hemorrhage, or meningitis, all of which require immediate medical management.

2. What Recommendations Can Help Reduce the Frequency of Exercise-Induced Headaches?

To reduce the risk of developing all types of headaches, it is important for athletes to eat 3 to 6 balanced meals per day and to follow appropriate hydration guidelines. Lack of sleep or changes in caffeine intake may also precipitate headaches.

It is believed that proper breathing techniques can be used to minimize the Valsalva maneuver during weight-lifting routines, and thus decrease the occurrence of BEHs.[1] Prophylactic propranolol or ergotamines may be helpful for prevention,[1] although the practitioner should use propranolol and other beta-blockers with caution in the athletic population (see question 4).

Cervicogenic headaches may be treated with physical therapy that is focused on neck motion and teaching proper weight-training technique.

Effort-associated migraines seem to be very sensitive to sleep, hydration, and nutritional status, similar to common migraines, so the previously mentioned guidelines for meals and hydration should be followed. A number of prophylactic medications can be used, including non-steroidal anti-inflammatory drugs (NSAIDs), aspirin, calcium channel blockers, tricyclic antidepressants, or selective serotonin reuptake inhibitors (SSRIs).[4]

Equipment-induced headaches, such as "goggle headaches," can be prevented by having appropriately fitting equipment. Coaches or athletic trainers should be involved in the fitting of helmets to ensure that they are fitted correctly.[5]

3. Some Patients Will Not Wear Helmets Because They Cause Headaches. What Are Some Sensible Helmet-Fitting Recommendations?

A properly fitted helmet should not produce a headache. Parents or coaches should be taught to properly fit helmets, and encourage their appropriate use. Athletes should be reminded that wearing a properly fitted helmet may protect them from serious injuries such as skull fractures.

- Proper fit should follow the manufacturer's recommendations for all helmet types.
- The first step is to use a cloth measuring tape to measure the circumference around the largest part of the skull. Use this measurement to select the appropriate-sized helmet from the manufacturer (if the athlete measures between sizes, always choose the smaller size).
- For football helmets, proper helmet height should be ensured.
  - The front of the helmet should be approximately ¾ to 1 inch above the player's eyebrows.
  - When fitting a football helmet, an inflation needle should be used to fill all air chambers so that the helmet fits snugly.
- To check for proper fit, the forehead skin should move with the front pad if the helmet is rotated from side to side. As it is twisted, the helmet and the head should move as one.
- During participation in sports, all straps should be secured, including the chin strap.[5]

4. For the Management of Migraine Headaches in Pediatric Patients, Which Prophylactic Medications May Have Adverse Exercise Consequences, and Which Medications Might Be More Favorable?

- Abortive medications are typically tried first, and include NSAIDs and those in the triptan family (eg, sumatriptan). Both of these types of medications have little or no sedative effect and would be appropriate for use in pediatric athletes. Narcotic medications would be contraindicated because of sedative effects, and because they are potentially banned by all athletic governing bodies.
- Prophylactic medication is typically considered if abortive medicine is ineffective or if the patient is having more than two migraines per month.
  - Beta-blockers are frequently used for migraine prophylaxis in the general population. However, in athletes, these medications reduce maximum heart rate, decrease exercise tolerance, and may worsen exercise-associated asthma, making them a poor choice.
  - Any medication containing caffeine should also be used with caution, because high levels may trigger a positive drug screen.
  - Calcium channel blockers (eg, verapamil) are very effective, and side effects should not affect athletic performance.
  - Other medications such as tricyclic antidepressants, SSRIs, and monamine oxidase inhibitors are more commonly used in adult athletes with migraines.[4,6]
- Prophylactic regimens of two natural substances have also shown promise in reducing the occurrence of migraine headaches. Two hundred milligrams of riboflavin and/or magnesium citrate twice daily may be an effective vitamin regimen to prevent migraines in athletes.[4]

5. How Common Is a Headache After a Patient Sustains a Concussion, and Should Athletes Be Allowed to Return to Play After a Concussion While They Have a Headache?

Headache is the most common symptom occurring with a concussion. In fact, studies have shown that more than 90% of athletes with concussions report having headaches.[7] Athletes should not be allowed to return to play (RTP) after a concussion while they are still experiencing any signs or symptoms, including headache. Athletes who RTP prior to concussion resolution may continue to be bothered by prolonged signs and symptoms that may linger for weeks, months, or even years. These athletes also experience a lower threshold for suffering a subsequent concussion.[7] Full resolution of all concussion-associated signs and symptoms should occur before an athlete is allowed to RTP. A graduated RTP protocol should be followed after the concussion has resolved.[8]

6. Are Athletes With a Personal or Family History of Recurrent Headaches More at Risk for Experiencing Complicated Concussions?

Athletes with a history of prior nonmigraine or migraine headaches are not at increased risk for prolonged recovery from concussion (>21 days).[2] However, a history of any type of frequent headaches, including migraines, can make RTP decisions more complicated. It is difficult to discern if a headache in a concussed athlete is secondary to the head injury or to the underlying headache issue. It is important to find out from the athlete the nature of the current headache, change in frequency and length of symptoms as it compares with his or her "typical" headache. Neurologists and neuropsychologists may need to be involved in RTP decisions if the headache persists when all other signs and symptoms of the concussion have resolved.

7. Football Players Routinely Report Headaches With Contact. How Can One Differentiate This More "Common" Headache From a Postconcussive or More Concerning Presentation?

Concussed high school football athletes have demonstrated rates of headache as high as 86% to 94%.[9] General headaches are a common report among athletes, with prevalence estimates ranging from one-third to one-half of athletes.[10] Specifically, headache is common in athletes who play contact sports. In a 2000 study, Sallis et al found that 85% of football players reported previous headache related to hitting in football.[9] Sabin et al found that the report of headache alone after contact was not associated with increased reporting of concussion symptoms, or altered sideline neurostatus or balance.[10] Therefore, headache is a common complaint after contact sports and, as a sole symptom after head trauma, appears to be a poor predictor for concussion.

In the absence of other symptoms, athletes reporting headache do not appear to show neuropsychologic changes consistent with a diagnosis of concussion. However, concussed athletes frequently demonstrate an increase in symptoms and severity in a variable time course following injury. Lovell et al demonstrated a significant increase in symptom scores and decline in memory 36 hours after sustaining an injury in concussed teenage athletes who had initially experienced complete resolution of symptoms within 15 minutes.[11] The resolution of symptoms, including headache, needs to be considered carefully. In the context of an obvious head injury, the report of a headache should be treated as a concussion, and the athlete should be removed from play and observed.

8. Can Neck Tightness or Spasm Lead to Headaches, and How Should One Evaluate and Manage Such Injuries?

Neck pain is frequently referred to the head, leading to the sensation of a headache, usually a cervicogenic headache or a tension headache. Any of the structures within the neck, including the musculature, ligaments, joints, and disks, may refer pain to the head due to the convergence of the nocioceptive pathways of the head and neck.[1] Therefore, it is important to discuss with the athlete the potential injury mechanisms of the neck or history of neck pain. It is also important to evaluate the loss of strength or sensation in the upper extremities, which may indicate an issue with the cervical spine. On examination, always assess neck range of motion and strength, and perform a complete neurologic examination of the upper extremities, including the testing of strength, sensation, and reflexes. The Spurling maneuver (Figure 11-1) tests for cervical nerve root

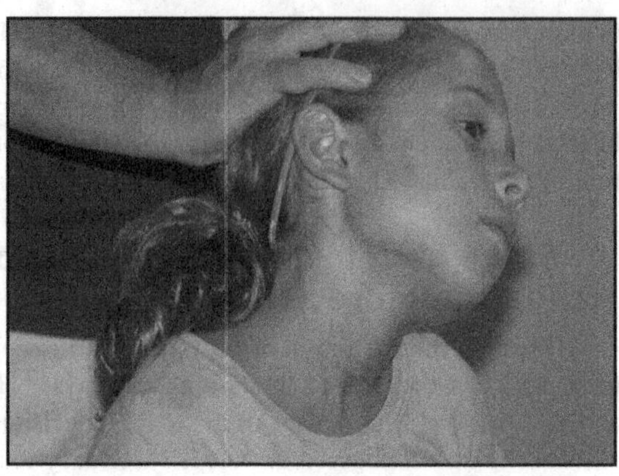

Figure 11-1. The Spurling maneuver.

compression by having the patient extend and rotate his or her neck to each side while the examiner applies a downward pressure (axial load) on the head. If the patient experiences radiation of pain or radicular symptoms past the ipsilateral shoulder, the test is positive.

If any part of the history or physical examination is concerning for potential cervical injury, further imaging should be pursued. Plain radiographs may show vertebral fractures, loss of disk height, and osteoarthritis. Loss of the normal cervical lordosis is concerning for cervical muscle spasm. Magnetic resonance imaging is useful for assessing for occult vertebral fractures, nerve root injuries, disk bulges/herniations, ligament injuries, and ruling out cervical stenosis.

Physical therapy is key in the treatment of neck pain. Manipulation, massage, and cervical traction have been shown to alleviate pain. Additionally, physical therapists can try electrical stimulation (ie, transcutaneous electrical nerve stimulation unit), heat, or ice therapy.

References

1. Rifat S, Moeller J. Diagnosis and management of headache in the weightlifting athlete. *Curr Sports Med Rep.* 2003;2(5):272–275.
2. Lau B, Kontos A, Collins M, et al. Which on-field signs/symptoms predict protracted recovery from sport related concussion among high school football players? *Am J Sports Med.* 2011;39(11):2311–2318.
3. Jacobson RI. More "goggle headache"; supraorbital neuralgia. *N Engl J Med.* 1983;308:226–227.
4. Swain R, Kaplan B. Diagnosis, prophylaxis, and treatment of headaches in the athlete. *South Med J.* 1997;90(9):878–888.
5. Fitting instructions and helmet care [package insert]. Elyria, OH: Riddell Inc; 2011.
6. Nadelson C. Sport and exercise induced migraines. *Curr Sports Med Rep.* 2006;5(1):29–33.
7. Marar M, McIlvain NM, Fields SK, et al. Epidemiology of concussions among United States high school athletes in 20 sports. *Am J Sports Med.* 2012 Apr;40(4):747–755.
8. McCrory P, Meeuwisse W, Johnston K, et al. Consensus statement on Concussion in Sport 3rd International Conference on Concussion in Sport held in Zurich, November 2008. *Clin J Sport Med.* 2009;19(3):185–200.
9. Sallis RE, Jones K. Prevalence of headaches in football players. *Med Sci Sports Exerc.* 2000;32(11):1820–1824.
10. Sabin MJ, Van Boxtel BA, Nohren MW, Broglio SP. Presence of headache does not influence sideline neurostatus or balance in high school football athletes. *Clin J Sport Med.* 2011;21(5):411–415.
11. Lovell MR, Collins MW, Iverson GL, Johnston KM, Bradley JP. Grade 1 or "ding" concussions in high school athletes. *Am J Sports Med.* 2004;32(1):47–54.

12 Gastrointestinal and Abdominal Issues

Michele LaBotz, MD, FAAP, CAQSM

1. What Causes Cramping in the Abdomen, and What Advice Can Be Given to Reduce the Incidence of Cramping? When Should a Clinician Be Concerned?

Abdominal discomfort with sports may come from either the gastrointestinal system (often the stomach) or the surrounding abdominal wall and supporting structures. In the pediatric athlete, these can be difficult to sort out.

Abdominal wall cramping

- Cramping emanating from the abdominal wall and its supporting structures is often perceived as a "side stitch." There is no clear consensus on the etiology of side stitches, but they are likely due to some combination of the following:
  - Decreased blood flow to the mesentery and diaphragm.
  - Mechanical traction on abdominal organs and the supporting ligaments with physical activity, especially running.
- Side stitches are most common in young and deconditioned athletes. Symptoms often improve as training continues and fitness increases. Treatment for an acute episode includes the following:
  - Support or pressure on the involved side, either with the athlete's hand or a wrap.
  - Changing the breathing pattern (a common pattern is to inhale on three strides and exhale rapidly on the fourth),[1] or breathing through pursed lips.

Gastrointestinal cramping

- Vigorous exercise decreases blood flow to the splanchnic bed and appears to delay gastric emptying.[2] Therefore, food and fluids that are ingested shortly before or during exercise take longer to empty, and the residual stomach volume can create a sense of nausea or cramping with physical activity.
- Gastrointestinal cramping is mainly experienced with running or high-intensity exercise.
- The following steps may minimize these symptoms by hastening stomach emptying. (Please note that there is a lot of individual variability in gastric tolerance, so there is often some trial and error involved in trying to minimize these symptoms; therefore, these steps should always be trialed in practice before competition.):
  - Stay well hydrated.
  - Take small, frequent sips of fluid during exercise.
  - Ingest fluids with relatively low levels of carbohydrates rather than plain water. This includes beverages that are 6% to 8% carbohydrate. This is found in most commercial

Koutures C, Wong V.
Pediatric Sports Medicine: Essentials for Office Evaluation (pp 71-78)

sports drinks or can be made by mixing equal volumes of water and nonacidic fruit juice (eg, apple).

- Drink tepid rather than ice cold fluids.
- Experiment with carbohydrate sources; it is important to note, however, that fructose may cause discomfort in some athletes.
- Avoid hypertonic fluids before exercise (eg, soda, fruit juices).
  - Decrease the amounts of fat, protein, and fiber in preexercise meals; preexercise meals should consist mainly of carbohydrates.
- Overall, most abdominal cramping with exercise is functional. Other possible pathology must be considered if symptoms persist after exercise or increase in severity as fitness improves.
- Endurance runners may develop an exercise-induced gastritis, which can lead to gastrointestinal blood loss. This should be considered in any athlete who presents with persistent symptoms or evidence of blood loss anemia.

2. Diarrhea Is Common in Endurance Athletes. Are There Any Recommendations to Reduce Frequency? Which Presentations Are More Concerning and Require Urgent Evaluation?

- Diarrhea during or after exercise, also known as "runners trots," can be disruptive and embarrassing to some young athletes. Exercise-induced diarrhea most commonly occurs in the young athlete as he or she increases the intensity of his or her workouts.
- Running appears to be particularly provocative of intestinal distress, which may be due to changes in both gastrointestinal blood flow and local hormonal secretion.[1]
- The majority of athletes will resolve symptoms by reducing the intensity of training until they are symptom-free, then gradually building back up to previous levels of exertion.[2] In addition, the following steps may reduce the frequency/severity of exercise-induced diarrhea:
  - Maintain appropriate hydration throughout the exercise period.
  - Avoid ingesting spicy or fiber-rich foods or beverages before exercise.
  - Avoid caffeinated and hot beverages before exercise.
  - Some athletes may be sensitive to particular sugars and should consider dietary elimination trials. Frequent offenders include the following:
    - Lactose
    - Fructose (common sweetener used in sports drinks and processed foods)
    - Sorbitol (found in some artificially sweetened gums and food products)
  - Avoid tight-fitting clothes around the abdomen.
  - Choose foods that tend to constipate, such as white rice, bread, and bananas.
  - Defecate before exercise, or schedule a planned bathroom stop early during activity.
- Any athlete who presents with bloody or mucus-filled diarrhea, weight loss, undue fatigue, or whose symptoms persist in spite of activity reduction should be evaluated for inflammatory, infectious, or other possible lower gastrointestinal pathology, as well as for possible blood loss anemia.
- Endurance athletes performing intense activity for multiple hours will often develop gastrointestinal mucosal damage, which leads to blood loss. This is typically occult, but stools may become frankly bloody after a particularly strenuous effort.
  - Athletes with occult or frank blood in their stools should have follow-up testing to assure resolution and should be screened for possible blood loss anemia.

3. Is There a Connection Between Gastroesophageal Reflux Disease and Asthma? Between Gastroesophageal Reflux Disease and Endurance Athletes? Are There Suggestions for the Prevention of Gastroesophageal Reflux Disease in These Athletes?

- The distinction between gastroesophageal reflux disease (GERD) and asthma can be difficult in young athletes, as both may present with chronic cough and dyspnea. While there appears to be significant overlap between patients with asthma and patients with GERD, the relationship between these two diagnoses is still uncertain. GERD may also be a factor in vocal cord dysfunction.
- Activities most commonly associated with GERD are as follows[2]:
  - Running or other high-intensity activity
  - Supine activity (eg, weight lifting)
  - Contact sports and sports that produce abdominal strain (eg, Valsalva maneuver)
- The prevention and treatment of GERD includes the following[2]:
  - Avoid exercising for several hours after eating
  - Keep any pre-exercise meals small, and avoid foods/beverages that are fatty, spicy, acidic, or caffeinated
  - Minimize Valsalva maneuvers with training
  - Consider decreasing the intensity of training or cross train to avoid GERD-producing activity
  - Avoid tight-fitting clothing or equipment
  - Try chewing gum or sucking on lozenges during exercise
  - For some athletes, a brief trial of medication may produce benefit (Table 12-1)
- Any athlete with persistent symptoms or who presents with additional symptoms such as weight loss or fatigue should have further evaluation.

4. What Is the Cause of Abdominal Muscle Strains, and When Can an Athlete Return to Play After Sustaining a Strain? Is Rehabilitation Necessary?

- Strains of the abdominal muscles occur when the muscles are rapidly shortened from a stretched starting position. Injury patterns include the following:
  - *Rectus abdominis strains*—Most common in tennis, particularly during the serve when the athlete transitions rapidly from maximal trunk extension to flexion.
  - *Oblique muscle strains*—Occur in sports requiring trunk rotation, such as basketball, gymnastics, figure skating, golf, baseball/softball, and other throwing sports.
- Treatment for abdominal strains follows the usual principles of PRICE (protection, rest, ice, compression, elevation; for further information please see Chapter 24, question 1). However, it is very difficult to rest the abdominal musculature, and sometimes an elastic brace or wrap can be beneficial. Formalized physical therapy will often help the athlete return to full sports participation more quickly, but many athletes can successfully rehabilitate themselves at home with appropriate guidance and the following progressive exercise regimen:
  - Relative rest until activities of daily living are relatively pain free.
  - Begin gentle stretches (extensions, side bends, and twisting). These should be performed slowly and in a pain-free fashion.
  - Begin isometric contractions of the abdominal muscles with the athlete laying supine with his or her knees flexed. The athlete then draws the umbilicus toward the back and pushes the lower back into the floor.

Table 12-1. Medications That May Be Helpful in Managing Symptoms of Gastroesophageal Reflux Disease in Young Athletes

DRUG CLASSES (SAMPLE GENERIC AND BRAND NAMES)	*DOSAGE*	*TIMING*	*DURATION*	*COMMENTS*
Proton Pump Inhibitors				
Omeprazole (eg, Prilosec OTC)	10–<20 kg: 10 mg PO once daily ≥ 20 kg: 20 mg PO once daily	15 to 30 min before breakfast daily	Initial trial 4 weeks	Proton pump inhibitors are the most effective drug class, particularly for frequent symptoms.
Lansoprazole (eg, Prevacid)	<30 kg: 15 mg qd >30 kg: 30 mg qd or bid			
Esomeprazole (eg, Nexium)	1 to 11 yo: 10 mg/day >12 yo: 20 to 40 mg/day			
H2 Receptor Antagonists				
Cimetidine (eg, Tagamet)	5 to 10 mg/kg q 6hrs (max 300 mg/dose)	1 hr before activity	12-week maximum	Effective with intermittent use.
Famotidine (eg, Pepcid AC)	>20 kg: 20 mg BID			
Ranitidine (eg, Zantac)	5 to 10 mg/kg/day ÷q 8 to 12 hrs			
Antacids				
Aluminum+/– magnesium hydroxides (eg, Maalox liquid, Mylanta)	Preparations vary. Follow labeled directions	Before activity or when symptoms occur	2 to 4 weeks	Antacids are convenient and the fastest acting for symptomatic use. Best used for occasional symptoms. Aluminum formulations may be constipating. Magnesium may have laxative effect.
Calcium carbonate (eg, Tums, Maalox tablets)	6 to 11 years old: 800 mg/dose > 11 years old: 1000 to 3000 mg/dose			

Dosage data compiled from Lee CKK, Tschudy, MM, Arcara, KM. Drug doses. In: Tschudy, MM, Arcara, KM, eds. *The Harriet Lane Handbook: A Manual for Pediatric House Officers*. Philadelphia, PA: Mosby Elsevier; 2012.

- Begin concentric exercises. There are many good options for a graduated abdominal-strengthening program; however, many young athletes have a difficult time performing these exercises correctly. Pointing the young athlete toward a Pilates (or similar) mat program, or exercises that utilize a stability ball or foam roller can be helpful.

- After full range of motion and no pain with abdominal muscle testing, athletes may then begin sports drills in a controlled setting with instructions to avoid rotation and rapid trunk flexion or extension.
- As long as the athlete remains pain free, they may gradually progress to full activity.

Rectus sheath hematomas—Unusual injuries that may present similarly to an abdominal strain. These hematomas occur when disrupted epigastric arteries bleed into the sheath of the rectus abdominis muscle, and may be due either to direct trauma or to mechanisms that are similar to those described previously for strains.

- Findings often include a firm, painful mass underlying the rectus musculature.
  - On examination, this remains palpable and becomes more painful as the muscles are tensed by having the supine patient raise his or her head or legs off of the table.
- The evaluation should include diagnostic ultrasonography or computed tomography (CT) scan to confirm the diagnosis and complete blood count (CBC) to assess the degree of bleeding into the hematoma.
  - Hematomas that are intramuscular, do not appear to be expanding, AND with normal vital signs and CBC can be managed with PRICE.
  - Hematomas that do not meet the above criteria warrant close observation and possible surgical intervention.

5. How Should Suspected Abdominal Injuries Be Evaluated in the Young Athlete?

- Although abdominal injuries in sports settings are relatively uncommon, they are frequently missed, and the potential for serious consequences requires a high index of suspicion for these injuries in the young athlete. The most common sideline scenario is a blunt injury or a sudden deceleration injury producing abdominal discomfort. Injuries in contact/collision sports are most common, but there are several patterns worth particular note:
  - Snowboarders appear to be uniquely susceptible to splenic trauma
  - Falls onto bicycle handlebars may produce severe injury, particularly of the duodenum and hollow viscera
- A close eye should be kept on any young athlete with post-traumatic abdominal pain. Sideline evaluation should determine the following:
  - Symptoms of diaphragmatic irritation producing right shoulder pain in liver injuries or left shoulder pain in spleen injuries (Kehr's sign)
  - Symptoms that worsen with time
  - Signs of peritoneal irritation (local tenderness, guarding, rigidity)
  - Possible hemodynamic instability (blood pressure, pulse, perfusion)

If any of these are present on the sideline, transportation should be arranged for the athlete to a local emergency facility where observation, imaging, and laboratory testing can be performed. These injuries can have a delayed presentation; therefore, those with persistent symptoms presenting in the office after abdominal trauma should be considered for evaluation as well.

Additional evaluation may include the following:

- Imaging
  - Focused assessment by ultrasonography for trauma (FAST)—Available in many emergency facilities; can help detect intraperitoneal fluid or blood.[4]
    - There is some concern that FAST may not be as sensitive in the pediatric population as compared with adults. Accuracy of FAST (as well as other ultrasonographic assessments) is also decreased in the obese patient.
  - CT scanning with contrast remains the gold standard for the diagnosis and staging of abdominal injuries.

Table 12-2. Recognition and Evaluation of the Most-Common Intra-Abdominal Injuries in Young Athletes			
	INJURY LOCATION		
	Spleen	**Liver**	**Kidney**
Mechanism	Blunt trauma to LUQ, sudden deceleration	Blunt trauma to RUQ, sudden deceleration	Blunt trauma to back, sudden deceleration
Symptoms	LUQ pain, left shoulder pain	RUQ pain, right shoulder pain	Dull back or diffuse abdominal pain
Examination	LUQ tenderness, guarding, rebound, serial assessment of hemodynamics (increased pulse, decreased blood pressure)	RUQ tenderness, guarding, rebound, increased pulse, decreased blood pressure	Costovertebral ecchymosis, evidence of associated bony or soft-tissue injury to spine, thorax, or pelvis
Evaluation	FAST and/or abdominal CT with IV contrast; CBC/serial hemograms	FAST and/or abdominal CT with IV contrast; CBC/serial hemograms, liver function tests	Urinalysis; imaging choices vary upon local preference, but most typically include CT with IV contrast and/or renal ultrasonography (if local expertise)
Treatment	Surgical only if hemodynamically unstable, otherwise, strict bed rest and monitoring	Surgical if hemodynamically unstable, otherwise, strict bed rest and monitoring	Ultrasonography (if local expertise) Bed rest and close monitoring for lower-grade injuries (contusions, nonexpanding hematoma, and small lacerations) • Vital signs • Hemograms • Urine output Higher-grade injuries may warrant intervention

CBC, complete blood count; CT, computed tomography; FAST, focused assessment by ultrasonography for trauma; IV, intravenous; LUQ, left upper quadrant; RUQ, right upper quadrant.

- Radiation exposure is of additional concern.

- Laboratory
  - CBC and serial hemograms, electrolytes, liver function tests, amylase, lipase, and urinalysis.

6. When Should a Splenic Contusion/Laceration Be Suspected in an Athlete, and What Is the Work-Up? Should This Type of Injury Be Referred to a Specialist? When Can the Athlete Return to Play?

Injuries to the spleen are the most common intra-abdominal injuries after blunt trauma in pediatric patients. See Table 12-2 for information on the recognition and assessment of these injuries. Athletes with acute or chronic splenomegaly appear to be at increased risk for injury. For more information, see Chapter 3, question 6. Splenic injuries are described by CT staging to determine the following:

- The size of any subcapsular hematoma and/or tears of the capsule and parenchyma.
- The disruption of trabecular or hilar blood vessels.

Table 12-3. Proposed Guidelines for Resource Utilization in Children With Isolated Spleen or Liver Injury				
	CT Grade			
	I	**II**	**III**	**IV**
ICU stay (day)	None	None	None	1
Hospital stay (day)	2	3	4	5
Predischarge imaging	None	None	None	None
Postdischarge imaging	None	None	None	None
Activity restriction (weeks)*	3	4	5	6

*Return to full-contact, competitive sports (eg, football, wrestling, hockey, lacrosse, mountain climbing) should be at the discretion of the individual pediatric trauma surgeon. The proposed guidelines for return to unrestricted activity include "normal" age-appropriate activities. (Reprinted with permission from Stylianos S and APSA Trauma Committee. Evidence-based guidelines for research utilization in children with isolated spleen or liver injury. *J Pediatr Surg*. 2000;35:165-169.)

Although most splenic injuries stop bleeding spontaneously, up to 10% of patients will rebleed.[5] Therefore, all athletes suspected of splenic injury should be monitored closely for changes in hemodynamics and perfusion. Hemodynamic instability is the main determinant for surgical intervention, however, over 90% of spleen injuries in pediatric patients are successfully managed nonoperatively.[5] Table 12-3 reflects the treatment expectations depending upon the CT grade of injury.[5]

7. When Should a Liver Contusion/Laceration in an Athlete Be Suspected? When Should This Type of Injury Be Referred to a Specialist? When Can the Athlete Return to Play?

Liver injuries commonly occur after blunt trauma to the upper right abdomen.

- Significant or persistent pain after abdominal trauma should produce a low threshold for additional evaluation.[6]
  - See Table 12-2 for additional information on evaluation.

Although most liver injuries in the pediatric population will cease bleeding spontaneously, these injuries are the most common cause of fatal hemorrhage in this population.[5] The decision for surgical intervention is largely guided by the presence of hemodynamic instability.

- Delayed presentation or recurrence of bleeding is not uncommon.
  - See Table 12-3 for information on the treatment recommendations/expectations in liver trauma.[5]

8. When Should I Suspect a Kidney Injury in an Athlete? When Should This Type of Injury Be Referred to a Specialist? When Can the Athlete Return to Play?

Detailed information on the evaluation and treatment of kidney injuries can be found in Table 12-2. The primary issues of concern in renal injuries include (and evaluation should delineate the presence of) the following:

- Bleeding—Most isolated renal injuries will stop bleeding spontaneously.
- Urinary extravasation and tissue devascularization.

In adults, hematuria and hypotension are highly predictive of renal injury; however, in children, these measures are less sensitive.[4] In addition, anomalous kidneys appear to be at increased risk for traumatic injury. (See Chapter 3, question 6, for additional information on sports participation with renal abnormalities.)

- Decisions on additional evaluation should be based on history and clinical suspicion.
- Patients with blunt trauma who meet the following criteria merit additional evaluation[6].
  - High-velocity or deceleration injury.
  - Hematuria with > 50 red blood cells/high-power field.
  - Microscopic hematuria associated with shock.

CT staging I to V can assist with treatment decision making.[4]

- Grades I to II injuries are treated conservatively.
  - These include renal contusions, nonexpanding hematomas, and lacerations < 1 cm.
- Although there is a trend toward nonoperative intervention in the hemodynamically stable patient with grades III to V injuries, over 50% of these injuries will require some form of intervention (often angiographic, endoscopic, or percutaneous techniques).[4]
  - Grades III to V injuries include lacerations > 1 cm or injuries to the collecting system or renal vasculature.

9. How Can Parents and Athletes Prevent Abdominal Injuries During Sports?

The most important aspect of abdominal injury prevention is attention to rules and fair play. Athletes who are "risk takers" or who are particularly aggressive in their style of play are at increased risk for injury. Football, ice hockey, and other sports that require protective gear typically leave the abdomen relatively uncovered and vulnerable. Although abdominal protection is available, athletes may perceive padding over that region as restrictive and uncomfortable.

Protective gear is sport specific and must fit properly and be in good condition to be optimally effective.

- *Football*—Flac jackets, rib guards, back plates, and padded shirts may provide additional abdominal protection.
- *Ice hockey*—Pants may protect the lower abdomen and pelvis; some shoulder pads may include abdominal and rib pads.
- *Lacrosse*—US lacrosse recommends rib pads for all boys; goalies in both boys and girls lacrosse need to wear chest and abdominal protection.
- *Field hockey*—Goalies should wear chest and abdominal protection.

References

1. Simons SM, Shaskan GG. Gastrointestinal problems in distance running. *Int Sport Med J.* 2005:(6):162–170.
2. Paluska S. Current concepts: recognition and management of common activity-related gastrointestinal disorders. *Phys Sports Med.* 2009; (37):54–63.
3. Lee CKK, Tschudy, MM, Arcara, KM. Drug doses. In: Tschudy, MM, Arcara, KM, eds. *The Harriet Lane Handbook :A Manual for Pediatric House Officers.* Philadelphia, PA: Mosby Elsevier; 2012.
4. Avarello JT, Cantor RM. Pediatric major trauma: an approach to evaluation and management. *Emerg Med Clin N Am.* 2007;(25):803–836.
5. Stylianos S; APSA Trauma Committee. Evidence-based guidelines for research utilization in children with isolated spleen or liver injury. *J Pediatr Surg.* 2000;35:165–169.
6. Husmann DA. Pediatric Genitourinary Trauma. In: Wein AJ, Kavoussi LR, Novick AC, Partin AW, Peters CA, eds. *Campbell-Walsh Urology.* 10th ed. Philadelphia, PA: Elsevier Saunders, 2012.

13 Hematology and Oncology Issues

Katherine M. Fox, MD and Holly J. Benjamin, MD, FAAP, FACSM

1. What Recommendations Can Be Made to Patients With Hemophilia for Sport/Activity Selection, the Monitoring of Factor Levels, Risks of Recurrent Bruising or Bleeding Into Joints, and the Potential Use of Medications to Boost Factor Levels for Sport Participation?

Hemophilia constitutes a group of bleeding disorders resulting from a deficiency of coagulation factors with an incidence of 1 in 5000 newborns. The clinical presentation varies greatly due to individual differences in functional plasma factor levels.[1]

- Hemarthrosis, synovitis, and bruising are frequent complications. Repeated joint hemorrhage leads to arthropathy, stiffness, and chronic pain. In the most severe phenotypes (only 1% to 2% or less of normal factor levels), individuals may have significant bleeding with little to no trauma. Given the risk of severe joint damage and life-threatening bleeds, the health care provider must appropriately educate the patient and his or her parents on safe participation in sports and physical activity.
- A sedentary lifestyle leads to weakness and joint instability, along with muscle atrophy, which can also contribute to pain and immobility. Regular exercise has been shown to reduce the frequency of bleeding episodes in select groups of children.[2]
- For many years, patients with hemophilia were turned away from full-contact sports, but these limitations have been lifted for many patients, depending on disease severity and control. Children with hemophilia who exercise have fewer bleeding episodes than those who do not exercise.[1] Aside from obvious cardiovascular benefits, greater muscle strength protects joints from hemarthrosis, increases joint stability, and reduces musculoskeletal injury risk. There are also obvious social and psychological benefits, adding to the reasons why patients with hemophilia should engage in sports and exercise.

Although sport restrictions placed on individuals with hemophilia have lessened with time, there are still risks involved, and patients need to be aware of them.

It is evident that collision or contact events can lead to a severe bleed.[1] The actual risk depends on the individual child's bleeding history, current treatment regimen, and use of coagulation factor prophylaxis. These risks and choice of sport must be assessed on a case-by-case basis. The American Academy of Pediatrics classifies sports into contact, limited contact, and noncontact.[3]

- Children should be closely assessed from both a hematologic and musculoskeletal standpoint before participating in contact sports. Consultation with a pediatric hematologist and a sports medicine physician is helpful.
- Children should receive appropriate factor prophylaxis to reduce the risk of bleeding. Prophylactic physical therapy may be appropriate to prevent injury. Parents and coaches must vigilantly enforce the use of protective equipment. A written plan for the prevention

Koutures C, Wong V.
Pediatric Sports Medicine: Essentials for Office Evaluation (pp 79-86)

and treatment of bleeding episodes should be shared between the physician, parents, coaches, and school officials. This plan may include factor replacement, ice, splinting, and rest to manage acute bleeds. The patient must abstain from physical activity until his or her joint pain or swelling resolves.

2. What Symptoms Suggest Iron Deficiency Anemia, and Who Might Be at the Highest Risk?

Iron is a component of hemoglobin (transports oxygen and carbon dioxide in the blood) and also a part of myoglobin (extracts oxygen from hemoglobin in muscle tissue). Iron also serves important roles in the electron transport chain and DNA synthesis.

To reach peak performance, the athlete needs maximal oxygen delivery to exercising skeletal muscle. VO_2 max (maximal rate of individual aerobic capacity/oxygen utilization with exercise) decreases in iron deficiency anemia (IDA).[4] There is also a decreased transport of oxygen to exercising tissue and a decrease in erythropoiesis, both of which impact performance.[4]

IDA is defined as a microcytic (low mean corpuscular volume [MCV]) and hypochromic anemia. The following are some possible symptoms of IDA, which are vague and often nonspecific:

- May or may not include fatigue, pallor, lightheadedness, and dizziness.
- Severe presentations may include tachycardia, tachypnea, and marked lethargy.
- Vegetarians are at particularly high risk for IDA. Meat and poultry are higher in iron than vegetable sources and are better absorbed.
- A general lack of adequate dietary iron commonly contributes to IDA (limited meat intake often due to individual choice or relative higher cost compared with other foods).
- Adolescents tend to have a higher dietary content of fat and carbohydrates rather than protein, placing them at increased risk for IDA, as protein enhances iron absorption.[4]
- Blood loss from menstruation is another common cause of IDA.
- Athletes at periods of peak growth are at increased risk due to increased iron demands.

Although IDA typically is a nutritional issue, it is important to perform a thorough and appropriate work-up to not miss chronic and systemic illness. Blood loss from gastrointestinal sources should be considered in the differential diagnosis for these patients. Athletes in general have a higher rate of nonsteroidal anti-inflammatory drug use, which may increase their risk for a gastrointestinal bleed.

3. Can Iron Deficiency Without Frank Anemia Cause a Reduction in Exercise Capabilities? Should We Treat Athletes Who Are Not Anemic for Iron Deficiency?

Iron deficiency without frank anemia is a complex issue, especially when considering the implications for athletics. There is evidence in the medical literature arguing both for and against iron supplementation in the nonanemic, iron-deficient athlete.[5-8] It is not clear if supplementing an iron-deficient, but nonanemic, individual improves performance. In most studies, iron supplementation does not improve VO_2 max rates or overall athletic performance.[6] Iron parameters may be low immediately after exercise, but this has not been shown to correlate with performance.[6] Supplementing with iron in nonanemic, iron-deficient individuals improves iron parameters and subjective performance in some cases. Given the mixed available evidence, iron deficiency without anemia is not a clear indication for supplementation.

An important point for the practitioner to be aware of is the risk of uncontrolled iron supplementation. Athletes, coaches, and parents may be tempted by the allure of college scholarships and financial success to "try anything" to improve performance. Elevated total body iron stores have been shown to be a risk factor for liver malignancy[6] and the development of hemochromatosis. The genetics of hemochromatosis are quite complex, with polymorphism and incomplete penetrance. An overconsumption of iron may induce pathology in an otherwise asymptomatic individual. Another risk of iron consumption is the masking of chronic and/or systemic underlying medical problems.

Treating a nonanemic athlete with iron supplementation should be done only after careful consideration. Some athletes with a relative anemia may have a normal hemoglobin level. If ferritin levels are low, a supervised trial of iron therapy may benefit the patient. In these cases, follow-up blood work would show an increase in iron indices and a rise in hemoglobin level from the individual's normal baseline level. A decrease in performance may be a manifestation of iron deficiency. After ruling out other causes of diminished performance, supplementing an iron-deficient athlete may prove beneficial in some cases. It is important to discuss the risks and benefits with the athlete and his or her parents so that they have a clear understanding that iron supplementation should not be unlimited and unrestricted. It is also important to educate the parents, athletes, and coaches that iron supplementation may not improve performance. Training methods, overall nutritional status, rest periods, and psychological factors should all be considered.

4. What Laboratory Tests Are Commonly Ordered in the Evaluation of Iron Deficiency Anemia, and How Are They Interpreted?

Understanding the approach to the diagnosis and screening for this condition is essential.

- A complete blood count (CBC) is the initial laboratory test to evaluate for IDA. The definition for anemia varies based on age and sex (Table 13-1).[9] If the initial CBC is consistent with these parameters, one should pursue more specific testing for iron deficiency.
- Additional laboratory tests commonly ordered in the evaluation of IDA include the following:
  - Ferritin is frequently used as the standard indicator of iron stores, although there is some debate as to whether it most accurately reflects total body iron stores, since it is an acute phase reactant that may vary in some conditions, including exercise. A commonly used cut off for normal ferritin is 30 to 35 ng/mL, which is appropriate for clinical practice. However, athletes with ferritin levels as low as 12 ng/mL have demonstrated normal performance.[5] In contrast, upregulation of iron absorption has been documented in athletes with ferritin levels as high as 60 ng/mL.[5] This adds to the confusion of which patient is most appropriate to supplement with iron therapy.
  - Transferrin and serum iron have high day-to-day variability and do not accurately reflect total body iron stores.
  - The soluble transferrin receptor (sTfr) mediates iron transfer from transferrin protein into red blood cells. It is a direct indicator of functional iron levels; sTfr circulating levels increase when iron stores are depleted and iron turnover is stimulated. sTfr has a significant advantage over traditional ferritin testing, since it is not impacted by acute inflammatory reactions. The traditional ferritin test is still widely used and accepted as an accurate diagnostic tool for IDA. However, sTfr is important to be aware of, as significant research has been done to assess its clinical utility, especially in regard to athletes.[10]

5. What Are the Best Ways to Correct Iron Deficiency: Iron-Rich Food Choices, Oral Iron Supplements (Pill Versus Liquid), or Even Injected Iron?

It is more effective to obtain iron from natural dietary sources than commercially prepared supplements. Iron is classified into two dietary types: heme and nonheme iron.

- Heme iron is obtained from meat sources (beef, turkey, chicken, tuna, crab, and pork), and animal sources contain more iron than nonheme or plant sources of iron and are more effectively absorbed.
- Nonheme iron sources include cereals, beans, spinach, and whole-wheat bread. It is possible to enhance the absorption of nonheme iron by consuming it with meat protein and vitamin C (ascorbic acid).

Table 13-1. Definition of Anemia by Hemoglobin Value		
	Hemoglobin Value	
	World Health Organization	**Centers for Disease Control and Prevention**
Infants/children 0.5 to 4.9 years	-	< 11 g/dL (110 g/L)
Children 5.0 to 11.9 years	-	< 11.5 g/dL (115 g/L)
Menstruating women	< 12 g/dL (120 g/L)	-
Pregnant females in first or third trimester	< 11 g/dL	< 11 g/dL
Pregnant women in second trimester	< 11 g/dL	< 10.5 g/dL (105 g/L)
Males	< 13 g/dL (130 g/L)	-
Adapted from U.S. Preventive Services Task Force. Screening for iron deficiency anemia—including iron prophylaxis. In: *Guide to Clinical Preventive Services*. 2nd ed. Baltimore, MD: Williams & Wilkins; 1996:231-246.		

- The absorption of heme iron is approximately 15% to 35% per meal compared with 2% to 20% for nonheme iron.[5] Iron storage levels impact iron's rate of absorption.
- Products that decrease the absorption of iron include tannins (found in teas), calcium, polyphenols (wine and tea), and phytates (found in whole grains).

The National Institutes of Health's Dietary Supplement Fact Sheet on iron is available at www.ods.od.nih.gov/factsheets/iron.asp, and is a good resource for patients and parents.[11]

Commercially prepared iron supplements are available if an individual cannot correct iron deficiency through iron-rich food sources alone.

- Ferrous iron salts such as ferrous sulfate or ferrous gluconate are better absorbed than ferric iron. Dosing varies based on age, weight, and sex and should be reviewed on an individual basis before initiating therapy. Higher supplement doses confer an increased risk of gastrointestinal side effects such as nausea, vomiting, diarrhea, constipation, and dark-colored stools.
- Intravenous forms of iron are reserved for severe presentations, including chronic uncontrollable bleeding, intolerance to oral iron, severe anemia, or intestinal malabsorption.

An individual's hemoglobin level should respond to iron therapy in about 2 or 3 weeks after initiating treatment. Iron storage levels are much slower to respond, and this may take up to 4 to 6 months. Gastrointestinal symptoms are a common reason for nonadherence to treatment, and need to be discussed when starting therapy and readdressed if nonadherence is suspected. Also, reviewing substances that enhance absorption (vitamin C and meat protein), as well as those that inhibit absorption (milk, tea, wine, and seeds), allows maximal improvement of iron stores with supplementation.

6. How Can I Tell the Difference Between Iron Deficiency and Other Forms of Microcytic Anemia, Such as Thalassemia? What Is Pseudoanemia of Sports?

As previously stated, IDA is a microcytic anemia with a low ferritin level. If an individual presents with microcytic anemia but a normal or high ferritin level, consider other diagnoses (Table 13-2).

- Thalassemia trait is another common cause of microcytosis, especially in children.
    - Beta-thalassemia is a genetic condition with underproduction of the normal beta-globin chains of hemoglobin. The beta-thalassemia trait occurs when an individual is heterozygous for this condition. Clinical manifestations include mild anemia with a low MCV. Hemoglobin electrophoresis will show an increase in hemoglobin A2, confirming the diagnosis.

Table 13-2. Laboratory Tests to Evaluate Common Causes of Microcytic Anemia			
TEST	*IDA*	*ANEMIA OF CHRONIC DISEASE*	*THALASSEMIA*
Ferritin	Decreased	Normal to increased	Increased
Serum iron level	Decreased	Normal to decreased	Normal to increased
Total iron-binding capacity	Increased	Slightly decreased	Normal
Transferrin saturation	Decreased	Normal to slightly decreased	Normal to increased
Red blood cell distribution width	Increased	Normal	Normal to increased
Adapted from Hematologic diseases, In: Wallach, J. *Interpretation of Diagnostic Tests.* 8th ed. Boston, MA. Little Brown and Company; 2006:385-419.			

- Other less common forms of microcytic anemia in children include other hemoglobinopathies, lead poisoning, anemia of chronic disease, and sideroblastic anemias. Laboratory testing can help to confirm each of these diagnoses.[12]
  - Hemoglobin electrophoresis will confirm a hemoglobinopathy such as sickle-cell disease or trait.
  - At-risk children with microcytic anemia that does not fit the pattern for IDA should have their serum lead level checked.
  - Anemia of chronic disease is characterized by normocytic or microcytic anemia with low ferritin levels. It is distinguished from IDA by low total iron-binding capacity (TIBC). In IDA, the TIBC is elevated.
  - Sideroblastic anemia is a group of disorders in which iron is deposited in bone marrow erythrocytes. This is less common than the other diagnosis mentioned, and it is diagnosed by bone marrow biopsy.

Pseudoanemia of sports is a physiologic response to training that occurs in many athletes, especially endurance athletes. It consists of an adaptive increase in plasma volume where athletes subsequently develop an increased rate of erythropoiesis and thus a rise in hemoglobin. The pseudoanemia develops as the rate of rise in hemoglobin is slightly less than the increases in plasma volume. Thus, the athlete would appear anemic or relatively anemic from his or her baseline on routine testing. These athletes will not have a microcytosis and iron studies would not be consistent with IDA. These changes will resolve once the training period is over. This is a normal adaptive and physiologic response, and treatment is not indicated.

7. What Is Sickle-Cell Trait, and When Might It Have Adverse Effects on Sport Participation?

Sickle-cell trait (SCT) is the inheritance of one gene for sickle hemoglobin and one for normal hemoglobin. SCT should not be confused with sickle-cell disease. SCT is more commonly found in persons whose ancestry is from African, South American, Central American, Saudi Arabian, Indian, and Mediterranean or Caribbean countries.[13] SCT traditionally had been considered a possible clinical risk factor for exertional collapse, acute rhabdomyolysis, and vascular dysfunction related to strenuous physical activity participation in hot and/or humid environments due to sickling of red blood cells[14] (Table 13-3). Recent studies have further investigated the risks of sport participation by SCT athletes to evaluate the frequency, epidemiology, and clinical profiles of SCT-related deaths in competitive athletes. Factors that were identified with increased risk of exertional collapse included participation in football, being African American and male, extreme

Table 13-3. Major Factors That Trigger Red Blood Cell Sickling	
1. Severe hypoxemia	3. Muscle hyperthermia
2. Metabolic acidosis	4. Red blood cell dehydration

exertion early in the season usually during conditioning drills, and high ambient temperatures. These recent studies looked at data from college athletes.[15-17] No studies exist that have examined similar risk stratifications in youth or high school athletes.

8. What Are the Controversies for the Universal Screening for Sickle-Cell Trait in Athletes?

Universal screening for SCT has been debated by various sports organizations and governing bodies as to whether it is a useful mechanism to improve the health and safety of athletes. It is noteworthy that routine newborn screening for infants born in the United States began in the 1980s and has been performed in all 50 states since 2006; therefore, the vast majority of young athletes have already been screened. However, there has traditionally been a lack of consistency in ensuring that patients and families are aware of sickle-cell status. It is recommended that this information be provided to families when the results of newborn screening become known.

With regard to universal screening in the athletic population, three ethical issues arise:

1. Risks of targeted screening require the ability to identify high-risk populations, which is extremely difficult.
2. Cost issues.
3. An athlete's right to consent or waive out of screening, as well as potential confidentiality issues.

Pro arguments for universal screening support the position that all athletes should know individual status and can therefore be better educated on the risks associated with SCT and sport participation. This might be effective in decreasing future morbidity and mortality risks. Universal screening eliminates the concerns for discrimination associated with targeted screening, although it does not eliminate the potential for discrimination resulting from disclosure or identification of an SCT athlete.

Con arguments against universal screening point out that universal precautions for heat-related illness and injury prevention in high-risk situations replace the need for screening as all athletes benefit from improved safety in playing conditions.[13] Arguments against universal screening are also tied to costs of screening tests, concerns for discrimination, and the fact that many athletes have already been tested and should be able to identify SCT status through newborn medical records. Finally, it is recommended that all athletes be educated on following universal precaution strategies, therefore obviating the need for universal screening.[14]

9. What Are Sensible Sport Recommendations for Patients With Sickle-Cell Trait?

SCT is not a contraindication for sport participation at any level, and no athlete should be disqualified from sport participation simply because he or she is identified as an SCT carrier. Recommendations for sport participation for SCT athletes include the following:

- All athletes should know their SCT status.
- Known SCT athletes should participate in a gradual preseason conditioning program and progressively build the intensity as tolerated.
- Highest-risk situations include early portions of practice cycles (first fall football workouts, after winter break) and early parts of a workout.
- Adequate hydration should be maintained at all times, and adequate rest and recovery breaks during training should be planned.

- Use additional caution in high-heat and humidity environments.
- If travelling to high altitudes, plan for altitude acclimatization. A change in altitude of more than 2000 feet may require modifications in training to allow for acclimatization.
- Avoid maximizing extreme bouts of exertion beyond 2 to 3 minutes.
- Avoid stimulants, supplements, or other drugs or medications when possible that can increase a risk of dehydration or exertional collapse.[13]
- Use caution or refrain from highly strenuous exercise when experiencing acute illness such as fever, gastrointestinal disturbances, or an asthma attack.

If certain symptoms occur, such as severe muscle pain, abnormal fatigue or weakness, chest pain or shortness of breath, dizziness or change in mental status (confusion, delirious), increasing body temperature, decreased ability to sweat, or at any time an athlete feels unable to continue to participate, he or she should immediately stop and notify a coach, parent, athletic trainer, or other supervising personnel and seek prompt medical attention.[17,18]

10. Are There Particular Screening or Monitoring Tests That Should Be Done for Patients Who Wish to Return to Play After Chemotherapy?

Clearance for sport participation following chemotherapy treatment for malignancy must be performed on an individual basis. Decisions are usually made by consultation with oncologists and any other specialists who must evaluate the long-term or permanent deleterious effects of chemotherapy treatment on the various organ systems. Lower-extremity numbness and pain, easy fatigability, generalized weakness, and memory and concentration deficits are just some of the residual effects of cancer treatment in children.[19] Common screening tests that are performed prior to receiving clearance for high-strenuous or contact sport participation are electrocardiograms or echocardiography, CBCs, and/or metabolic panels. It is important to note that even during chemotherapy treatment, many pediatric oncologists encourage low-strenuous, noncontact exercise, depending on the patient's current health status.[19]

11. What Findings on History or Examination May Suspect Malignancy Rather Than a Sports Injury?

Pain at rest, nighttime pain, or migrating pain may be signs of a systemic disease rather than a classic sports-related orthopedic injury and must be thoroughly evaluated. With regard to leukemias and lymphomas, vague or systemic symptoms such as bone pain, fatigue, fever, weight loss, or any sign of abnormal bleeding, lymphadenopathy, hepatosplenomegaly, or other palpable unexplained masses should signal a high index of suspicion and a prompt thorough evaluation involving laboratory screening, and appropriate imaging should be urgently performed. Central nervous system tumors may cause signs of increased intracranial pressure, nerve abnormalities, and/or seizures. Renal tumors may present with symptoms of hypertension, abdominal pain, and/or hematuria. Health care providers who routinely care for sports-related injuries and who perform sports physicals should always carefully review the patient's history, perform a complete physical examination, and remain vigilant to unusual or prolonged signs and symptoms of injury or illness that may lead to a prompt diagnosis of a serious health problem other than an orthopedic sports-related injury. Overtraining syndrome, anemia or other eating disorders, rheumatologic conditions, diabetes, cardiac disease, pulmonary conditions, and psychologic conditions such as depression and anxiety are other concerns that can present with subtle signs and symptoms and must be differentiated from malignancies.[20]

12. Are There Any Limits to HIV-Positive Patients Participating in Sports?

There are no limitations to sport participation for known HIV-positive athletes.[21] However, universal precautions must be strictly and consistently utilized when handling blood or body fluids with visible blood. The risk of transmission to other athletes appears minimal; therefore, all sports may be played by HIV-positive athletes as long as their current health state is adequate for the demands of the sport. It is important to note that the mandatory HIV testing of athletes is not justified and is not currently recommended by any of the major governing sports bodies at any level of sport participation.[22] The decision to disclose HIV status is at the athlete's discretion. Clearance for sport participation can be determined by the athlete's physician, and at all times, strict confidentiality guidelines should be followed.[23] A viral load that is low or undetectable is reassuring but not mandatory for sport participation. There is some concern with certain contact sports such as boxing, wrestling, martial arts, and football in which frequent skin breaks occur; participation should be avoided in those athletes with high viral loads and approached with caution in general for HIV-positive patients.[22]

References

1. Philpot J, Houghton K, Luke A. Physical activity recommendations for children with specific chronic health conditions: juvenile idiopathic arthritis, hemophilia, asthma, and cystic fibrosis. *Clin J Sports Med.* 2010;20(3):167–172.
2. National Hemophila Foundation. *Playing it Safe: Bleeding Disorders, Sports and Exercise.* New York, NY: National Hemophila Foundation; 2005.
3. American Academy of Pediatrics Committee on Sports and Fitness. Medical conditions affecting sports participation. *Pediatrics.* 2001;107: 1205–1209.
4. Suedekum N, Dimeff R. Iron and the athlete. *Curr Sports Med Rep.* 2005;4(4):199–202.
5. Rodenberg R, Gustafson S. Iron as an ergogenic aid: ironclad evidence? *Curr Sports Med Rep.* 2007;6(4):258–264.
6. Zoller H, Vogel W. Iron supplementation in athletes—first do no harm. *Nutrition.* 2004;20:615–619.
7. Hinton PS, Giordano C, Brownlie T, Haas JD. Iron Supplementation improves endurance after training in iron-depleted, nonanemic women. *J Appl Physiol.* 2000;88:1103-1111.
8. Tsalis, G. Nikolaidis MG, Mougios V: Effects of iron intake through food or supplement on iron status and performance of healthy adolescent swimmers during a training season. *Int J Sports Med.* 2004;25:306-313.
9. U.S. Preventive Services Task Force. Screening for iron deficiency anemia—including iron prophylaxis. In: *Guide to Clinical Preventive Services.* 2nd ed. Baltimore, MD: Williams & Wilkins; 1996:231–246.
10. Schumacher Y, Schmid A, Konig D, Berg A. Effects of exercise on soluble transferrin receptor and other variables of the iron status. *Br J Sports Med.* 2002;36:195–200.
11. National Institutes of Health. Dietary Supplement Fact Sheet: Iron. Office of Dietary Supplements Web site. http://ods.od.nih.gov/factsheets/Iron-HealthProfessional/. Updated August 24, 2007. Accessed March 23, 2013.
12. Vranken M. Evaluation of microcytosis. *Am Fam Physician.* 2010;82(9):1117–1122.
13. Koopmans J, Cox LA, Benjamin HJ, Clayton EW, Ross LF. Sickle cell trait screening in athletes: pediatricians' attitudes and concerns. *Pediatrics.* 2011;128(3):477–483.
14. American College of Sports Medicine. Current comment: sickle cell trait. www.acsm.org/docs/current-comments/sicklecelltrait.pdf. Accessed March 23, 2013.
15. Maron BJ, Harris KM, Haas TS. Sickle cell trait causing sudden death in competitive athletes: observations from the 30-year US national sudden death in young athletes registry free. *J Am Coll Cardiol.* 2011;57(14s1):1198.
16. Harmon KG, Drezner JA, Klossner D, Asif IM. Sickle cell trait associated with a RR of death 37 times in national collegiate athletic association football athletes: a database with 2 million athlete-years as the denominator. *Br J Sports Med.* 2012;46(5):325–330.
17. Harris KM, Haas TS, Eichner ER, Maron BJ. Sickle cell trait associated with sudden death in competitive athletes. *Am J Cardiology.* 2012;110(8):1185–1188.
18. American Academy of Pediatrics Council on Sports and Fitness. Climatic heat stress and exercising children and adolescents. *Pediatrics.* 2011;128;(3):741–747.
19. Berg C, Neufeld P, Harvey J, Downes A, Hayashi RJ. Late effects of childhood cancer, participation and quality of life of adolescents. *OTJR: Occupation, Participation and Health.* 2009:29;(3):116–124.
20. Young G, Toretsky JA, Campbell AB, Eskenazi AE. Recognition of common childhood malignancies. *Am Fam Physician.* 2000;61(7):2144–2154.
21. American Academy of Pediatrics Council on Sports and Fitness. Medical conditions affecting sports participation. *Pediatrics.* 2008;121;(4):841–848.
22. American Academy of Pediatrics, Committee on Sports Medicine and Fitness. Human immunodeficiency virus and other blood-borne viral pathogens in the athletic setting. *Pediatrics.* 1999;104(6):1400–1403.
23. American Medical Society for Sports Medicine and American College of Sports Medicine. Human immunodeficiency virus (HIV) and other blood borne pathogens in sports. *Am J Sports Med.* 1995;23:510–514.

14 Rheumatology Issues

Jeremy Ng, MD and Matthew Grady, MD, FAAP

1. Can Children With Juvenile Idiopathic Arthritis Participate in Sports? Are There Any Precautions?

Yes, children with juvenile idiopathic arthritis (JIA) can participate in sports, but a few general concepts should guide their sports participation:

- Decreased aerobic and anaerobic exercise capacity is common, so exercise needs to match their level of fitness.
- Weight bearing and aquatic exercises are safe and do not exacerbate arthritis.
- The extent of participation will be dictated by the severity and duration of illness.
- Exercise has many potential health benefits (Table 14-1).

JIA includes a wide spectrum of disorders (Table 14-2). Distinguishing between the subtypes helps in sports participation recommendations. The polyarticular rheumatoid factor-positive individuals have the worst overall prognosis.

The following precautions to participation will be related to the underlying disease involvement:

- *Temporomandibular joint involvement*—May benefit from mouth guards.
- *Cervical spine involvement*—Increased risk for spinal cord injury from contact/collision sports, need C1 to C2 x-rays and clearance from orthopedics.
- *Uveitis*—Consider eye protection.
- *Periods of active joint disease*—Limit/avoid highly competitive contact sports due to potential risk for damage to the joint surface and growth plate.
- *Systemic involvement (myocarditis/pericarditis)*—Limits based on extent of organ involvement.

JIA-affected individuals

- Decreased aerobic and anaerobic exercise capacity, usually related to the duration (> 2 yrs) and not severity of the disease.
- Diminished exercise capacity can be present in athletes whose JIA is in remission.
- Cochrane Review in 2007 found exercise programs did not exacerbate arthritis and should be considered safe.[1]
- Short-term benefits from exercise programs have been demonstrated.[1]
- Long-term benefits of exercise on quality of life and function remain unclear.

Exercise recommendations for children and adolescents with JIA:

- Encouraged to be physically active and participate in moderate fitness and strengthening exercises.
- Titrate activities to tolerance, recognizing that decreased aerobic and anaerobic exercise capacity is common.

Koutures C, Wong V.
Pediatric Sports Medicine: Essentials for Office Evaluation (pp 87-95)

Table 14-1. Benefits of Exercise
• Psychologic benefits of participating in normal childhood activities • Optimizing bone mineral density • Reduced loss of proteoglycans and cartilage damage • Lower obesity risk in active children (less load on the joints) • Increased muscle strength from weight-bearing exercises • Increased range of motion and fitness from aquatic exercises with less strain on joints

Table 14-2. Juvenile Idiopathic Arthritis Subgroups and Their Descriptions
SYSTEMIC (20% TO 30%)
• Fever • Salmon-colored rash • Small and large joint involvement
POLYARTICULAR (25% TO 35%)
• 5 ≥ joints involved • Small and large joints involved • Rheumatoid factor-positive group has the worse prognosis
OLIGOARTICULAR (45%)
• 4 ≤ joints involved in first 6 months, mostly knees and ankles • Called persistent oligoarticular JIA if 4 or fewer joints involved • Called extended oligoarticular JIA if 5 or more joints involved after 6 months
PSORIATIC ARTHRITIS (2% TO 15%)
• Arthritis plus two of the following: ◦ Dactylitis ◦ Nail abnormalities ◦ Psoriasis or positive family history of psoriasis
ENTHESITIS-RELATED ARTHRITIS
• Form of spondyloarthropathy • Arthritis plus two of the following: ◦ Sacroiliac joint tenderness/inflammatory lumbosacral pain ◦ Positive HLA B27 ◦ Arthritis in boy age 6 or older ◦ Acute anterior symptomatic uveitis ◦ First-degree relative with history of ankylosing spondylitis, enthesitis-related arthritis, reactive arthritis, sacroiliitis with irritable bowel syndrome, or acute anterior uveitis

- Can participate in competitive contact sports if their disease is well controlled and they have adequate training and physical capacity.
- In individuals with severe disease, individualized training in a group exercise format has both physical and social benefits.

2. What Is Hypermobility Syndrome? What Are the Challenges in Sports Participation in an Athlete That Has This Entity?

Joint Hypermobility

- Joints that move beyond the normal physiologic range.
- May be a benign finding in 5% to 10% of general pediatric population.[2]
- Children and female athletes have higher percentages of hypermobile joints.
- Joints that are hypermobile put additional strain on surrounding soft tissues (joint capsule, ligaments, tendons, muscles) that serve as joint stabilizers.
- Hypermobile joints may not have any associated joint pain or instability.

Hypermobility Syndrome (Benign Joint Hypermobility Syndrome)

- Condition that includes hypermobile joints and associated joint pain or recurrent dislocations.
- Considered a benign connective tissue disorder, inherited in a multifactorial pattern.
- Although it shares similar joint findings, it is distinct from osteogenesis imperfecta, Marfan syndrome, and Ehlers-Danlos syndrome.
- Joint pain is not associated with underlying rheumatologic disease.
- The Beighton score (Table 14-3) can be used to assess joint hypermobility.
- The Brighton criteria (Table 14-4) can help one make the diagnosis of hypermobility syndrome.

Athletes With Hypermobile Joints

- Are at increased risk for ligament tears and joint dislocations, especially patella and glenohumeral dislocations.
- During vigorous physical activity, stress on the surrounding soft tissue may exceed the capacity of the soft tissues and cause pain.
- Strength training may decrease but will not eliminate these risks.
- Participation in contact/collision sports should be individualized based on risk of injury.

Treatment of Hypermobile Joint Pain

- Physical therapy focused on strengthening muscles groups and improving joint proprioception.
- Orthoses to limit range of motion (ROM), such as an ankle brace or orthotics, may be helpful.
- Affected individuals should avoid "party tricks" that deliberately stretch the joint capsule, since this may lead to further joint instability.

3. What Is the Work-Up for a Suspected Infected Joint?

Primary

- Labs—Complete blood count (CBC), erythrocyte sedimentation rate (ESR), C-reactive protein (CRP), Lyme immunoglobulin G (IgG)/immunoglobulin M (IgM), blood culture.
- Joint fluid analysis—Cell count, glucose (ratio fluid to serum, 0.8:1.0), Gram stain and culture +/– crystal analysis, DNA polymerase chain reaction and synovial tissue biopsy.
- X-ray.
- Ultrasonography (especially of hip).

Table 14-3. Beighton Score
1 POINT EACH FOR LEFT AND RIGHT SIDE, TOTAL POSSIBLE SCORE IS 9
• > 10 degrees hyperextension of the elbow
• Ability to passively touch forearm with the thumb while the wrist is flexed
• > 90 degrees extension of the fifth finger (see Figure 14-1)
• > 10 degrees hyperextension of the knee (genu recurvatum)
• Ability to touch the floor with palms of hands while standing with knees straight

Figure 14-1. Gorling's sign: ability to passively extend 5th digit 90 degrees or more.

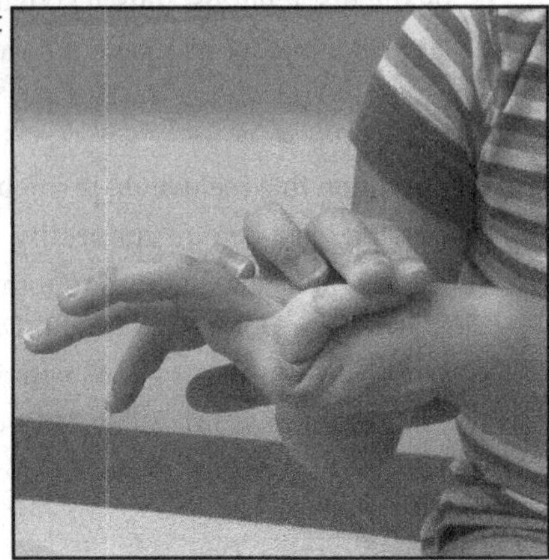

Table 14-4. Brighton Criteria
MAJOR
• Beighton score of 4/9 currently or in the past
• Arthralgia in 4 or more joints for more than 3 months
MINOR
• Beighton score of 1 to 3
• Arthralgia in 1 to 3 joints for more than 3 months or back pain for < 3 months
• Dislocation or subluxation of more than 1 joint or in 1 joint 2 or more times
• < 3 lesions of soft-tissue lesions (includes epicondylitis, tenosynovitis, bursitis)
• Marfanoid habitus in the absence of Marfan syndrome (arm span to height ratio > 1.03, upper body to lower body ratio < 0.89, arachnodactyly, tall thin build)
• Abnormal thin skin with striae, hyperextensibility, and abnormal scarring
• Drooping eyelids or myopia
• Varicose veins, hernia, rectal/uterine prolapse
• Mitral valve prolapse
DIAGNOSIS OF HYPERMOBILITY SYNDROME (ANY ONE OF THE FOLLOWING)
• 2 major criteria
• 1 major plus 2 minor
• 4 minor criteria
• Minor criteria plus one affected first-degree relative

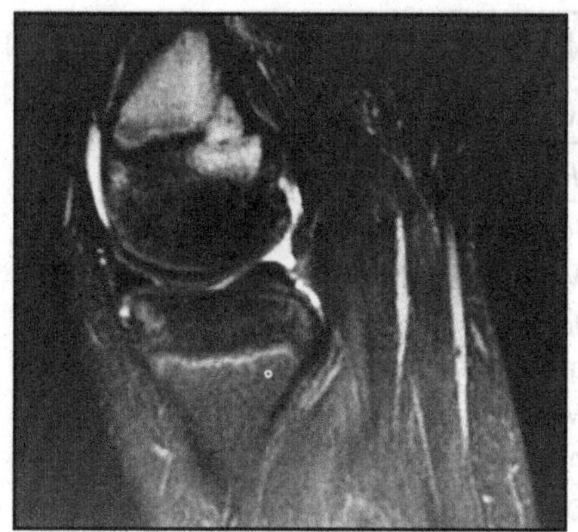

Figure 14-2. MRI knee demonstrating osteomyelitis of the distal femoral metaphysis.

Secondary

- Magnetic resonance imaging (MRI) with and without contrast.
- Computed tomography (CT) scan with and without contrast.

The hip joint is the most commonly infected joint in children. Ultrasonography is very good at detecting joint effusions and should be ordered for suspected hip infection. In children with open growth plates, osteomyelitis in the distal metaphysis may have a similar presentation as a septic joint (Figure 14-2). Often, the labs will be borderline normal. X-rays and MRIs are helpful in making the diagnosis of osteomyelitis. CT scans are best to evaluate bony architecture and may be ordered by an orthopedic surgeon if a biopsy is needed.

4. What Is the Work-Up for a Joint That Should Be Evaluated by a Rheumatologist?

Preliminary Lab Work-Up

- CBC, ESR, CRP, antinuclear antibody (ANA), rheumatoid factor (RF) (more helpful in teens/multiple joint involvement), Lyme IgG/IgM in Lyme-endemic area.

Additional Labs Based on Clinical Suspicion

- JIA: anti-cyclic citrullinated peptide antibodies; enthesitis/spondyloarthritides: HLA B27, lupus: anti-double-stranded DNA (anti-dsDNA); anti-Smith antibodies; viral: parvo B19 IgG/IgM; and rheumatic fever: antistreptolysin O titer, anti-DNase B, and anti-strep hyaluronidase tests.

5. Fatigue or General Malaise Is a Common Report Among Athletes. Which Presentations May Suggest a Rheumatologic Condition, and What Evaluation Is Recommended?

The differential diagnosis of fatigue in an athlete is extensive. Practical considerations dictate a limited evaluation for life-threatening conditions and a system-focused evaluation based on history and physical examination. The presentation of rheumatologic conditions (JIA, lupus, psoriatic arthritis, spondyloarthropathy, and inflammatory bowel disease with joint involvement) can be varied. Table 14-5 lists the common signs and symptoms of fatigue with rheumatologic involvement.

The evaluation of fatigue with suspected rheumatologic involvement includes preliminary rheumatology screening labs plus common conditions that may mimic rheumatology involvement.

- Rheumatology—See question 4.
- Thyroid-stimulating hormone and CMP to evaluate thyroid, renal, and liver function.
- Food and exercise diary to evaluate caloric intact versus output and possible overtraining.

Table 14-5. Common Signs and Symptoms of Fatigue With Rheumatologic Involvement	
SIGNS	*SYMPTOMS*
• Joint warmth, erythema, effusion • Synovial thickening • Pain on passive joint ROM • Decreased joint ROM • Diffuse (not localized) joint pain in the absence of trauma • Muscle atrophy around involved joints • Systemic involvement includes rash, fever, weight loss, subcutaneous nodules, oral or nasal ulcerations, gastrointestinal symptoms • Uveitis (generally asymptomatic) • Psoriasis, nail abnormalities, dactylitis • Enthesitis, sacroiliac joint tenderness	• Joint symptoms longer than 6 weeks • Morning stiffness • Joint stiffness after a period of no joint motion (gel phenomenon) • Multiple joints involved • Afternoon fatigue • Decreased aerobic or anaerobic exercise capacity (decline in performance)

6. An Athlete Presents With Pain After an Injury That Is Lasting Much Longer Than Anticipated or Is Greater in Amplitude Than May Be Expected. What Are the Potential Causes, and How Should the Primary Care Provider Evaluate and Refer Such Cases?

- The potential causes of unanticipated pain after an injury are as follows:
  - Complex regional pain syndrome (CRPS)/reflex sympathetic dystrophy/causalgia (Table 14-6).
  - Osteomyelitis/septic arthritis.
  - Occult fracture/stress fracture.
  - Malignancy (pathological fracture or leukemia).
  - Osteoid osteoma.
  - Joint hypermobility syndrome with slow soft-tissue healing.
  - Peripheral neuropathy (brachial plexus injury).
  - Tarsal coalition/abnormal foot mechanics for foot and ankle pain.
- History is a crucial part of the evaluation of CRPS.
  - Minor injury, a fracture, or a medical problem (JIA flare) precipitates the abnormal neuropathic response.
  - Pain typically gets worse 1 to 2 weeks after the athlete sustains the injury.
  - Both CRPS 1 and CRPS 2 produce a similar constellation of signs and symptoms (see Table 14-6).
  - Classic features include expanding border of pain, which gets worse with immobilization.
  - Significant psychologic/psychosocial history, including home or school stressors.
  - Individuals (80% are female) with CRPS type 1 often have common traits: people pleasers, and motivated, achievement-oriented, perfectionists.[3]
- Complex regional pain syndrome type 1 (previously called reflex sympathetic dystrophy)
  - CRPS Type 1 is described as a pathologic nerve response to a real injury. Injury is usually minor.

Table 14-6. Signs and Symptoms of Complex Regional Pain Syndrome	
SIGNS	*SYMPTOMS*
Early • Overall well appearing • Cold clammy extremity • Secondary changes in local blood flow **Late** • Muscle atrophy (often secondary to disuse) • Changes in the hair, nails, and skin	• Progressive neuropathic pain • Hyperpathia (exaggerated pain response to painful stimuli) • Hyperalgesia (exaggerated pain response to nonpainful stimuli) • Cutaneous allodynia (pain to light touch) • Pain that worsens with immobilization

- Normal nerve conduction pattern from skin/peripheral nerve to spinal cord to brain is altered and an *aberrant loop* develops.
- Signal from the spinal cord is directed both to the brain and to the local neurovascular (sympathetic) system, which feeds back to the site of injury. The signal from the spinal cord is directed both to the brain and to the local neurovascular (sympathetic) system, which feeds back to the site of injury.
- Neurovascular response is peripheral vasoconstriction, which causes a localized hypoxia and lactic acidosis, further triggering a pain response.

- Complex regional pain syndrome type 2 (previously called causalgia)
  - CRPS type 2 is less commom and associated with actual peripheral nerve injury.

The treatment of CRPS involves attempting to break this aberrant loop. Intensive physical therapy includes constant tactile stimulation with a variety of objects (hot, cold, soft, rough) to "flood the system and cause it to reset." The inpatient therapy produces the best results and includes intensive physical therapy (5 to 6 hours/day) with or without psychotherapy (biofeedback, behavioral modification). Other therapies include sympathetic blocks, transcutaneous electrical nerve stimulation, and medications (tricyclics, anticonvulsants, opioids, glucocorticoids).

- Outpatient treatment—Start the following immediately:
  - Daily tactile stimulation (desensitization) for 3 hours a day to the affected body part.
  - Desensitization is painful and frequently requires parent participation and support.
  - Formal physical therapy is required.
  - Joint immobilization or disuse is counterproductive and should be avoided.
  - Pain medications should be minimized or avoided.
  - Psychosocial stresses should be identified and addressed.
  - Many individuals respond to 1 month of outpatient therapy, with those identified earlier in the process recovering faster.
  - Individuals who are not progressing with 1 month of outpatient treatment need referral to a regional pain center.

Evaluation for Prolonged or Excessive Pain

- Exclude significant structural abnormalities or conditions first.
- Evaluation includes a focused history and physical examination and plain x-rays (Table 14-7).
- **CRPS is a diagnosis of exclusion.**
- Additional imaging such as a bone scan, CT scan, or MRI, and labs including CBC and ESR are guided by the initial evaluation when CRPS is not suspected.

TABLE 14-7. EVALUATION OF PROLONGED/EXCESSIVE PAIN: HISTORY, PHYSICAL EXAMINATION AND PLAIN FILMS		
HISTORY (KEY FACTS)	*PHYSICAL EXAM*	*X-RAYS*
Mechanism of Injury • Minor versus major trauma • Osteomyelitis can develop a few weeks after focal bone injury **Timing of Onset and Progression of Symptoms** • Improving: more likely soft-tissue injury • Worsening: CRPS **Associated Constitutional Symptoms** • Fever, weight loss, decreased appetite: associated with leukemia/infection **Area of Pain** • Remaining focal: more likely structural • Expanding: more likely CRPS	**Focal Pain** • More likely to be structural (stress fracture or soft-tissue injury) **Pain to Light Touch of Skin** • Almost always CRPS **Overlying Skin Changes** • Warm/erythema: infectious or inflammatory process • Cold/clammy: CRPS	**Periosteal Reaction** • Healing fracture, malignancy, osteoid osteoma **Lucency in Bone** • Brodie abscess, bone cyst, pathologic fracture **Structural Bone Abnormality** • Tarsal coalition

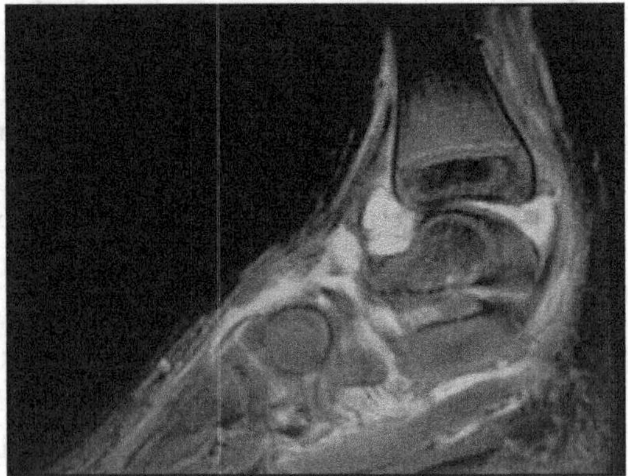

Figure 14-3. MRI ankle demonstrating ankle joint effusion.

7. Swollen and Painful Joints in Athletes May Have Causes That Are Nonsports or Trauma Related. Which History, Examination, or Diagnostic Findings Might Suggest a Nonsports- or Trauma-Related Injury?

Figure 14-3 shows a swollen ankle joint in a patient with JIA.

HISTORY

- Joint pain/swelling for more than 4 to 6 weeks
- Night pain and/or morning stiffness
- Pain out of proportion to examination
- Minor trauma-producing pain (pathologic fracture)
- Multiple joint involvement

Physical Examination

- Diffuse joint pain
- Red, warm joint
- Decreased ROM actively or pain with passive range of motion
- Enthesitis
- Allodynia
- Joint effusion
- Inability to bear weight/altered gait
- Skin bruising/petechiae
- Lymphadenopathy

Diagnostic Findings

- X-rays may show periosteal reaction, a bony lucency, or soft-tissue calcifications.
- Labs may show CBC abnormalities (anemia, low platelets, abnormal white blood cell count), ESR/CRP elevation, positive ANA, or positive RF.
- CT scan may show cortical bone destruction, indicating a malignancy or infiltrative process (eosinophilic granuloma).
- MRI may show joint effusion, synovial hypertrophy (pigmented villonodular synovitis), arteriovenous malformation, metaphyseal osteomyeleitis, or cortical bone involvement.

References

1. Takken T, Van Brussel M, Engelbert RH, Van Der Net J, Kuis W, Helders PJ. Exercise therapy in juvenile idiopathic arthritis: a Cochrane Review. *Eur J Phys Rehabil Med.* 2008 Sep;44(3):287-97.
2. Grahame R, Bird HA, Child A. The revised (Brighton 1998) criteria for the diagnosis of benign joint hypermobility syndrome (BJHS). *J Rheumatol.* 2000;27:1777–1779.
3. Sherry DD, Malleson PN. The idiopathic musculoskeletal pain syndromes in childhood. *Rheum Dis Clin North Am.* 2002;28(3):669–685.

Suggested Readings

Biro F, Gewanter HL, Baum J. The hypermobility syndrome. *Pediatrics.* 1983;72:701–706.

Klepper SE. Exercise and fitness in children with arthritis: evidence of benefits for exercise and physical activity. *Arthritis Rheum (Arthritis Care & Research).* 2003;49(3):435–443.

Klepper SE. Effects of an eight-week physical conditioning program on disease signs and symptoms in children with chronic arthritis. *Arthritis Care Res.* 1999;12:52–60.

Philpott J, Houghton K, Luke A; Canadian Paediatric Society, Healthy Active Living and Sports Medicine Committee, Canadian Academy of Sport Medicine, Paediatric Sport and Exercise Medicine Committee, Physical activity recommendations for children with specific chronic health conditions: juvenile idiopathic arthritis, hemophilia, asthma and cystic fibrosis. *Paediatric Child Health.* 2010;15(4):213–218.

Recommendations for the diagnosis and management of juvenile idiopathic arthritis. *2009 The Royal Australian College of General Practitioners.* www.racgp.org.au/guidelines/juvenileidiopathicarthritis. Accessed May 1, 2012

Ross J, Grahame R. Joint hypermobility syndrome. *BMJ.* 2011:342:c7167.

Seckin U, Sonel Tur B, Yilmaz O, Yagci I, Bodur H, Arasil T. The prevalence of joint hypermobility among high school students. *Rheumatol Int.* 2005;25:260–263.

Singh-Grewal D, Wright V, Bar-Or O, et al. Pilot study of fitness training and exercise testing in polyarticular childhood arthritis. *Arthritis Rheum.* 2006;55:364–372.

Takken T, Van Der Net J, et al. Aquatic fitness training for children with juvenile idiopathic arthritis. Rheumatology (Oxford). 2003;42:1408–1414.

Work group recommendations: 2002 Exercise and Physical Activity Conference, St. Louis, Missouri. Session V: evidence of benefit of exercise and physical activity in arthritis. *Arthritis Rheum.* 2003;49:453–454.

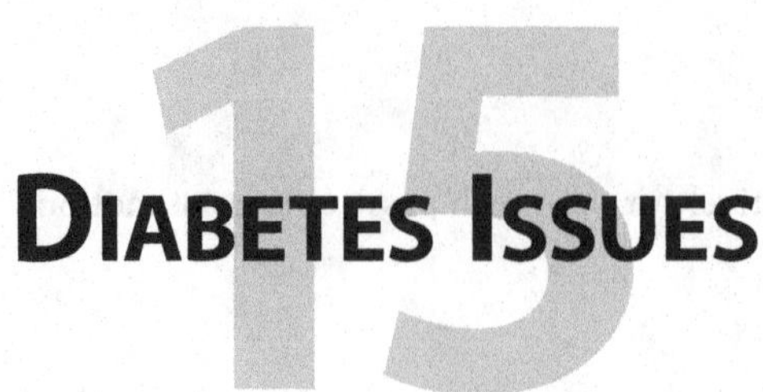

Diabetes Issues

David Wang, MD; Suriti Kundu Achar, MD; and Suraj Achar, MD, FAAFP

1. What Levels of Preactivity Blood Glucose Suggest a Risk for Hypoglycemia, and How Should a Patient Respond to These Levels and Potentially Modify Activity?

- A preactivity blood glucose level of < 100 mg/dL may increase the risk of hypoglycemia.
- To prevent hypoglycemia, the basal dose of insulin can be reduced and carbohydrate intake can be increased to ensure a high enough preactivity blood glucose level (usually 150 to 250 mg/dL).
- If the patient's blood sugar level is < 100 mg/dL prior to activity, carbohydrates should be consumed and vigorous or prolonged exercise should be avoided.[1]
  - If carbohydrate supplementation is able to achieve a stable blood glucose of > 140 mg/dL, the athlete can proceed with activity but must monitor his or her blood sugar at least every 30 minutes while exercising.
- Signs and symptoms of hypoglycemia usually develop in those with a blood glucose level of < 70 mg/dL.

2. What Levels of Preactivity Blood Glucose Suggest a Risk for Hyperglycemia, and How Should a Patient Respond to These Levels and Potentially Modify Activity?

- Many athletes intentionally begin exercise with an elevated blood sugar (150 to 250 mg/dL) in an attempt to prevent exercise-induced hypoglycemia.[2]
- If the patient's blood sugar is above the renal glucose reabsorption threshold of 180 mg/dL (findings may include glycosuria with symptoms of polyuria and polydipsia), athletes should avoid fluids with carbohydrate, as these may lead to increased urination, fluid loss, and dehydration.[1]
- If the patient's preactivity blood glucose level is ≥ 250 mg/dL, then urine or blood should be tested for ketones.[1]
  - If ketones are present, exercise is contraindicated.[1]
  - If ketones are not present, exercise is not contraindicated but should be performed with caution.[1]
- Rigorous exercise will bring down the blood glucose level 40 to 60 mg/dL every 30 minutes.
- If the patient's preactivity blood glucose level is ≥ 300 mg/dL without ketones, exercise can be performed, but with caution and frequent blood sugar monitoring.[1]
- Insulin should be administered to correct the hyperglycemia, and the athlete should maintain excellent hydration.

Koutures C, Wong V.
Pediatric Sports Medicine: Essentials for Office Evaluation (pp 96-102)

- If the patient has persistent hyperglycemia, especially with short-duration, intense activities, an increase in the basal insulin rate or small insulin boluses can be considered.[1]

3. What Are Some Common Exercise Effects on Insulin Needs, and How Can Athletes Modify Dosing/Food Intake Accordingly?

Exercise Effects on Insulin Needs

- Metabolic adjustments that maintain normoglycemia during exercise are mainly hormonally mediated.[3]
- During the first few minutes of moderate-intensity exercise, glycogen is the major fuel source for skeletal muscle. As exercise continues, the predominate sources of energy become blood glucose and non-esterified fatty acids. A hormonal and autonomic response causes a decrease in circulating insulin concentrations and a rise in counter-regulatory hormones to match this demand, increasing hepatic glucose production and tissue uptake, as well as mobilizing fatty acid from adipose tissue.
- After exercise, the body is basically in a fasting state. There are low glycogen stores in both the liver and muscle, with increased hepatic glucose production. Levels of counter-regulatory hormones remain high for quite some time, resulting in hyperglycemia and hyperinsulinemia.
- Injury or trauma suffered during exercise will result in a hyperglycemic state.
- For subcutaneously injected insulin, the absorption rate increases during exercise due to increased subcutaneous and skeletal muscle blood flow and increased body temperature.[1]

Athletes' Modifications

- In general, insulin requirements are less in athletes, often between 0.2 and 0.6 U/kg/day.[4]
- Children may be prone to greater variability in blood glucose, and in the case of adolescents, hormonal changes can contribute to the difficulty in controlling blood glucose levels.[3]
- Every athlete is different, requiring trial and error to determine personal response to exercise and appropriate insulin modifications. At the beginning of a new season, testing blood glucose levels often during the 12-hour postexercise period can help establish insulin requirements.[5]
- It is important for the athlete to have consistent training regimens that mimic competition to establish an appropriate adjustment to his or her insulin regimen.
- Meals should be taken 3 to 5 hours before exercise given delayed gastric emptying in diabetes.[4]
- If exercise is brief (< 30 minutes) and mild in intensity (< 70% VO_2max), minimal adjustment needs to be made to the patient's insulin regimen.
- If moderate morning activity is planned, the prior night's basal insulin dose should be reduced by 20% to 50%.
- The morning short-acting insulin dose prior to exercise should be decreased by 30% to 50%.[4]
- If exercise is high intensity (eg, a marathon, triathlon, rugby, football, hockey), insulin doses may require a reduction of 70% to 90%.[4]
- If an insulin pump is used, reduce the basal rate by 20% to 50% 1 to 2 hours before exercise, reduce the bolus dose up to 50% at the meal prior to exercising, and suspend or disconnect the insulin pump at the start of exercise. It is important to note that pumps should not be disconnected for longer than 60 minutes without supplemental insulin.[1]

- Doctors and parents can also reduce the insulin infusion rate by half and give the other half of the long acting insulin (glargine) once daily. The children can then remove the pump if heavily involved in sports or swimming frequently.
- After exercise, 60 to 120 g of carbohydrate should be consumed to restore muscle and liver stores of glycogen, and insulin doses should be reduced by 25% to 50%—even though the body is in a hyperglycemic state—to reduce the risk of late-onset hypoglycemia.[4]
- If the exercise is unexpected and an adjustment in insulin dosing cannot be made, carbohydrate supplementation should be used instead. A patient should consume 20 to 30 g of carbohydrates at the onset of exercise and then every 30 minutes following completion of exercise.[4]
- Once the patient establishes a stable exercise/training and insulin regimen, most adjustments to prevent exercise-induced hypoglycemia will be made by carbohydrate dietary supplementation.[2]
- Typically, 15 to 60 g of carbohydrates in the form of drinks containing 5% to 10% carbohydrate will match the losses during exercise.[2] During times of injury, athletes should have increased blood glucose monitoring and appropriate adjustments to their insulin dosages to counter the hyperglycemic effects.
- Insulin should never be administered intramuscularly because muscle contraction with activity will accelerate insulin absorption.
- The injection site should not be exposed to heat (including whirlpools, hot packs, and ultrasonography) or cold (including ice baths and ice) for up to 4 hours after injection because this can accelerate or slow absorption, respectively.

4. What Are Some Recommendations for a Diabetic Action Plan for Activity Designed for Coaches, Athletic Trainers, Physical Education Teachers, and Other Adult Supervisors?

Every athlete with diabetes should have a written care plan for games and practices prepared and agreed upon by parents, school nurses, medical providers, and key activity/sport supervisors.

- The care plan should include guidelines for the frequency of the monitoring of blood glucose and urine ketones with specific values at which participation is excluded.
- Guidelines for insulin therapy, including the type of insulin, doses, adjustments depending on the type and severity of activity, and a correctional scale for hyperglycemia, should also be included.
- The entire team caring for the athlete, including doctors, coaches, trainers, and parents, must be prepared for variances in length of competitions, environmental conditions, emotional stress and excitement, and absorption of insulin and dietary supplements.
- The care plan should also include the athlete's medication list, which should include nondiabetes-related medications.
- Guidelines for recognizing hypoglycemia and appropriate treatment options, including when and how to use glucose tabs (4 g of carbohydrates each), glucose tube (15 g of carbohydrates each), and a glucagon injection kit, should also be included. Consider taping glucose tablets and/or hard candy to a clipboard for ready access if symptomatic hypoglycemia is observed.
- The care plan should include guidelines for recognizing hyperglycemia and appropriate treatment options.

Emergency contact information for parents and physicians, as well as consent for medical treatment (for minors) and the identification of specific trained personnel who are able to carry out the action plan, should also be included.

- Medication alert tag should be present with the athlete with diabetes at all times.
- All necessary testing equipment/supplies should be in a first aid pack.

5. What Are Common Situations or Signs of Hypoglycemia That Might Be Seen on the Athletic Field, and What Would Be Appropriate Responses?

Common Situations of Hypoglycemia

- Often, hypoglycemia is the result of excess insulin use.
- Male patients and adolescents are at a higher risk of suffering an episode of severe hypoglycemia.[1]
- Due to counterregulatory hormone responses, the risk of hypoglycemia is greater when exercise is performed in the afternoon, involves more lower-extremity activities and if it is prolonged rather than in short bursts.[6]
- A previous hypoglycemic episode puts the athlete at a higher risk of suffering another episode in the following days due to resulting impaired release of counterregulatory hormones.[1]
- Late-onset hypoglycemia can occur after exercising, even while the athlete is sleeping; exercise's effects on improving insulin sensitivity in skeletal muscle and depleting glycogen stores can last for several hours to days after exercise.

Signs of Hypoglycemia

- As glucose levels drop to below 65 mg/dL, counterregulatory hormones are released and symptoms of hypoglycemia develop.
- Autonomic symptoms—Tachycardia, sweating, palpitations, hunger, nervousness, headache, trembling, and dizziness.[1]
- Neurogenic symptoms (as glucose continues to fall to below 30 to 40 mg/dL)—Blurred vision, fatigue, difficulty thinking, loss of motor control, aggressive behavior, seizures, convulsions, loss of consciousness, and eventually brain damage and death.[1]

Treatment of Hypoglycemia

Hypoglycemia is considered mild if the athlete is conscious and can follow directions and swallow. It is considered severe if the athlete is unconscious or unable to follow directions, including swallowing or eating.[1]

- The treatment of mild hypoglycemia is as follows[1]:
  - Administer 10 to 15 g of fast-acting carbohydrates (4 to 8 glucose tablets or 2 T of honey)
  - Wait about 15 minutes and then recheck the patient's blood sugar.
  - If the blood sugar remains low, administer another 10 to 15 g of fast-acting carbohydrates and then recheck the patient's blood sugar in another 15 minutes.
  - If the blood sugar does not return to the normal range after the second supplement, activate emergency medical services.
  - When the blood glucose does return to the normal range, the athlete should consume a snack.
- The treatment of severe hypoglycemia is as follows[1]:
  - Activate emergency medical services immediately.
  - Prepare and inject one vial of glucagon. The athlete should awaken within 15 minutes. The glucagon may cause the athlete to vomit, so turn him or her onto his or her side after administration.

- When the athlete is conscious and able to swallow, provide him or her with a snack.

An evening snack or reduced evening dose of insulin after activity may be necessary to avoid late-onset hypoglycemia.

6. Can Insulin Pumps Be Padded During Contact Sports, and if so, How Can This Be Done?

A disadvantage of an insulin pump is its susceptibility to damage during contact sports. If the athlete decides to wear the pump during activity, it should be protected as described below:

- Take a piece of padding about ¼-inch thick that is just larger than the size of the pump, and cut a hole the size of the pump into it.
- Place this piece over the pump.
- Put a second pad the same size as the first, but without a hole cut into it, on top.
- Secure the padding with a wrap or compression clothing.[7]

If the pump is to be worn during contact sports, a backup pump or insulin supply must always be available in case it is damaged.

For athletes who wear patch pumps, a neoprene sleeve from a cut-up wetsuit or an ace wrap can be placed around the athlete's limb where the patch pump is located. While this will help prevent dislodging, it typically will not survive a direct or side impact blow. If this is to occur, the patch pump will need to be changed out for a new one.

7. What Type of Athlete or Set of Findings Suggest a High Risk for Type 2 Diabetes Mellitus?

As many as 80% of individuals with type 2 diabetes are overweight.[8] However, obesity is not the only risk factor for diabetes. Metabolic syndrome (hypertension, impaired glucose metabolism, central obesity, low high-density lipoprotein levels, and elevated triglyceride levels) increases the risk of type 2 diabetes. Although type 2 diabetes is extremely rare in competitive athletes,[2] athletes are not immune to developing metabolic syndrome or type 2 diabetes. One study of 70 collegiate football linemen identified 34 as having metabolic syndrome, and 9 had elevated HbA1c values.[9] Athletes who gain an advantage by being larger than their opponents have the potential for developing central obesity. Athletes with a waist circumference >40 inches should be evaluated for other risk factors for metabolic syndrome and type 2 diabetes.[9]

8. Are There any Limits to Sport Participation in Athletes With Type 2 Diabetes Mellitus?

- The young athlete with diabetes who is in good metabolic control can safely participate in most activities.[3]
- The following situations are exceedingly rare for children with type 2 diabetes, since they require a longer duration of diabetes:
  - Patients with type 2 diabetes with proliferative diabetic retinopathy should avoid strenuous activity including anaerobic exercise, straining, or Valsalva-like maneuvers, as these can precipitate vitreous hemorrhage or traction retinal detachment.[3]
  - Patients with type 2 diabetes with overt nephropathy should be discouraged from high-intensity exercises.[3]
  - Significant peripheral neuropathy is an indication to limit weight bearing exercise given the risk for ulcer formation and fractures. Activities such as the using the treadmill, prolonged walking, jogging, and step exercises are contraindicated. Recommended activities for those with significant peripheral neuropathy include swimming, biking, rowing, chair exercises, arm exercises, and other nonweight-bearing exercises.[3]

- Patients with diabetes with autonomic neuropathy should avoid exercise in hot or cold environments given their difficulty with thermoregulation.[3]
- Patients on metformin can generally perform most—if not all—exercise programs. There is a theoretical increase in lactic acidosis with intense exercise.
- Patients on sulfonylurea therapy should perform vigorous exercise with caution given the risk of hypoglycemia.[8]

9. What Are Some Common Recommendations for Athletes With Type 2 Diabetes Mellitus?

- Exercise should be discussed in every encounter with a patient with type 2 diabetes.
- Exercise has been shown to improve insulin sensitivity and assist in decreasing blood sugar, including an improvement of HbA1c levels by 10% to 20% from baseline.[3]
- Physical activity recommendations for healthy adults and for patients with type 2 diabetes are quite similar.[2]
- Patients with type 2 diabetes who were previously sedentary should aim to accumulate a minimum energy expenditure of 1000 kcal/week, which equates to a minimum of 30 minutes of accumulated moderate-intensity activity on 5 days of the week.[6]
- To decrease cardiovascular risk, it is recommended that 150 min/week of at least moderate intensity and/or 90 min/week of vigorous activity be performed, with the addition of resistance training 3 times per week encouraged.[6]
  - Resistance exercises should involve all muscle groups, and patients should perform 8 to 10 repetitions per set for a total of 3 sets.[6]
- Exercise should be performed on at least 3 days per week, with no more than 2 consecutive days without training.[6]
- Both aerobic and resistance training are equally beneficial for glycemic control, although aerobic training has a greater effect on body composition, and combining the two is twice as effective for glycemic control.[4]
- The American College of Sports Medicine and the American Diabetes Association recommend aerobic exercise at an intensity of 40% to 70% VO_2 max, and anaerobic exercise for a minimum of one set of 10 to 15 repetitions using 8 to 10 resistance exercises.[2]
  - This is intended to minimize the contribution of the anaerobic energy systems and allow individuals an extended period of time to be active (20 to 60 minutes) to allow for an adequate stimulus to increase or maintain aerobic capacity and to expend sufficient calories to assist with weight control.[2]
- In terms of medication: prior to starting exercise training, patients with multiple blood sugar readings of < 80 mg/dL or with more than two symptomatic hypoglycemic episodes in a week should have their dosages cut by 50% to 100%. If they have modest control, the dose can be cut by 25% to 50%. If their blood sugars are generally above 100 mg/dL, they should have no or minimal change in their dosages.[4]

References

1. Jimenez CC, Corcoran MH, Crawley JT, et al. National Athletic Trainers' Association Position Statement: management of the athlete with type 1 diabetes mellitus. *J Athl Train*. 2007;42(4):536–545.
2. Hornsby WG, Chetlin RG. Management of competitive athletes with diabetes. *Diabetes Spectrum*. 2005;18(2):102–107.
3. American Diabetes Association. Diabetes mellitus and exercise: position statement. *Diabetes Care*. 2002;25(1):S64–S68.
4. Peirce NS. Diabetes and exercise. *Br J Sports Med*. 1999;33(3):161–173.
5. Silverstein J, Klingensmith G, Copeland K, et al. Care of children and adolescents with type 1 diabetes: a statement of the American Diabetes Association. *Diabetes Care*. 2005;28:186–212.

6. Gallen I. The management of insulin treated diabetes and sport. *Practical Diabetes Int.* 2005;22(8):307–312.
7. Philbin R. Smart pumps and sports: to wear the pump or Not? Children with Diabetes. www.childrenwithdiabetes.com/sports/sp-disconnect.htm. Accessed March 24, 2013.
8. Marwick TH, Hordern MD, Miller T, et al. Exercise training for type 2 diabetes mellitus: impact on cardiovascular risk: a scientific statement from the American Heart Association. *Circulation.* 2009;119:3244–3262.
9. Buell JL, Calland D, Hanks F, et al. Presence of metabolic syndrome in football linemen. *J Athl Train.* 2008;43(6):608–616.

Acknowledgment

The authors wish to give special thanks to Kimberly Krenek for her advice and support as a mother with a child with type 1 diabetes mellitus.

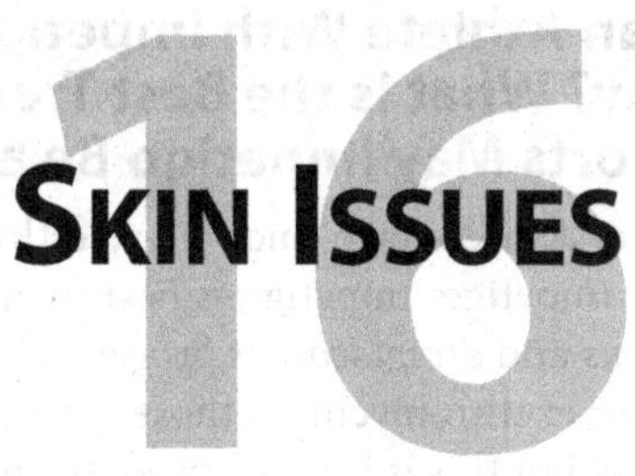

Skin Issues

Mark Halstead, MD

1. What Are Some Methods to Prevent Methicillin-Resistant *Staphylococcus aureus* Colonization and Infection in Athletes, and What Is the Best Way to Clean Equipment to Minimize Its Colonization?

The prevention of methicillin-resistant *Staphylococcus aureus* (MRSA) infection and colonization starts with adequate hand washing and personal hygiene. Showering after practice or competition should occur as soon as possible. Towels, razors, bar soaps, and clothing should not be shared. Clothing should be laundered in hot water after activity.

Educating athletes as to what may represent a MRSA lesion may allow for earlier reporting and subsequent withholding of athletes with active draining lesions from practice or competition to help reduce the spread of infection.

Equipment should be cleaned on a regular basis, preferably before and after use. Cleaning may be accomplished with many commercially prepared solutions or with a dilute bleach solution. However, there have been no definitive studies consistently implicating equipment as a major source of transmission.[1,2]

2. What Are Some of the Best Ways to Prevent Blisters/Calluses? What Is the Best Treatment for Healing and to Enable Return to Play With Minimal Discomfort?

Blisters and calluses develop through repetitive rubbing forces to the skin. To adequately prevent a blister or callus, reducing or eliminating the rubbing force is paramount. This may be accomplished through the use of materials that reduce excessive skin moisture, such as antiperspirants, powders, and chalk. Moisture-wicking clothing can be used, and avoiding cotton clothing may also help to reduce the friction.

When a small blister occurs, the roof of the blister should be left intact. Larger blisters may benefit from draining the fluid from the edge and leaving the roof intact. Various commercially available adhesive barrier products exist to cover and reduce pressure on the area of the blister. These options may allow the athlete to return to play (RTP) with minimal discomfort.

Calluses may be best treated with the application of a donut pad over the callus to reduce excessive pressure on the lesion. The use of a pumice stone following soaking the area may help to reduce the overall size of the callus.[3]

Koutures C, Wong V.
Pediatric Sports Medicine: Essentials for Office Evaluation (pp 103-107)

3. When Should an Athlete With Impetigo Be Allowed to Return to Play? What Is the Best Treatment, and in What Sports May Impetigo Be a Concern?

Any sport with direct skin-to-skin contact, such as wrestling, football, and rugby, would raise concern for an athlete with impetigo. Impetigo is best treated with a 10-day course of oral antibiotics that cover both *S aureus* and *Streptococcus pyogenes*. This may include the penicillins, a first-generation cephalosporin, or erythromycin for those with a penicillin allergy. Topical treatment with mupirocin may be used, but this is best reserved for small lesions.

Criteria for RTP include the following:

- Resolution of the crusted, exposed areas.
- No new lesions for at minimum 48 hours.
- A minimum of 72 hours of antibiotic treatment.
- Nonactive lesions can be covered with nonporous bandaging for participation.[3]

4. When Should an Athlete With Folliculitis Be Allowed to Return to Play? What Is the Best Treatment for Folliculitis? In What Sports May Folliculitis Be a Concern?

Folliculitis is commonly caused from either *S aureus* or *Pseudomonas aeruginosa*. *P aeruginosa* folliculitis infections are commonly produced from contaminated water, most frequently from water sports or hot tubs. *S aureus* folliculitis infections are typically from an infected hair follicle, which may occur from shaving or in sports for which helmets or chinstraps are used.

Treatment is usually with either topical or oral antibiotics with coverage for *S aureus*, such as penicillin, first-generation cephalosporins, or erythromycin if the patient has a penicillin allergy. *P aeruginosa* folliculitis is typically self-limited and does not usually need treatment.

For *S aureus* folliculitis, the National Collegiate Athletic Association does not allow RTP until there have been no new lesions for 48 hours and the athlete has been treated for 72 hours. The athlete with *P aeruginosa* folliculitis does not need to be withheld from participation.[3]

5. What Is Acne Mechanica, and How Does It Occur? What Is the Best Treatment, and How Can It Be Prevented?

Acne mechanica is a common problem typically found in athletes who play sports where heavy equipment, such as pads or helmets, is used. It may be due to excessive heat, occlusive clothing, and excessive pressure or friction to the skin from the equipment or clothing.

The best treatment and prevention is through reducing the stress and pressure on the skin, using soaps or cleansers that contain benzoyl peroxide, and using moisture-wicking materials in clothing and equipment.[3]

6. What Are Some Possible Treatments for *Molluscum contagiosum*? In What Sports Is *Molluscum Contagiosum* a Possible Concern?

Molluscum contagiosum is an infection caused by the poxvirus. It is more likely to spread among athletes who play in sports with direct skin-to-skin contact, such as football, rugby, and wrestling. Treatment is traditionally focused on destructive methods such as curettage, the use of liquid nitrogen, and topical treatments such as cantharidin.[3] Athletes may return to contact or collision sports if the molluscum can be covered with an occlusive dressing.

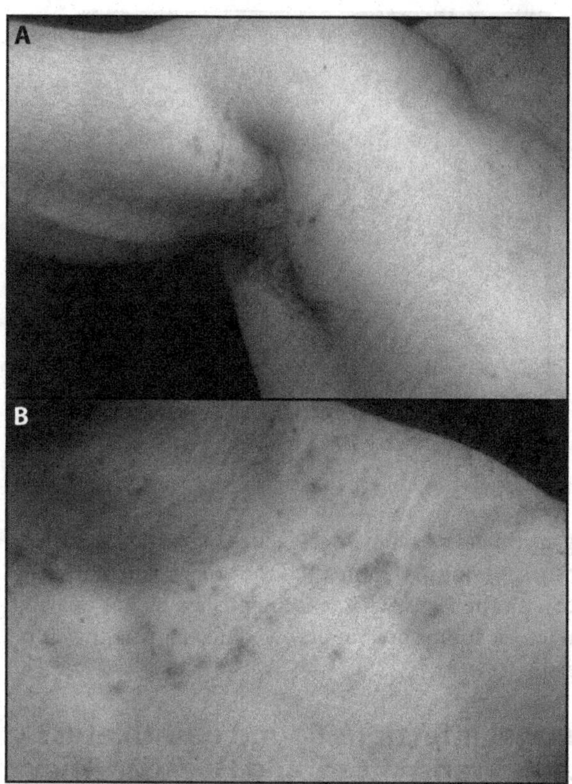

Figure 16-1. *Herpes gladiatorum* (A) under the arm and (B) on the chest. (Reprinted with permission of Gary Williams, MD.)

7. When Should an Athlete With a Herpes Simplex Virus Outbreak Be Allowed to Return to Play? In What Sports Is a Herpes Simplex Virus Outbreak a Concern? What Is the Best Treatment for a Herpes Simplex Virus Outbreak, and Is There a Prophylaxis Regimen?

Herpes simplex virus (HSV) infections have been a big concern in the sport of wrestling, although rugby players have also had outbreaks of HSV infections. Commonly referred to as *Herpes gladiatorum* (Figure 16-1) due to its frequency in wrestlers, there are other types of herpes infections, such as cold sores and genital herpes.[3]

During an outbreak, antiviral agents such as acyclovir, valacyclovir, and famciclovir can be used for treatment. Drying agents such as alcohol also have been used to help hasten healing. Prophylaxis with valacyclovir has been demonstrated to reduce infections in several studies of wrestlers.[4,5]

Since HSV infections are highly contagious, an athlete should be withheld from participation until all of his or her lesions are crusted over. It has also been recommended that the crusted lesions be covered when RTP occurs.

8. How Do Athletes Get Plantar Warts, and How Do Plantar Warts Affect Athletic Play? What Are Some Methods for the Treatment of Warts, and How Can They Be Prevented?

Plantar warts are caused by the human papilloma virus and generally enter the skin through a macerated area, often from frequently sweaty feet. Athletes who participate in impact sports may develop pain while running, especially with larger warts. These lesions often have pinpoint black dots surrounded by a well-circumscribed region of skin maceration or breakdown.

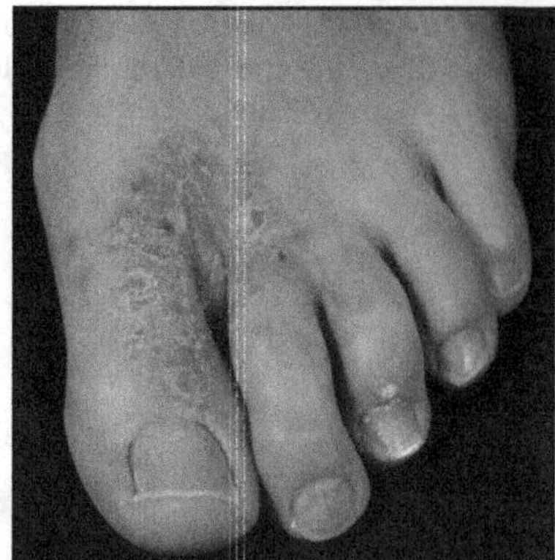

Figure 16-2. Tinea pedis. (Reprinted with permission of Gary Williams, MD.)

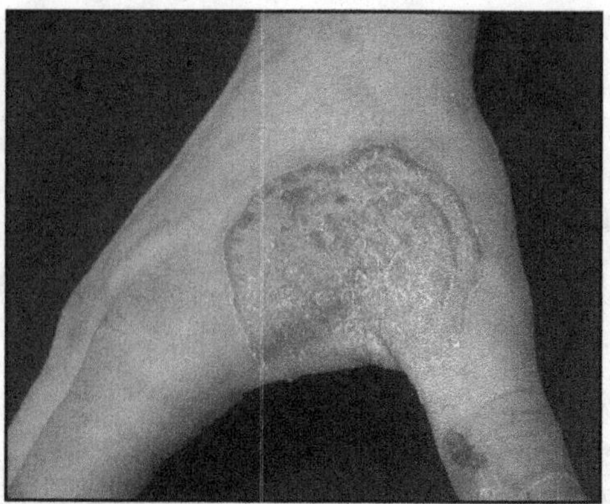

Figure 16-3. Tinea corporis. (Reprinted with permission of Gary Williams, MD.)

Various treatment options exist, including cryotherapy, salicylic acid, curettage, and laser treatments. None have been found to be consistently superior in treatment to the others. Currently, the only preventive measures are to avoid contact with the virus. This is accomplished by not wearing wet shoes, not going barefoot (particularly in locker rooms or showers), and not sharing towels or clothing (such as socks and shoes) with others.[3]

9. What Are Some Common Fungal Infections Found on Athletes? How Are Fungal Infections Usually Transmitted, and How Can They Be Prevented? In What Sports May Fungal Infections Be a Concern? What Is the Best Cleanser to Use for Infections?

The most common fungal infections in athletes are cutaneous dermatophyte infections that are named based on their location on the body.

- Foot—Tinea pedis (Figure 16-2)
- Groin—Tinea cruris
- Body—Tinea corporis (Figure 16-3)
- Head—Tinea capitis

These can be transmitted through direct contact with the infected skin or, less commonly, through contact with surfaces in a warm and moist environment. Tinea infections are of particular concern in wrestlers given the frequent skin-to-skin contact that occurs in this sport.

Prevention is best achieved through avoiding contact with the skin of an infected athlete. Proper screening programs before events such as wrestling tournaments can be helpful to identify athletes who may need to be treated and restricted from competition. Studies have found efficacy and safety in once-a-week or every-other-week oral antifungal prophylaxis for wrestlers.[6,7]

A minimum of 72 hours of topical antifungal treatment is generally recommended before contact/competition is allowed. Consider the use of a 10- to 14-day course of oral antifungal medication for multiple or difficult-to-eradicate tinea lesions. Tinea capitis often needs several weeks to months of oral therapy and restriction from direct contact with other athletes.

Most commercially available disinfectants will effectively kill the dermatophyte on fomites.[3]

10. What Is Black Heel? How Do I Manage This Condition?

Black heel, otherwise known as talon noir (Figure 16-4), develops by a sheering force to the skin. This is produced from quick stopping and planting in sports. Capillaries underneath the epidermis are traumatized, causing petechiae to develop on the heel. No specific management is needed, as these lesions will resolve without treatment within a few weeks.[3]

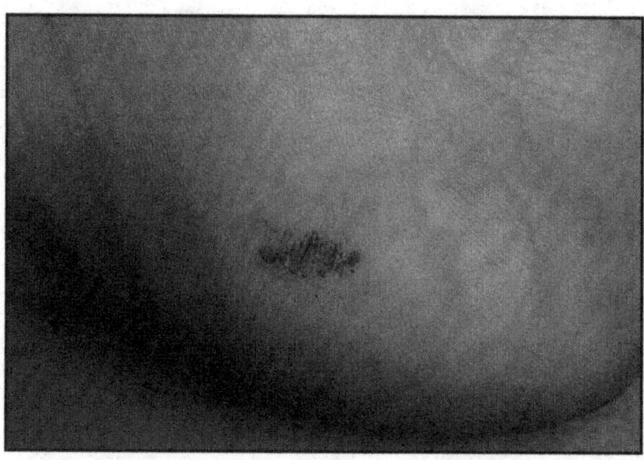

Figure 16-4. Talon noir (also known as "black heel"). (Reprinted with permission of Gary Williams, MD.)

11. What Is Pitted Keratolysis? How Do I Manage This Condition?

Pitted keratolysis is an infection caused by *Corynebacterium* that leads to multiple "pits" and desquamation typically around main pressure-bearing areas such as the heel, ball of the foot, or the palms of the hands.

Treatment is through the use of topical antibiotics such as erythromycin, clindamycin, or mupirocin. Also, limiting the use of tight footwear and considering the use of moisture-wicking socks may help.[3]

12. Is Scabies an Issue With Athletes?

Sports are not a major source of scabies; however, an athlete with scabies should be withheld from competition. Treatment is typically with 5% permethrin cream.[3]

References

1. Kirkland EB, Adams BB. Methicillin-resistant Staphylococcus aureus and athletes. *J Am Acad Dermatol.* 2008;59:494–502.
2. Cohen PR. The skin in the gym: a comprehensive review of the cutaneous manifestations of community-acquired methicillin-resistant Staphylococcus aureus infections in athletes. *Clin Dermatol.* 2008;26 :16–26.
3. Cordoro KM, Ganz JE. Training room management of medical conditions: sports dermatology. *Clin Sports Med.* 2005;24:565–598.
4. Anderson BJ. Prophylactic valacyclovir to prevent the outbreaks of herpes gladiatorum at a 28-day wrestling camp. *Jpn J Infect Dis.* 2006; 59(1):6-9.
5. Anderson BJ. The effectiveness of valacyclovir in preventing reactivation of herpes gladiatorum in wrestlers. *Clin J Sport Med.* 1999;9(2):86-90.
6. Brickman K, Einstein E, Sinha S, Ryno J, Guiness M. Fluconazole as a prophylactic measure for tinea gladiatorum in high school wrestlers. *Clin J Sport Med.* 2009;19(5):412-414.
7. Kohl TD, Martin DC, Nemeth R, Hill T, Evans D. Fluconazole for the prevention of tinea gladiatorum. *Pediatr Infect Dis J.* 2000;19(8):717-722.

Acknowledgment

The author and editors would like to express their gratitude to Gary Williams, MD for the pictures used in this chapter.

17

Female Athlete Concerns

Kate E. Berz, DO and Teri M. McCambridge, MD, FAAP

1. What Are the Three Components of the "Female Athlete Triad," and Which Types of Athletes/Sports Might Be at Highest Risk?

Each of the three components should be thought of as a continuum that ranges from normal healthy behavior to disorder, and each may occur alone or in combination with the others.

- *Energy availability*—The athlete must consume adequate energy to maintain her body weight given the metabolic demands of sport. An athlete may inadvertently fail to meet the required caloric intake for sport, or she may have a frank eating disorder.
- *Menstrual function*—Spectrum of dysfunction includes eumenorrhea, oligomenorrhea, and amenorrhea. The mechanism is not completely understood. Low-energy availability may disrupt luteinizing hormone and gonadotropin-releasing hormone pulsatility.
  - *Primary amenorrhea* is the absence of menses at age 15 years in the presence of normal growth and secondary sexual characteristics. High-risk athletes are cheerleaders, divers, and gymnasts.
  - *Secondary amenorrhea* is the absence of menses for more than 3 cycles or 6 months in females who previously had normal menstrual cycles. High-risk athletes are dancers and distance runners.
  - *Pregnancy* is the most common cause of secondary amenorrhea.
- *Bone mineral density*—Bone health ranges from optimal to osteoporosis and is affected by many factors, including diminished caloric intake, amenorrhea, and genetics.

Triad concerns can be seen in any postpubertal through premenopausal female athlete. Research indicates that those at greatest risk participate in weight class sports, disciplines that favor leanness, or those that include subjective scoring (62% of gymnasts had triad concerns in one study; in other studies of endurance athletes, aesthetic sport athletes, and weight class sport athletes, 25% to 31% had triad concerns versus 5% to 9% in controls).[1] Additional "at-risk" athletes include those with psychologic stressors such as injury, family dysfunction, or a history of abuse. Athletes who have a restrictive diet (eg, vegan or vegetarian) may struggle to consume adequate calories. Preoccupation with weight and food can be a red flag for coaches and parents.[1] Additional unhealthy behaviors that may be clues to presence or risk of an eating disorder include avoidance of eating in front of others, meticulous counting of calories or fat, and laxative use.

2. What Are Some of the Most Common Nutritional Deficiencies Seen in Female Athletes, and How Can They Be Managed?

Usually, inadequate intake is the underlying issue; however, malabsorption must be considered in the case of an athlete who may be using laxatives or inducing vomiting. The cure may be as

Koutures C, Wong V.
Pediatric Sports Medicine: Essentials for Office Evaluation (pp 108-116)

TABLE 17-1. COMMON NUTRITIONAL DEFICIENCIES IN FEMALE ATHLETES AND RECOMMENDATIONS FOR MANAGEMENT		
DEFICIENT ITEM	*COMMON CAUSES*	*RECOMMENDATIONS*
Magenesium/Zinc	Inadequate meat, nuts, and vegetables	More meat, nuts, and vegetables
Vitamin B_{12}/Folate	Low animal products and leafy green vegetables	More meat and leafy green vegetables
Vitamin D/Calcium	Indoor sports (low sun exposure); vegan	Increase sun; supplements (1200 to 1500 mg calcium; 800 IU Vitamin D)
Iron	Low meat intake; menstrual losses	See Table 17-3
Energy	Avoidance of dairy, fat, and protein	Increase calorie-dense foods

TABLE 17-2. RECOMMENDED DIETARY ALLOWANCES OF COMMONLY DEFICIENT VITAMINS AND MINERALS							
AGE (YR)	*IRON (MG)*	*CALCIUM (MG)*	*FOLATE (MCG)*	*B_{12} (MCG)*	*MAGNESIUM (MG)*	*VITAMIN D (IU)*	*ZINC (MG)*
9 to 13	8	1300	300	1.8	240	600	8
14 to 18	15	1300	400	2.4	360	600	9
19 to 30	18	1000	400	2.4	310	600	8
Values listed in units per day. Value for calcium is the recommended amount for adequate intake.							

simple as increasing intake to meet daily expenditure or adding an avoided food group to her diet. The athlete should use vitamin and mineral supplements to increase levels in a controlled manner. See Table 17-1 for common nutritional deficiencies. See Table 17-2 for information on vitamins and their recommended dietary allowance and see Table 17-3 for a list of good sources of iron and calcium.

3. In Female Athletes Suspected of Having Energy Availability or Potential Eating Disorders, What Are Some Common Evaluations and Specialty Referrals?

A dietician can calculate energy availability. The gold standard for calculating energy availability is to track a 3-day food and activity diary, which includes 2 weekdays and 1 weekend day and to weigh food portions. The athlete wears an accelerometer to determine caloric expenditure. A list of helpful specialties includes a sports physician, sports dietician, and psychologist or behavioral medicine specialist specializing in eating disorders. In addition, the support of family, coaches, and friends is important.[2] See Table 17-4 for suggested laboratory evaluations for assessment of nutritional status and Table 17-5 for interpretation of laboratory evaluations.

Other studies to consider include the following:

- For persistent amenorrhea >6 months, dual energy x-ray absorptiometry (DXA) to evaluate bone mineral density (BMD)
- Electrocardiogram in an athlete with presyncope or syncope to investigate for arrhythmias and bradycardia. Additional potential abnormal findings in eating disorders include low voltage changes, prolonged QTc interval, and T-wave inversions.

TABLE 17-3. DIETARY SOURCES OF CALCIUM AND IRON	
AMOUNT OF FOOD	*CALCIUM CONTENT (MG)*
8 oz milk or 6 oz yogurt	300
1 oz Swiss cheese	272
2 oz sardines with bones	240
6 oz cooked turnip greens	220
3 oz almonds	210
1 oz cheddar cheese	204
8 oz broccoli	178
8 oz cottage cheese	155
AMOUNT OF FOOD	*IRON CONTENT (MG)*
3 oz canned clams drained	23.8
3 oz cooked oysters	10.2
3 oz cooked organ meat (liver, giblet)	5.2 to 9.9
4 oz canned white beans	3.9
1 T Blackstrap molasses	3.5
4 oz cooked lentils or fresh spinach	3.2 to 3.3
4 oz cooked kidney beans or chickpeas	2.4 to 2.6
3 oz cooked ground beef	2.2

TABLE 17-4. RECOMMENDED LABS FOR A GENERAL EVALUATION OF NUTRITIONAL STATUS		
Serum electrolytes*	25, OH vitamin D	CRP ESR
CBC with differential	Ferritin	Urinalysis
*See Table 17-5 for information about electrolyte abnormalities. CBC, complete blood count; CRP, C-reactive protein; ESR, erythrocyte sedimentation rate.		

- Unhealthy behaviors that may be clues to the presence or risk of an eating disorder include limiting food intake, constant weighing, avoidance of eating in front of others, counting calories or fat, and laxative use.

4. Is There Any Evidence That Starting the Oral Contraceptive Pill in Cases of Amenorrhea/Hypomenorrhea Will Enhance Long-Term Bone Development?

Oral contraceptive pills (OCPs) can be used to restore menses by providing estrogen, which may prevent or slow further bone demineralization. Since the problem is energy intake, metabolic factors that impair new bone formation will not normalize with hormone replacement. Increases in BMD are more related to increases in weight rather than use of OCPs per se. Returns of menses through caloric increases, weight gain, or a decrease in exercise are the best mechanisms for increasing bone density. If nonpharmacologic treatment has failed in an athlete with hypothalamic functional amenorrhea over the age of 16 years, then consider OCPs to prevent further bone loss. Bisphosphonates have no proven efficacy in premenopausal women and may cause harm in future pregnancies.[3]

An athlete with amenorrhea deserves further evaluation (Table 17-6).

Table 17-5. Evaluation of Electrolyte Abnormalities Using a Serum Metabolic Panel	
LABORATORY VALUE	*CLINICAL IMPLICATIONS*
Glucose	Decreased in poor nutrition, increased in insulin deficiency
Sodium	Decreased with increased water intake or laxative use
Potassium	Decreased in vomiting, laxative or diuretic use, refeeding syndrome
Chloride	Decreased in vomiting, increased with laxative use
Bicarbonate	Increased in vomiting, decreased in laxative use
BUN	Increased in dehydration
Creatinine	Increased in dehydration or renal dysfunction, falsely elevated due to low muscle mass
Calcium	Decreased or normal in poor nutrition with bone breakdown
Phosphate	Decreased in poor nutrition or refeeding
Magnesium	Decreased in poor nutrition, laxative use, refeeding syndrome
Total Protein Albumin	Increased in early malnutrition due to muscle breakdown
Aspartate Aminotransaminase (AST) Alanine Aminotransaminase (ALT)	Increased in liver dysfunction
Amylase	Increased in vomiting and pancreatitis
Lipase	Increased in pancreatitis
Adapted from Academy for Eating Disorders Report 2011. *Critical Points for Early Recognition and Medical Risk Management in the Care of Individuals with Eating Disorders.* www.aedweb.org	

Table 17-6. Work-Up for Amenorrhea	
hCG to exclude pregnancy	FSH/LH can be low in ovarian failure or eating disorder
TSH	Free testosterone and DHEAS if signs of masculinization
Physical exam and ultrasonography: evaluate anatomic abnormalities in the case of primary amenorrhea	Serum Prolactin
hCG, human chorionic gonadotropin; TSH, thyroid stimulating hormone; FSH, follicle stimulating hormone; LH, luteinizing hormone; DHEAS, dehydroepiandrosterone sulfate.	

5. How Do You Determine When to Restrict From Play Versus Allowing Continued Sports Participation and Modifying Unhealthy Eating Behaviors?

The female athlete triad should be treated like an injury, with rehabilitation consisting of increasing energy availability or decreasing energy expenditure. The athlete should receive an outline of clear and concise expectations, as well as attainable goals to maintain participation or to return to play. A contract is often a useful tool (Table 17-7).

TABLE 17-7. ELEMENTS OF A CONTRACT IN EATING DISORDER MANAGEMENT
• Frequency of follow-up appointments: usually once per week until weight stabilizes • Frequency of labs: initial visit and then every 6 to 8 weeks until trend of steady weight gain is established • Names of practitioners who will evaluate the athlete: nutritionist, psychologist, physician • Expected weight gain per week: 0.5 to 1 lb • Minimum acceptable weight (<85% of expected weight for height/age is DSM-IV-TR criteria for anorexia nervosa) • Goal Body Mass Index (<18.5 or <5th percentile on a growth chart is considered underweight • Weight at which the athlete must stop physical activity or that requires hospitalization • Statement that failure to comply will result in restriction from sport • Statement that the athlete's family may be contacted as necessary if condition worsens • Statement that all initial labs and screening tests must be completed in a certain time frame—usually 1 to 2 weeks
A contract is a useful tool when working with an athlete with energy availability problems including disordered eating. Components of a contract should include clearly outlined expectations for return to play or continuation of play.

- Mechanisms for modifying unhealthy behavior.
  - Shift obsession from calories to portions.
  - Create concrete objectives, such as adding 100 kcals/week or adding an avoided food group.
  - Address underlying issues, such as individual/family therapy or medications.
- Contraindications for participation.
  - Body mass index below 17 or weight that crosses two lines on the growth chart.
  - Failure to meet targeted weight gains.
  - Hospitalized for dehydration, severe/symptomatic bradycardia, or electrolyte issues.

6. What Are Some Common Breast Issues With Female Athletes?

- *"Jogger's nipple"*—Abrasions from poorly fitted bras or shirts and repetitive motion that become irritated when jogging.
- *"Bicyclist's nipple"*—Same definition as above; may develop after a period of riding in cold wind.
- Synthetic, moisture-wicking materials in sports bras, along with barrier creams/adhesive bandages, can reduce chafing and protect open wounds.
- Females with larger breasts may have shoulder discomfort from bra straps, breast pain from increased motion during sport, and back pain. Athletes should wear a well-fitting bra or two sports bras, if necessary. Shoulder straps can be padded to provide more comfort.
- In contact sports, proper technique and protection should be emphasized. For example, a proper soccer chest trap does not involve the breast, but rather the superior portion of the sternum. Chest protection is used in certain athletes participating in high-risk collision sports, such as field/ice hockey and lacrosse goaltenders or softball catchers.
- It is important to ask the question, "Do you have breast discomfort during exercise?" in order to offer solutions or investigate underlying etiologies.

7. How Common Is Stress Urinary Incontinence in Young Athletes, How Is It Differentiated From More Serious Issues, and What Can Be Done to Treat It?

Urinary incontinence is the involuntary loss of urine occurring in the absence of detrusor contraction; it is likely underreported due to perceived embarrassment. One study found the prevalence during sport among young, nulliparous, elite athletes to vary between 0% in golf and 67% in gymnastics.[4] Risk factors include increasing age, increased parity, heavy physical activity, high-impact sport, hypoestrogenic amenorrhea, and obesity. The pathophysiology is not completely understood, but the incontinence occurs when the intravesical pressure exceeds the urethral pressure. Proposed mechanisms include weak pelvic floor muscles and the role of catecholamines produced during exercise. Common contributing causes include constipation and urinary tract infections.

A pelvic examination can rule out anatomic variants and assess the integrity of the pelvic floor. An abdominal mass should warrant an abdominal ultrasonography to look for a mechanical cause, such as a tumor. A magnetic resonance image of the lumbar spine without contrast to rule out spinal cord involvement should be investigated in the presence of other neurologic symptoms. In the case of isolated stress incontinence that does not respond to conservative measures, use a renal and bladder ultrasonography to look for anomalies of the urinary tract. A physical therapist can design a pelvic floor-strengthening program that would include Kegel exercises and thoracoabdominal activation. Other management tips include voiding on a schedule and using a sanitary napkin for exercise. Biofeedback, imipramine, and pseudoephedrine hydrochloride have been used for prevention. Gynecologist or urologist referrals are appropriate for athletes who do not respond to physical therapy or education.[4,5]

8. What Possible Factors Explain the Fact That Adolescent and Young Adult Female Athletes Playing At-Risk Sports Have a Higher Risk of Anterior Cruciate Ligament Tears Than Male Athletes of the Same Age and Sport?

Table 17-8 illustrates multiple potential intrinsic risk factors for anterior cruciate ligament (ACL) tears in female athletes, which include increased valgus knee position during landing from jumping (Figures 17-1 and 17-2). Potential extrinsic factors include motion perturbations such as contact with another player and shoe-surface interaction (Table 17-9).

9. Are There Any Proven Interventions That Might Reduce the Risk of Anterior Cruciate Ligament Tears in Female Athletes?

Neuromuscular training programs focusing on proper lower-extremity alignment, especially with jumping and turning, have been shown to reduce the incidence and risk of noncontact ACL injuries. The following programs must be performed more than one time per week for a minimum of 6 weeks (multicomponent programs showing better results than single component programs):

- Plyometrics train the muscles, connective tissue, and proprioceptors to work effectively while focusing on proper technique and body mechanics.
- Balance training includes a balance board protocol and functional balance exercises including hopping forward, landing on one leg, and holding the landing for a period of time.
- The biofeedback component utilizes a trained observer, coach, or athletic trainer to give feedback on correct body positioning during exercise. In addition, mirrors and video recording may be used to visualize correct technique.
- Strength training includes hamstring and quadriceps strengthening to provide knee stability and reduce knee mechanical load, and hip and core strengthening to provide postural stability and proper alignment.[6,7]

Table 17-8. Intrinsic Factors for Anterior Cruciate Ligament Tears in Female Athletes

ANATOMICAL
• Femoral notch and ACL size
• Increased Q angle due to wider female pelvis
• Increased knee joint laxity
• Foot pronation and navicular drop
• Increased hamstring flexibility
• Increased anterior tibial translation
• Increasing body mass index with increasing age
• Estrogen receptors on the ACL
NEUROMUSCULAR
• Imbalances in the quadriceps and hamstrings functional relationship
• Muscle fatigue
• Decreased trunk proprioception
BIOMECHANICAL
• Knee abduction
• Lateral trunk motion
• Tibial rotation

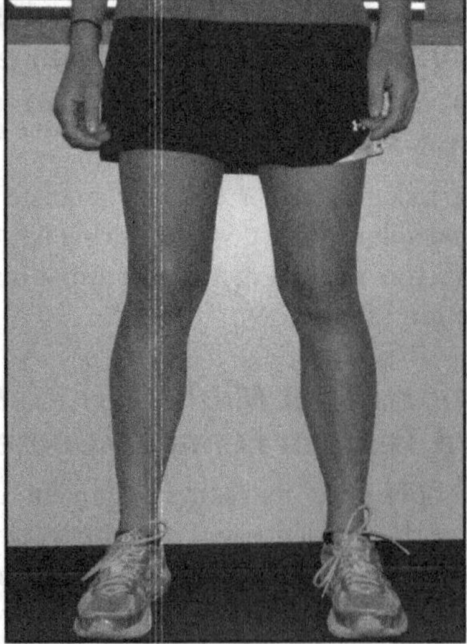

Figure 17-1. Landing with hips, knees, and feet in good alignment.

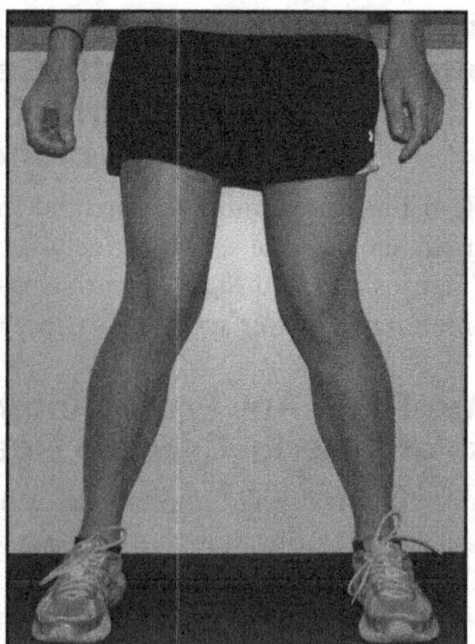

Figure 17-2. Landing with excessive knee valgus.

10. Are Female Athletes at Greater Risk for Stress Fractures? How Many Stress Fractures Must One Sustain Before You Do a Work-Up, and Which Sports Are at Greatest Risk?

Female athletes are at greater risk than male athletes for a stress fracture resulting from an underlying medical cause. Common medical causes include genetic factors, estrogen deficiency, excessive glucocorticoid exposure, and hyperparathyroidism. At-risk athletes are those involved in lean body building or subjective scoring sports, such as gymnastics, ballet, figure skating, and

Table 17-9. Extrinsic and Modifiable Risk Factors for Noncontact Anterior Cruciate Ligament Injuries
• Weather and surface conditions
• Artificial turf versus natural grass
• Balance of hamstring and quadriceps strength and recruitment
• Core strength and proprioception
• Muscle fatigue which alters neuromuscular control
• Landing technique (Figures 17-1 and 17-2)
• Shoe-ground interface
• Footwear—cleat number, length, and placement

Table 17-10. Definition of Clinically Significant Stress Fracture
ONE OR MORE OF THE FOLLOWING:
• Long bone fracture of the lower extremity
• Vertebral compression fracture
• Two or more long bone fractures of the upper extremity

distance running. One stress fracture warrants screening for the female athlete triad or any of its components, but 3 stress fractures warrant BMD screening using DXA. In the case of children and premenopausal females, the International Society for Clinical Densitometry recommends using z-scores for BMD, which compare the individual to age-matched norms. It is generally accepted that diagnosing osteoporosis in children cannot be made on the basis of the DXA alone. The presence of a clinically significant fracture (Table 17-10) and low BMD are both required. Low BMD is defined as a z-score less than or equal to –2, and the low-normal range is between –1 and –2.

Female athletes with amenorrhea should take 1200 to 1500 mg of calcium per day plus 800 IUs of vitamin D. Appropriate weight training is another potentially effective therapy for low BMD. For other general risk factors for stress fractures, see Table 17-11.

11. What Advice Should Be Given to the Pregnant Female Athlete?

In general, exercise is not harmful to the pregnant female athlete or her fetus. Athletic performance may be altered due to bodily changes such as increased ligamentous laxity, increased breast size, weight gain, and altered center of gravity.

- Contraindications to exercise during pregnancy:
  - Bleeding in the second or third trimester
  - Intrauterine growth retardation
  - Pregnancy-induced hypertension
  - Premature rupture of membranes
  - History of preterm labor
  - Cervical incompetence
- Activities to avoid when pregnant:
  - Any new sport
  - Weight lifting
  - Scuba diving
  - Water sports (other than swimming)
  - Horseback riding

Table 17-11. General Risk for Stress Fractures	
• Secondary amenorrhea	• Increased training demands
• Low body weight	• Prior history of stress fracture
• Poor calcium intake	• Family history of osteoporosis/osteopenia
• Tobacco or excessive alcohol use	• Low vitamin D

- Strenuous aerobic exercise (if previously sedentary)
- Contact sports
- Competitive events
- Mechanical stress to the trunk
- Bicycling in the second and third trimesters

Return to sports postpartum is advisable at 4 to 6 weeks postvaginal delivery and 6 to 8 weeks after Cesarean section. Exercise while lactating is permitted, but the mother should wear a supportive bra and remain hydrated.

12. What Are the Risks and Issues With Body Piercings?

- Local infection with risk for MRSA. Clean piercings twice daily with an antibacterial soap and treat signs of cellulitis with topical bacitracin at the first sign of erythema or with trimethoprim/sulfamethoxazole (160 mg/800 mg) twice daily for 7 to 10 days (alternatives are clindamycin and doxycycline).
- Pain.
- Risk of forcible removal during contact sports.
- Irritation from equipment or clothing.
- Local allergic reaction.

Rules vary among sports regarding the allowance of piercing, although most sports restrict the wearing of visible jewelry. If body jewelry cannot be removed, then cover with athletic tape to avoid accidental removal or injury to herself or another athlete.

References

1. Nattiv A, Loucks AB, Manore MM, Sanborn CF, Sundgot-Borgen J, Warren MP. American College of Sports Medicine position stand. The female athlete triad. *Med Sci Sports Exerc.* 2007;39:1867–1882.
2. Medical Care Standards Task Force. Eating Disorders Critical Points for Early Recognition and Medical Risk Management in the Care of Individuals with Eating Disorders. *Academy for Eating Disorders*; 2011.
3. Liu SL, Lebrun CM. Effect of oral contraceptives and hormone replacement therapy on bone mineral density in premenopausal and perimenopausal women: a systematic review. *Br J Sports Med.* 2006;40:11–24.
4. Bo K. Urinary incontinence, pelvic floor dysfunction, exercise and sport. *Sports Med.* 2004;34:451–464.
5. Nygaard IE, Thompson FL, Svengalis SL, Albright JP. Urinary incontinence in elite nulliparous athletes. *Obstet Gynecol.* 1994;84:183–187.
6. Hewett TE, Myer GD, Ford KR. Anterior cruciate ligament injuries in female athletes: part 1, mechanisms and risk factors. *Am J Sports Med.* 2006;34:299–311.
7. Hewett TE, Ford KR, Myer GD. Anterior cruciate ligament injuries in female athletes: part 2, a meta-analysis of neuromuscular interventions aimed at injury prevention. *Am J Sports Med.* 2006;34:490–498.

Suggested Web Sites

Female Athlete Triad Coalition: www.femaleathletetriad.org
Academy for Eating Disorders: www.aedweb.org
Women's Sports Foundation: www.womenssportsfoundation.org
Athletes Targeting Healthy Exercise and Nutrition Alternatives (ATHENA): www.athenaprogram.com
Prevent injury and Enhance Performance (PEP): http://smsmf.org/files/PEPExercises.pdf
Knee Injury Prevention Program (KIPP®): www.childrensmemorial.org/depts/sportsmedicine/program.aspx
American Congress of Obstetricians and Gynecologists: www.acog.org/For_Patients

18

Athletes With Special Needs

Charmaine Sekona, MD and Valarie Wong, MD, FAAP

1. If an Athlete Has a Specific Disability (Amputation, Cerebral Palsy, Hydrocephalus With Shunt, Meningomyelocele, Spinal Cord Injury, Down Syndrome, Hearing and Vision Impairment), What Are the Concerns and Guidelines for Sports Participation?

- Every child athlete with special needs requires individualized care, and Table 18-1[1-5] can provide basic guidelines on the concerns health care providers should be aware of based upon the child's specific impairment.
- Further information can be found in the *Preparticipation Physical Evaluation Monograph*, 4th edition, Chapter 7 entitled "The Athlete With Special Needs."[6]

2. What Are the Special Olympics and Paralympics, and Who Can Participate?

- The Special Olympics is the largest sports organization worldwide for people with intellectual disabilities. It was inspired by Eunice Kennedy Shriver, who in 1962 founded Camp Shriver, a summer day camp for people with intellectual disabilities. The camp was later organized in 1968 into the first International Special Olympics in Chicago, Illinois.
    - People with intellectual disabilities who are age 8 years and older can participate. In 2012, almost 4 million people participated in the Special Olympics in over 170 countries. There is also a Young Athletes program for children with intellectual disabilities aged 2 to 7 years.[7]
- The Paralympics began as the Stoke Mandeville Games in England, which were founded in 1948 to help injured World War II servicemen with their physical therapy. It later became known as the Paralympic Games, the first of which was held in Rome, Italy, in 1960.[8] Now, the Paralympics are held right after the Olympic Games in the same venue.
    - Participants in the Paralympics are categorized based upon their impairment and the level of impairment. They are evaluated by a classification committee to determine if they meet 1 of the 10 impairment classifications (in alphabetical order)[8]:

        1. Ataxia
        2. Athetosis
        3. Hypertonia
        4. Impaired muscle power
        5. Impaired passive range of movement
        6. Intellectual impairment
        7. Leg length difference
        8. Limb deficiency
        9. Short stature
        10. Vision impairment

Koutures C, Wong V.
Pediatric Sports Medicine: Essentials for Office Evaluation (pp 117-123)

Table 18-1. Concerns for Athletes With Special Needs		
SPECIFIC DIAGNOSIS	*CONCERNS*	*GUIDELINES FOR SPORTS PARTICIPATION*
Amputations	• Proper wheelchair fit, if applicable	• Evaluate for areas of friction on hands and arms • Consult with orthotist
	• Pressure sores at sites of prostheses, if applicable	• Pressure sores need to have completely healed prior to returning to sport • Consult prosthetist as needed
	• As opposed to adults, children may have continued appositional growth of the limb bone	• Regular follow-up with a pediatric orthopedist is needed; limb may need revision[1]
	• Stress injuries to back and hips in lower-extremity amputations; overuse injuries	• Examine back and hips and use same guidelines for those without amputation; adapt to individual sport as needed
Cerebral palsy	• Impaired flexibility, contractures • Impaired hand-eye coordination • Impaired muscular control	• Evaluate the individual athlete to determine if a particular sport is safe for him or her[2] • Incorporate physical and occupational therapy as needed
	• Temperature control issues	• Educate the patient and the family on temperature control
Hydrocephalus with shunt	• The risk for shunt complications due to sports is < 1%[3]	• No restriction from noncontact sport • Controversial with contact sports • Wear appropriate head gear
Meningomyelocele	• Same concerns as for spinal cord injury • Easy fatigue	• Individualize risk for all sports • Safety of a particular sport may depend upon the level of the injury
Spinal cord injury	• Autonomic dysreflexia, also known as "boosting," can be life threatening	• See Question 4
	• Pressure sores	• Pressure sores need to have completely healed prior to returning to sport
	• Frequent urinary tract infection in those with bladder dysfunction or neurogenic bladder	• Regular voiding, adequate hydration, good bowel regimen, proper catheterization technique
	• Impaired thermoregulation in those with lesions above T8 (hypo- and hyperthermia) ◦ Due to impaired sweating with less body surface area for cooling, venous pooling, and lack of shiver response[3]	• Increased risk with anticholinergics • Maintain adequate hydration • Remove from sport at the first sign of issues

(continued)

Table 18-1 (continued). Concerns for Athletes With Special Needs

SPECIFIC DIAGNOSIS	*CONCERNS*	*GUIDELINES FOR SPORTS PARTICIPATION*
Down Syndrome	• Congenital heart disease (present in about 50%)[4,5]	• Follow disease-specific Bethesda Conference guidelines[5]
	• Atlantoaxial instability leading to spontaneous subluxation of the cervical spine	• See Question 3
	• Hypermobile (flat feet, joint laxity, hip subluxations, dislocations) and decreased pain sensation	• Screen for injuries, use orthotics as necessary
	• Vision/Hearing impairments	• See next 2 rows
Vision impaired	• At risk for injury due to fall and collision	• Promote development of motor skills with experience; the Paralympics and United States Association of Blind Athletes promote activities for the visually impaired • Guides can be used to aid the athlete, including sounds, other people or animals, and guide wires[3]
Hearing impaired	• Possible vestibular dysfunction	• May need to restrict from activities involving climbing, diving, jumping on trampolines, or tumbling[3]

3. What Is Atlantoaxial Instability, and Why Are There Differing Opinions on Screening Between the American Academy of Pediatrics and the Special Olympics?

- Atlantoaxial instability (AAI) refers to an increased atlantodens interval (ADI) between C1 and C2 (Figure 18-1). Approximately 15% of children with Trisomy 21 (Down syndrome) have this condition.[9] It is also seen in children with rheumatoid arthritis, Klippel-Feil syndrome, and achondroplasia. An ADI of greater than 4.5 mm is needed for the diagnosis of atlantoaxial subluxation in children. An ADI of greater than 3.0 mm is consistent with atlantoaxial subluxation in adults.[6]
- It is important for the general pediatrician to monitor for signs and symptoms of AAI in the pediatric patient with Down syndrome during routine visits. If a patient has neurologic signs and symptoms, he or she should immediately be referred to a spinal surgeon.
- Screening for AAI is controversial. The American Academy of Pediatrics (AAP) and the Special Olympics each have their own statements regarding how screening for AAI should be handled.
    - AAP: current evidence does not support performing routine screening radiographs for assessment of potential AAI in asymptomatic children.[4] If there is high suspicion for AAI, cervical spine flexion/extension films need to be taken.[4]

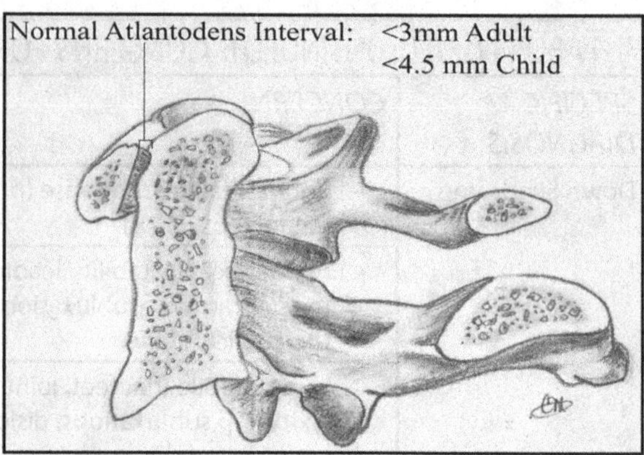

Figure 18-1. Atlantoaxial instability. (Graphite Pencil-Copyright © 2012 Cora Maglaya, PT, ATC, CSCS.)

- Special Olympics: temporary restriction of athletes with Down syndrome is required from participation in certain activities that pose potential risk (see list below) until an "x-ray shows no evidence of instability on C1 vertebrae,"[7] and the patient is examined by a knowledgeable physician. If the athlete has AAI, the parents must be informed and two physicians must fill out the appropriate forms after examining the athlete. Activities that result in hyperextension, radical flexion, or direct pressure on the neck and upper spine include the following[7]:
    - Judo
    - Football (soccer)
    - Alpine skiing
    - Pentathlon
    - Snowboarding
    - Squat lift
    - Equestrian sports
    - Butterfly stroke and diving starts in swimming
    - Diving
    - High jump
    - Artistic gymnastics
    - Any warm-up exercise that places undue stress on the head and neck

4. How Do Athletes With Spinal Cord Injuries Enhance His or Her Performance in Sports?

- All patients with spinal cord injuries (SCIs) are at risk for autonomic dysreflexia (AD), which is the lack of proper complementary sympathetic and parasympathetic control to ensure the correct regulation of cardiovascular control, heat regulation, and bowel and bladder control. Most people with SCIs experience orthostatic hypotension, which can make exercise and athletic training more difficult for them.
- The intentional implementation of AD (also known as "boosting") by an athlete can potentially increase his or her peak heart rate, peak blood pressure, circulating norepinephrine levels, maximal oxygen uptake, and peak power relative to when nonboosted.[10] Athletes may use various means to induce AD, including intentionally distending one's bladder by clamping a foley, pinching oneself with a device in a leg that has no sensation, or even breaking a bone in a nonfunctional leg. Athletes with SCIs that are above the level of T6 are at the higher risk because that is where the critical area of the spine brings sympathetic control to the heart.[10]

- Due to the dangers of uncontrolled hypertension, the International Paralympic Committee has banned boosting from the Paralympics. Athletes are checked prior to competition for evidence of AD.
- The management of an episode of AD involves keeping the person in a sitting position, removing restrictive clothing, and managing any bowel or bladder issues. If these measures do not lower the arterial pressure below 150 mm Hg, then medications such as captopril, nifedipine, or topical nitrates can be used.[10]

5. What Are Some of the Concerns When an Athlete Is on Attention Deficit Hyperactivity Disorder/ Attention Deficit Disorder Medications?

- Stimulants may increase core temperature, leading to an increased risk of heat injury. Two studies suggested that these medications may mask symptoms of fatigue and lead to athletes exercising at dangerous body temperatures of >40°C for longer periods of time.[11] Athletes using stimulants need to take precautions and maintain adequate hydration.
- Resting and exercise heart rate are both potentially increased by methylphenidate.[11]
- Team physicians should refrain from prescribing stimulants to children with pre-existing heart disease or symptoms consistent with cardiovascular disease.[11]
- The American Heart Association (AHA) and the AAP differ on obtaining an electrocardiogram (EKG) screen for silent cardiovascular disease in patients taking attention deficit hyperactivity disorder (ADHD) medication. The AAP does not recommend a routine EKG prior to starting stimulant medication unless there is a clinical indication to obtain an EKG.[12] On the other hand, the AHA suggests performing a routine EKG prior to starting stimulant therapy.[13] The physician who cares for patients with ADHD and attention deficit disorder (ADD) should monitor their blood pressure, heart rate, and any symptoms associated with exercise.
- Most sudden cardiac deaths in athletes are due to a congenital cardiac condition, so concerns over sudden cardiac death due to medication use should not preclude a physician from treating an athlete who has ADHD. Rates for sudden death in athletes who are properly treated with stimulants do not differ from the rates of those in the general population.[11]
- Most of the stimulants that are used to treat ADHD and ADD are on the World Anti-Doping Agency Prohibited List for use during athletic competition. The athlete may apply for a Therapeutic Use Exemption which will allow him or her to use the stimulants during competition. Please refer to Chapter 6, question 9, for more information.

6. What Are the Potential Attitudes of Athletes With Attention Deficit Hyperactivity Disorder/Attention Deficit Disorder in Terms of Risk-Taking or Drug-Abusing Behavior?

Many students have admitted to using stimulants; surveys cited that anywhere from 5.3% to 34% of college students admitted using stimulants for reasons ranging from medical use to abuse, especially during periods of stress.[11] However, it has not been shown that patients who are taking medications for ADHD have an increased risk of drug abuse. In fact, those with ADHD who are properly treated are less prone to substance abuse.[11]

- Stimulants may enhance performance through improving "attention to task, peer relationships, or balance."[11]
- Stimulants may have ergogenic effects for athletes by helping with weight control and decreasing pain sensation, thereby leading to the possible abuse by athletes.[11]

7. Are Patients With Pre-Existing or Suspected Attention Deficit Hyperactivity Disorder/Attention Deficit Disorder More At Risk for Focus and Attention Issues After a Concussion? What Can Be Done to Help Manage These Athletes?

- Approximately 15% to 20% of children who experience moderate to severe traumatic brain injury (TBI) without a history of pre-existing ADHD have behavioral symptoms that meet the *Diagnostic and Statistical Manual of Mental Disorders, Fourth Edition*, criteria for ADHD 6 months after the injury.[14]
- Ideally, the athlete will be managed by an interdisciplinary team including the physician, neuropsychologist, psychologist, psychiatrist, trainer(s), coach(es), school officials (including counselors and teachers), and the family members. Many institutions have teams dedicated to caring for athletes with TBIs. Management may include increasing or restarting ADHD medications.

8. What Constitutes Appropriate Seizure Control, and Are There Certain Sports/Activities That Have to Be Modified in a Patient With New-Onset or Poorly Controlled Seizures?

- Exercise in people with epilepsy has many benefits, and every effort should be made to encourage safe and full participation.
- There is no consensus on what constitutes appropriate seizure control; this needs to be individualized.
- Most restrictions can be lifted if a child has been seizure free for 1 year or longer.[15]
- Sports where children can fall need to be modified. Swimming is safe for children who have good seizure control when appropriately supervised.
- The AAP recommends avoidance of the following noncontact sports in those with poorly controlled seizure disorders[2]:
  - Archery
  - Riflery
  - Swimming
  - Weightlifting
  - Power lifting
  - Strength training
  - Sports involving heights

References

1. Amputation. Pediatric Orthopaedic Society of North America Web site. www.posna.org/education/StudyGuide/amputations.asp. Accessed June 12, 2012.
2. Rice SG. Medical conditions affecting sports participation. *Pediatrics*. 2008;121:841–848.
3. Patel DR, Greydanus DE. Sport participation by physically and cognitively challenged young athletes. *Pediatr Clin North Am*. 2010;57(3):795–817.
4. Bull MJ, Committee on Genetics. Health supervision for children with down syndrome. *Pediatrics*. 2011;128;393-406.
5. Maron BJ, Zipes DP. 36th Bethesda Conference: Elegibility recommendations for competitive athletes with cardiovascular abnormalities. *J Am Coll Cardiol*. 2005;45(8):1313-1315.
6. Bernhardt DT, Roberts WO, eds. The Athlete with Special Needs. In: *American Academy of Pediatrics, Preparticipation Physical Evaluation Monograph*. 4th Edition. Leawood, KS: American Academy of Family Physicians; 2010:131-139.
7. Coach guides: participation by individuals with down syndrome who have atlantoaxial instability. Special Olympics Web site. http://sports.specialolympics.org/specialo.org/Special_/English/Coach/Coaching/Basics_o/Down_syn.htm. Accessed May 25, 2012.

8. International Paralympic Committee. Classification. Paralympic Movement Web site. www.paralympic.org/Classification/Introduction. Accessed May 25, 2012.
9. Pueschel, Scola FH. Atlantoaxial instability in individuals with Down syndrome: epidemiologic, radiographic, and clinical studies. *Pediatrics.* 1987;80(4):4555-4560.
10. Krassioukov A. Autonomic dysreflexia: current evidence related to unstable arterial blood pressure control among athletes with spinal cord injury. *Clin J Sport Med.* 2012;22(1):39–45.
11. Putukian M, Kreher JB, Coppel DB, Glazer JL, McKeag DB, White RD. Attention deficit hyperactivity disorder and the athlete: an American Medical Society for Sports Medicine position statement. *Clin J Sport Med.* 2011;21(5):392-401.
12. Perrin JM, Friedman RA, Knilans TK; Black Box Working Group; Section on Cardiology and Cardiac Surgery. Cardiovascular monitoring and stimulant drugs for attention-deficit/hyperactivity disorder. *Pediatrics.* 2008;122(2):451-453.
13. Vetter VL, Elia J, Erickson C, et al. Cardiovascular monitoring of children and adolescents with heart disease receiving medications for attention deficit/hyperactivity disorder [corrected]: a scientific statement from the American Heart Association Council on Cardiovascular Disease in the Young Congenital Cardiac Defects Committee and the Council on Cardiovascular Nursing. *Circulation.* 2008;117(18):2407-2423.
14. Levin H, Hanten G, Max J, et al. Symptoms of attention-deficit/hyperactivity disorder following traumatic brain injury in children. *J Dev Behav Pediatr.* 2007;28(2):108–118.
15. Howard GM, Radloff M, Sevier TL. Epilepsy and sports participation. *Curr Sports Med Rep.* 2004;3(1):15–19.

19 Concerns Among Obese and Overweight Athletes

Emelynn J. Fajardo, DO; Yasmin D. Deliz, DO; and Stephen G. Rice, MD, PhD, MPH, FAAP, FACSM

1. What Are Some Medical or Orthopedic Concerns That Are More Commonly Found in Obese/Overweight Athletes When They Exercise?

- Heat-related injuries—Obese or overweight people may encounter problems regulating body temperature when undergoing moderate to strenuous activity in warm climates.
  - Moving a larger body mass requires more heat generation, which may increase the risk of exercise-related heat injury, including heat exhaustion and heat stroke
  - Adipose tissue acts as "dead weight."
  - Dissipating heat may be more difficult in the obese individual.
  - Good hydration is vital, as thirst is a poor indicator of replacement fluid need.
  - Athletes should schedule water breaks regularly throughout the activity.
  - Pre-exercise hyperhydration is helpful in preventing dehydration and heat-related illness.
  - Hot, humid exercise conditions should be avoided.
- Extra mass increases the risk of exercise-related heat injury, including heat exhaustion and heat stroke.
  - Good hydration is vital, as thirst is a poor indicator of replacement fluid need. Athletes should schedule water breaks regularly throughout the activity. Pre-exercise hyperhydration is helpful in preventing dehydration and heat-related illness.
  - Hot, humid exercise conditions should be avoided.
- Joint-related conditions—Extra stress is placed on major weight bearing joints such as the hips, knees, and ankles in athletes who are obese or overweight.
  - The repetitive application of increased axial loading forces can cause the degeneration of articular cartilage and sclerosis of subchondral bone. Excess fat may have a direct metabolic effect on cartilage by enhancing irregular growth. Individuals may develop osteoarthritis at an early age.
  - Overweight adolescent boys are at increased risk for developing slipped capital femoral epiphysis (SCFE). This may develop as a slow gradual process or acutely due to a trauma or minor fall. Children with SCFE present with hip or medial thigh/knee pain with an intermittent limp and an externally rotated leg at the affected hip.
  - Blount's disease (tibia vara or varus deformity of knees and shins) is a growth disturbance to the medial tibial physis most commonly seen in obese males aged 10 to 14. The classic presentation involves an obese child with a progressive limp and unilateral

Koutures C, Wong V.
Pediatric Sports Medicine: Essentials for Office Evaluation (pp 124-129)

or bilateral bowing of the tibia. Clinical findings may include leg length discrepancy, tenderness at the medial tibial physis and tibial torsion associated with the tibia vara.[1]

- The maintenance of foot architecture and function is essential for comfortable and normal walking, running, and jumping. Excessive weight increases the energy forces that must be dissipated with each step, which can weaken tendons and ligaments that support the integrity of the arch of the foot. Chronic overload can possibly produce excessive pronation of the foot (pes planus), shin splints, heel spurs, and plantar fasciitis.
- Obese or overweight individuals are at an increased risk for sprains and strains of the lower extremities due to higher body mass and force.
- They are likely to have more extended and difficult recovery periods from injury due to the burden of extra weight and its stress on the body.

- Psychosocial complications—With high societal standards put on appearance and weight (thin and lean for women; muscular for men), overweight children and adolescents can feel as if they are inadequate or not of "normal appearance." Obesity can also affect the onset of puberty, which can also adversely influence self-image in obese females; puberty has been noted to occur earlier in obese girls than in nonobese girls, whereas in obese boys, puberty may occur later than in their counterparts.[2] Obese and unfit children and adolescents are often subject to bullying and also humiliation in gym class (eg, being picked last for teams or exposing their large physiques when wearing shorts, T-shirts, or bathing suits). The combination of negative self-image and societal pressure can lead to depression, anxiety, eating disorders, and acts of violence.

2. Can Obesity Cause Back Pain or Other Back Issues?

- Extra weight can put additional stress upon the vertebral column, leading to muscle spasms of the upper and lower back, vertebral disc herniation, and early degenerative disc disease.
- When standing, abdominal obesity moves the center of gravity forward, exaggerating the lordotic curve of the low back. Such continual stress increases the pressure on the facet joints and the pars interarticularis.
- When sitting, abdominal obesity can lead to the loss of normal lordotic curvature as the upper body leans forward, exerting extra pressure on the anterior portion of the vertebral discs, which may ultimately lead to disc herniation.

3. How Accurate Is the Body Mass Index in Children and Adolescents? How Does It Compare With Body Fat Analysis by Calipers, Impedance, or Hydrostatic Weighing?

Body mass index (BMI) is determined by using a child's weight and height with the following formula:

$$\frac{\text{mass(kg)}}{[\text{height(m)}]^2}$$

BMI is an estimate of body fat rather than a direct measure. However, it does correlate with hydrostatic weighing and caliper measurement. Although BMI is not a diagnostic tool, it is an inexpensive and easy option to screen children and adolescents for potential weight issues. For screening purposes, the American Academy of Pediatrics recommends that clinicians calculate and plot BMI once per year. BMI in children takes age and gender into account and is plotted on the Centers for Disease Control and Prevention charts to translate into a percentile (Table 19-1).[3]

Studies suggest that body fat measurement, particularly abdominal fat, is more predictive of cardiovascular health risk and metabolic morbidity and mortality than BMI.[4] Since BMI is calculated from only two measurements (height and weight), it does not deal directly with the

Table 19-1. Body Mass Index Interpretation in Children and Categories for Adults	
BMI INTERPRETATION IN CHILDREN[3]	
Weight Status Category	**Percentile Range**
• Underweight	• Less than the 5th percentile
• Healthy weight	• 5th percentile to less than the 85th percentile
• Overweight	• 85th to less than the 95th percentile
• Obese	• Equal to or greater than the 95th percentile
BMI CATEGORIES FOR ADULTS (KG/M²):	
• Underweight = BMI of < 18.5 • Normal weight = BMI of 18.5 to 24.9 • Overweight = BMI of 25 to 29.9 • Obesity = BMI of 30 or greater	

relationship of muscle mass and fat tissue. While those with significant percentages of body fat will always have a higher BMI, the BMI measurement is not always tantamount to obesity.

- The current gold standard for measuring body fat composition is air displacement plethysmography (ADP). This device may be best known as the Bod Pod (Life Measurements Inc, Concord, California). Access to such devices can be limited and expensive.
- Skin fold analysis (SFA) using calipers is the most reliable and comparable measurement of body fat, provided measurements are taken by trained personnel. Many formulas have been devised to convert the calipers measurements into body fat percentages; most of these were developed using modest-sized samples of relatively homogeneous Caucasian-descent populations; thus, the formula may not be accurate for all ethnic groups.
- Bioimpedance analysis (BIA) devices are also an economical, accessible, and popular choice for obtaining body fat measurements. Studies have shown that BIA devices can provide similar results to ADP; however, results may vary across different devices.[5] A limitation on the accuracy of BIA devices is the degree of hydration of the individual being measured. BIA devices may not be accurate enough to give precise, reliable body composition measurements based on a single measurement, but may be more practical and useful in longitudinal follow-up if trained personnel are not available for accurate sequential SFA measurements.[6]
- Hydrostatic (underwater) weighing has often been cited as the true "gold standard," but it entails expensive equipment for the whole body water tank and scale as well as ensuring that the individual has pushed the maximum amount of air out of the lungs while underwater. This method is generally found only in research facilities and at universities.

All methods for determining body fat percentages are accurate within a 2% to 3% margin of error.[6]

- This margin of error may have significant implications. For example, when used to determine the appropriate weight class for a wrestler, this range of imprecision could lead to placing the athlete in one whole weight class above or below his true weight class.
- Thus, these readings are estimates of body fat percentage.
- For an individual who is embarking on a weight management program, serial measurements may accurately reveal a trend in reduced body fat accompanying weight loss or a trend in increasing body muscle mass rather than body fat mass from a strength-training program.

4. What Are the Key Components of an Exercise Prescription?

- Frequency—How often is the exercise carried out?
- Intensity—How does the activity compare to maximal intensity?
- Duration—How many sets and repetitions does the individual complete? How long does the individual perform exercise?

It is recommended that children/adolescents be physically active for 60 minutes on most days of the week while playing or participating in sport-related activities or a structured physical education program.[7]

A specific prescription must be tailored to the patient's current state of physical fitness. The 5 components of physical fitness that should be evaluated are as follows:

1. Aerobic capacity
2. Muscle strength
3. Muscle endurance
4. Muscle flexibility
5. Body composition

To maximize improvement while minimizing the risk of an overuse injury, days of rest and varying intensities/body region exercised are essential parts of an exercise prescription.

- There should be 1 to 2 days of rest per week for the entire body.
- It is important to alternate hard and easy days and to vary the focus on upper- and lower-extremity exercises every other day.
- All exercise regimens should include a warm-up, the focused exercise, and a cool-down. Warm-up and cool-down periods should be at 50% of the focused exercise intensity, and are vital in improving performance and decreasing the risk of dangerous cardiac events. Cool-down decreases muscle soreness by helping to clear metabolic waste from skeletal muscle.[4]

5. When Introducing a Previously Sedentary, Overweight Child to an Exercise Program, What Activities May Allow More Immediate Success and a Reduced Risk of Injury?

The primary goal is to initiate a program of graduated physical activity in part by remembering the simple theory of inertia: bodies at rest tend to stay at rest, bodies in motion tend to keep moving. Exercise that limits or minimizes stress upon joints is preferred.

- Examples of low-impact activities are walking, the elliptical machine, biking, and swimming.
- Stretching and/or a gradual warm-up must always precede activity.
  - Static stretching has been found to be superior to ballistic (bouncing) stretching.[8]
  - Each stretch should be nonpainful and held for a minimum of 10 seconds, ideally 30 seconds or longer.
  - Greater flexibility can be attained by stretching immediately after a workout.

Virtually every individual is able to handle a 10% increase in workload per week with minimal risk of overuse injury. The 10% per week increase in workload guideline is essential in designing a fitness program. Using this guideline, it takes about 7 to 8 weeks to double one's workload. "Slow and steady" are key words of wisdom.

6. What Is the Role of Fitness Testing in Helping Monitor and Develop an Initial or Ongoing Exercise Program?

While exercise testing may be helpful in structuring an exercise program after the individual attains a modest level of fitness, in the beginning, emphasis on testing may be unproductive or provide a barrier to participation in the unfit, obese, sedentary child or adolescent.

Exercise testing demonstrates the body's response to physiologic stress.

- For aerobic workouts, 60% to 85% of maximal heart rate is generally recommended as the target work zone.
- Maximal heart rate may also be estimated using the following formula: 220–age.
- 85% of maximal heart rate should never be exceeded for a sustained amount of time.
- The cardiovascular system is insufficiently challenged when an individual is below 60% of max heart rate; however, all efforts at physical activity should be praised and encouraged, even if the threshold for quality benefits is not initially reached.[5]

Physical fitness testing can be divided into health-related and performance-related fitness.

- Health-related fitness is a description of an individual's cardiorespiratory fitness, muscular strength and endurance, flexibility, and body composition.
- Performance-related fitness is an assessment of the motor skills required to function in certain jobs or sports activities.
  - Includes agility, balance, coordination, power, reaction time, and speed.
- It is important to keep these differences in mind, since exercise programs designed for the simple maintenance and the development of health-related fitness will differ greatly from an exercise program designed to enhance athletic performance.[9] There are several different standardized test batteries, although criteria for physical fitness will vary across different age groups, gender, and function level. In some cases, it may be more beneficial to utilize a combination of separate components or multiple test batteries.[10]
  - FITNESSGRAM—Developed in 1993 by Cooper Institute for Aerobics Research, Association of Health, Physical Education, Recreation, and Dance (AAHPERD), and Human Kinetics Publishers is the most widely used comprehensive health-related physical fitness assessment program used in individuals from kindergarten through college age.
  - The test includes standards for ages 5 to 17, both genders, and adults. Assessment of physical fitness is accomplished through measurements of aerobic capacity, body composition, muscle strength, endurance, and flexibility.
  - Brockport Physical Fitness Test—Criterion-referenced assessment battery designed for individuals aged 10 to 17 with physical and/or mental disabilities; consists of 27 different tests.
  - President's Challenge—Administered to individuals aged 6 to 17, and consists of five tests (curl-ups, shuttle run, mile run/walk, pull ups/pushups/flexed arm hang, V-sit reach/sit and reach); awards are given to individuals based on the percentile scores attained on all tests.
  - AAHPERD Health-Related Physical Fitness Test—Assesses fitness in college students who are specifically enrolled in physical education classes but has shown usefulness in the general college population.
  - The Canadian Standardized Test of Fitness—Includes a Physical Activity Readiness Questionnaire, and standardized anthropometric measurements (height, weight, girth, body fat), aerobic fitness measurement, and assessment of muscular strength, flexibility, and endurance with gender and age appropriate norms for ages 15 to 69 years.

Studies have shown that children who participate in fitness programs will be more likely to develop and maintain practices that promote health and physical activity.[1]

7. What Are Some "Pearls" to Encourage an Overweight Child to Become More Physically Active?

- Obese children should limit sedentary screen time to no more than 7 hours per week.
- Increase time for unstructured play; encourage physical movement that burns calories.

- Finding enjoyable activities is key. Children have a greater enjoyment of sports when the emphasis is placed on skill development, cooperative play, and having fun.
- Confidence may affect overweight adolescents' exercise participation. A positive attitude and feedback from parents and coaches are essential.
  - Since they are often bigger than their peers, overweight children often find increased abilities to lift heavier and repetitive weights. Thus, weight-training can give a more immediate confidence and sense of satisfaction.
- Set attainable goals. Adolescents find it easier and more satisfying to fulfill small attainable goals. Taking "baby steps" is helpful.
- For overweight and mildly obese children and adolescents undergoing significant growth and development, the focus should be on weight maintenance rather than weight loss. For children and adolescents who are greater than the 97th percentile, a slow weight loss of 1 to 2 pounds per month can be a reasonable goal.

8. Can Activity-Related Video Games (Wii Fit [Nintendo Co, Ltd, Kyoto, Japan], Dance Dance Revolution [Konami Corporation, Tokyo, Japan]) Play a Significant Role in Weight Management?

Conflicting evidence exists regarding the efficacy of activity-related video games for weight loss.

- Video games have been found to be more effective in the laboratory setting than in home studies. The biggest problem is a dramatic drop in daily use after initial game play.
- Video games may not provide the cooperative play or social pressure of organized sports.
- Activity-related video games may therefore serve as a supplement, rather than a replacement, to other athletic activities.[11]

References

1. Madden C, Putukian M, McCarty E, Young C. *Netter's Sports Medicine*. Philadelphia, PA: Elsevier Saunders; 2010.
2. Wagner IV, Sabin MA, Pfäffle RW, et al. Effects of obesity on human sexual development. *Nat Rev Endocrinol.* 2012;8(4):246–254.
3. Council of Sports Medicine and Fitness and Council on School Health, American Academy of Pediatrics. Active healthy living: prevention of childhood obesity through increased physical activity. *Pediatrics.* 2006;117:1834-1842.
4. Centers for Disease Control and Prevention. Healthy weight: assessing your weight. www.cdc.gov/healthyweight/assessing/index.html. Accessed June 17, 2013.
5. Garber CE, Blissmer B, Deschenes MR, et al American College of Sports Medicine position stand: quantity and quality of exercise for developing and maintaining cardiorespiratory, musculoskeletal, and neuromotor fitness in apparently healthy adults: guidance for prescribing exercise. *Med Sci Sports Exerc.* 2011;43(7):1334–1359.
6. Peterson JT, Repovich WES, Parascand CR. Accuracy of consumer grade bioelectrical impedance analysis devices compared to air displacement plethysmography. *Int J Exer Sci.* 2011;4(3):176–184.
7. 2008 Physical Activity Guidelines for Americans. Chapter 3: Active Children and Adolescents. www.health.gov/paguidelines/guidelines/chapter3.aspx. Accessed June 17, 2013.
8. Alter MJ. Sports Stretch. Champaign, IL: Leisure Press; 1990.
9. Miller DK. *Measurement by the Physical Educator: Why and How.* Indianapolis, IN: Benchmark Press, Inc; 1988.
10. Tritschler K. *Practical Measurement and Assessment.* 5th edition. Philadelphia, PA: Lippincott Williams & Wilkins; 2000.
11. Baranowski T, Abdelsamad D, Baranowski J, et al. Impact of an active video game on healthy children's physical activity. *Pediatrics.* 2012;129(3):e636–e642.

Acknowledgment

The authors wish to thank medical student Jane Hur and pediatric resident Allison Sopko, MD, for their invaluable contributions.

General Radiology Imaging and Laboratory Testing
What to Order and When

20

Mohammed Mortazavi, MD and Quynh B. Hoang, MD

Imaging

1. What Are Some General Rules to Follow When Ordering X-rays?

- Conventional radiographs are sensitive and specific in detecting long bone fractures.
- They are indicated when there is a history of trauma (which may indicate that the patient needs immediate, further work-up), but in general x-rays should almost always be the initial imaging tool. Other indications for obtaining plain films can be found in Table 20-1.
- Because conventional x-rays compress images into two dimensions, it is essential to obtain a minimum of two views of the area of interest that are 90 degrees apart (eg, AP/lateral).
- X-ray interpretation becomes difficult when bones project upon one another and when they have irregular surfaces. This can be addressed by obtaining additional projections (eg, oblique) or special views.
- If there is a history of trauma, x-rays should include the joint above and the joint below the bone that is involved.

2. Should X-rays Be Ordered Before Asking for a More Advanced Imaging Modality?

Almost all imaging should begin with conventional radiography, especially if there is a history of trauma because x-rays are excellent in revealing long bone fractures. They also provide excellent contrast between bone and soft tissue. They are widely and readily available, inexpensive, and results can be known in a short period of time. Although advanced imaging modalities such as magnetic resonance imaging (MRI) and computed tomography (CT) scan can provide more diagnostic details, abnormal findings can sometimes be nonspecific. Thus, correlation with plain films is crucial for the correct interpretation of musculoskeletal abnormalities on advanced imaging modalities.

3. When Do I Need to Order Comparison Views on Plain X-rays?

- Physeal injury—Salter-Harris type I fractures or chronic physeal stress injuries (such as seen in gymnast wrist or little league shoulder) may show the subtle widening of the physis on radiographs, and it is not always apparent. Comparison views may be helpful in demonstrating the difference in the two sides (Figures 20-3 and 20-4).
- Accessory ossification center—Accessory ossicles can be incidental findings and are distinguished from fracture fragments by their smooth, round contours. A radiograph of the opposite side can sometimes be helpful, as there can be bilateral findings.

Koutures C, Wong V.
Pediatric Sports Medicine: Essentials for Office Evaluation (pp 130-137)

Table 20-1. Indications for Obtaining Plain Films	
• Bone or joint pain, especially pain worsening at night* • Bone infection, especially accompanied by fever, weight loss* • Radiopaque foreign body • Evaluating structural/developmental abnormalities	• Injury at apophyseal sites to rule out avulsion fracture • Bone or soft-tissue mass • Assessing for anatomic or ossification variants • Follow-up radiographs 14 to 21 days postinjury to diagnostically confirm an occult fracture (Figures 20-1 and 20-2)
*Potential "red flags" that may need immediate, further work-up.	

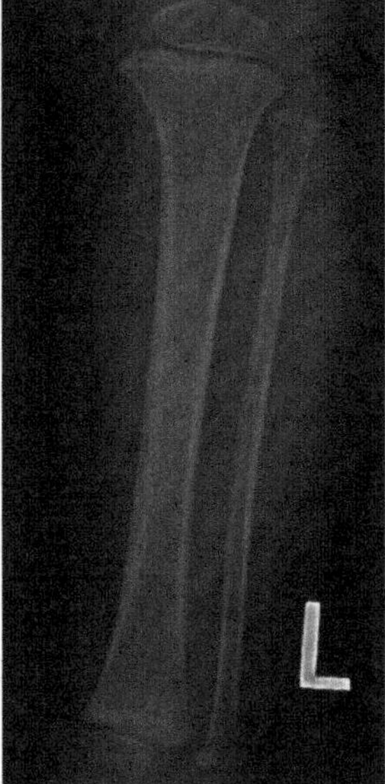

Figure 20-1. X-ray of a normal tibia in a child who refused to bear weight after an injury.

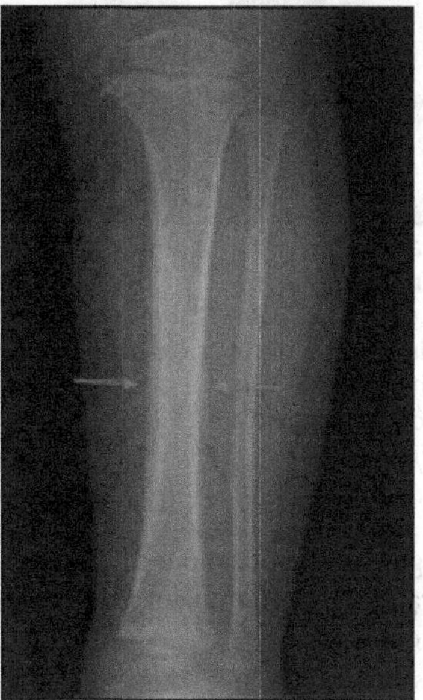

Figure 20-2. X-ray of a healing midshaft tibia fracture taken 3 weeks after the 2-year-old patient was treated in a long leg cast for an occult fracture; x-ray shows periosteal reaction along the tibia shaft, suggesting fracture healing.

- Apophyseal or ossification center variations—Fusion of apophyses and ossification centers may be variable and appear abnormal on x-rays, especially if there is incomplete fusion (Figure 20-5). When in doubt, obtaining comparison views can be helpful to rule out avulsions or fractures, as often times the findings of apophyseal or ossification variants are bilateral. This is also true for apophyseal injuries and injuries to ossification centers with little displacement.

4. Ultrasonography Is Best Used to Evaluate What Conditions?

Ultrasonography has the advantages of avoiding radiation exposure, being inexpensive and easily available, and allowing for dynamic imaging in real time. It has been widely used in diagnosing pediatric hip disorders. However, with its excellent soft-tissue contrast and advances in high-resolution ultrasonography, it is now well suited to evaluate the pediatric musculoskeletal

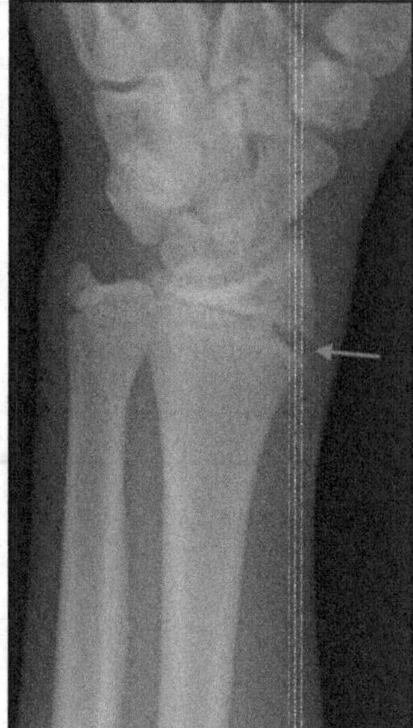

Figure 20-3. X-ray of a left distal radius physeal injury in a gymnast presenting with wrist pain; note the widening of the distal radius physis compared with the normal physis of the patient's right wrist (see Figure 20-4).

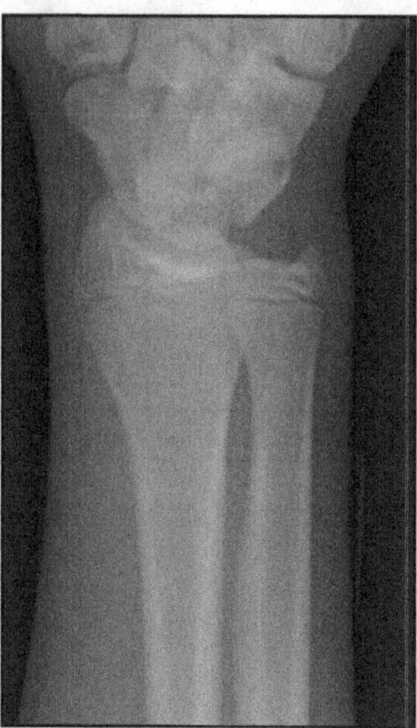

Figure 20-4. Normal x-ray of the same patient's right wrist shows no widening of the distal radial physis.

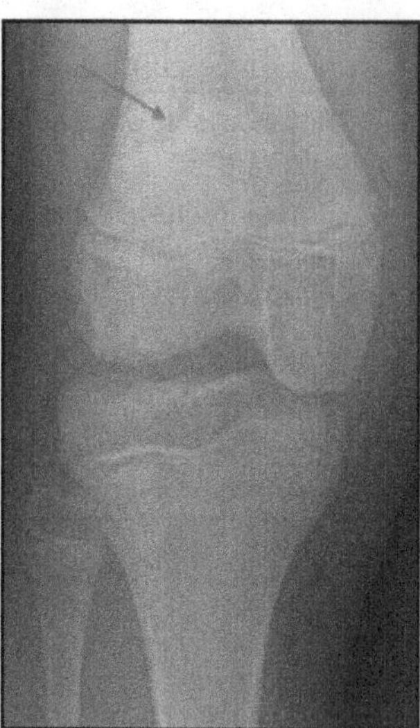

Figure 20-5. Normal x-ray findings showing a bipartite patella, which may commonly be mistaken for an acute fracture.

system. Although many applications for ultrasonography have been developed, it is most ideal for evaluation of traumatic, inflammatory, degenerative, and even infections or neoplastic conditions that affect the following:

- Tendons
- Muscles
- Joints (shoulder, knee, hip)
- Ligaments
- Peripheral nerves
- Soft-tissue foreign bodies

5. Computed Tomography Scan Is Best Used to Evaluate What Conditions?

CT provides the best imaging modality for investigation of bone. It provides clear details of fractures in terms of extent of the injury and the position of bony fragments, which may be necessary for decision making in terms of nonoperative management or surgical intervention. It can also assess for bony healing. CT is also the imaging modality of choice in trauma because it detects acute bleeding and can quickly provide details of bony anatomy in all dimensions. The following conditions are best evaluated with CT:

- Complex or intra-articular fractures
- Assessment of fracture and stress fracture healing, including the lumbar spine
- Acute head or abdominal/pelvic trauma

6. Bone Scan Is Best Used to Evaluate What Conditions?

Bone scan has an advantage over other imaging modalities in that it is highly sensitive to any bony pathology and can detect bone injury as early as 24 hours after a triggering event. The downfall is that it lacks specificity. Any abnormalities on bone scan will require further investigation with a more specific imaging modality to determine the etiology of the abnormality. Bone scan is best indicated as a screening tool for the evaluation of the following:

- Stress fractures
- Osteomyelitis; detecting occult infections or localizing the site of infection when an inflammatory process is present
- Generalized bone pain to detect presence of tumor
- Osseous metastases in neoplastic disease

7. Magnetic Resonance Imaging Is Best Used to Evaluate What Conditions?

MRI provides excellent soft-tissue contrast. It also has the ability to provide high-resolution images of the body in multiple planes. For these reasons, MRI is the ideal imaging modality for evaluating soft tissue, joints, and bones. The following conditions can be best assessed with MRI:

- Soft-tissue injury (muscle, ligament, tendon, meniscus, cartilage)
- Joint derangements
  - Shoulder (rotator cuff disease, glenoid labrum tear, acetabular labrum tear)
  - Knee (ligament injury, meniscal tear)
- Osteochondral injuries
- Occult fracture, especially physeal injuries
- Stress fractures
- Lower back pain
- Infection (osteomyelitis, abscess)
- Abnormalities of bone marrow
  - Infection (osteomyelitis)
  - Stress reaction or fracture
  - Bone contusion
  - Neoplasia
  - Devascularization (avascular necrosis)
- Bone and soft-tissue masses, tumors
- Spinal cord injury

8. Which Imaging Modalities Might Have Greater Radiation Exposure?

Radiation risk from diagnostic imaging is an area of concern, particularly in the pediatric population. These patients are more sensitive to radiation-induced cancer risk than adults. To this regard, MRI and ultrasonography are commonly being used because of their lack of ionizing radiation exposure. Of the remaining imaging modalities, CT has the greatest radiation exposure. Most epidemiologic studies on radiation exposure risk have been completed in cohorts who have been exposed to radiation treatment for benign diseases. Very few studies have looked at the cancer risk following diagnostic radiation exposure in children. In general, however, radiation doses are low for a single procedure unless the diagnostic procedure is performed multiple times. Studies have shown that high cumulative dose exposure over time can increase the risk of developing malignancies in a linear fashion, notably solid tumors and leukemia.[1]

Laboratory Testing

Laboratory considerations in ailing athletes are diverse and depend greatly on the working differential diagnosis of the physician. In general, labs are ordered in athletes when there is concern for an underlying medical condition such as infection, hematologic/oncologic disease, rheumatologic disease, endocrine abnormality, cardiac disease, metabolic disorders, or gastrointestinal disease. A large number of lab studies are available, so it is important to approach the sick athlete with considerations of his or her history, symptoms, and examination. More often than not, the history will indicate the direction of the work-up. For this reason, only order labs that are indicated after obtaining a thorough history and performing a thorough physical examination so as to minimize the risk of missing an ominous diagnosis. If the history and examination are normal, laboratory tests are usually unnecessary on the initial visit given their very low yield, but they can be considered if there is no improvement of symptoms over a 2- to 3-week period.[2]

9. What Tests Should Be Considered When Evaluating a Fatigued or Underperforming Athlete?

- Athletes may report symptoms of fatigue, a decline in training endurance or performance, or just feeling ill from training. Most of these athletes will be suffering from overtraining syndrome, which is associated with increased training intervals, intensity, duration, and decreased rest periods. Along with declining performance, a history of mood symptoms, muscle or joint pain, elevated resting heart rate, and sleep disturbance have been described.[3-5] For young athletes, fatigue and disinterest for competition are also common manifestations.[5] In overtraining syndrome, these symptoms typically persist beyond a 2-week period despite appropriate rest.[3,4] Although obtaining a thorough training history is essential to assess such athletes, overtraining must remain a diagnosis of exclusion until other medical conditions have been ruled out. If the patient's history does not seem to match up with overtraining alone, it is often warranted to evaluate for underlying medical conditions that may present with fatigue. Generalized laboratory tests may include complete blood count (CBC), ferritin levels, thyroid studies, and vitamin D levels. If the athlete is female, a pregnancy test may be warranted. Based on clinical history and physical examination, the following laboratory assessments can be considered, by system:
- Cardiovascular—Chest pain, syncope, or unusual dyspnea on exertion.
    - Evaluate for arrhythmias, valvular heart disease, and structural heart disease.[2,6,7]
        - Chest x-ray, EKG, echocardiogram.
- Female Athlete Triad—See Chapter 17, questions 1 to 3.
- Gastrointestinal—Nausea, vomiting, bloating, anorexia, and abnormal stooling patterns.
    - Consider food allergies, celiac disease, and inflammatory bowel disease.
        - Food allergy testing, fecal fat, stool cultures, celiac panel, and inflammatory bowel disease panel.
    - Consider infections, ischemic colitis.
        - CBC, comprehensive metabolic panel, lipase, hepatitis panel, stool culture, *Clostridium difficile* toxin, and stool O&P, stool guaiac, double contrast barium enema.
    - If gastrointestinal upset appears to be more gastric related, consider gastritis/ulcers.
- Infectious disease—Fever, malaise, and fatigue.
    - Chronic, indolent infections can present with vague symptoms of fatigue, fevers, and malaise.
    - Consider infectious mononucleosis.
        - Obtain Epstein-Barr virus titers.

- A thorough symptom history can guide specific laboratory testing for any suspected infection.
- General labs include CBC, C-reactive protein (CRP), erythrocyte sedimentation rate (ESR), and blood cultures.
- Specific antibody titers and cultures based on history.

- Oncologic—Fevers, fatigue, anorexia, weight loss, night sweats, and night pain.
  - Consider leukemia, lymphoma, sarcoma, germ cell tumors, and central nervous system tumors.
  - Ask the patient about constitutional symptoms.
  - CBC, ESR, CRP, and often a peripheral blood smear or focused imaging of the symptomatic region can be useful.
- Rheumatologic—Fatigue, fever, weight loss, rash, and joint pain.
  - Fatigue may be the initial presenting symptom prior to clinical manifestation of other more specific symptoms such as rash or joint pain.
  - Consider rheumatoid arthritis, systemic lupus erythematosus, sarcoidosis, dermatomyositis, and scleroderma.
  - CBC, CRP, ESR, rheumatoid factor (RF), creatine phosphokinase, and antinuclear antibody (ANA) titer are helpful initial lab tests followed by rheumatologic referral and more specific antibody testing, if needed.[6]

10. What Lab Tests Should I Order if I Suspect an Infected Joint?

- Septic joint: effusion, erythema, warmth, tenderness, and +/– fever.
- Rheumatologic disease, trauma, bleeding disorders, and oncologic processes should also be considered.[8]
- Obtain CBC, CRP, ESR, RF, ANA titer, and blood culture.
- Joint aspirate should be sent for cell count, Gram stain, and culture.[8]

11. Can Young Athletes Have Normally Elevated Labs?

It is important to keep in mind that certain labs are expected to be mildly elevated in the young active athlete, especially after recent exercise, and they should not draw concern for work-up. In particular, the specific labs discussed in Table 20-2 may be transiently elevated after vigorous activity and would need to be repeated in the rested state to confirm normalization.[7,9,11] Also, due to their larger muscle mass, athletes often have elevated baseline levels of labs pertaining to muscle metabolism.[9,10,12]

TABLE 20-2. COMMONLY ELEVATED LABS IN ATHLETES			
LAB	*ACCEPTABLE ELEVATIONS*	*APPROPRIATE FOLLOW- UP*	*COMMENTS*
Alkaline phosphatase	2 to 3 times adult levels in children with high growth velocity 2 to 3 times adult levels during pregnancy	None necessary	Normal adult range: 30 to 120 U/L Children: up to 350 U/L
Proteinuria	1 to 2+ proteinuria up to 48 hours postexercise	Repeat supine morning sample 48 hours postexercise	If repeat sample abnormal: obtain 24 hours urine protein/ creatinine
Hematuria[11,12]	Microscopic hematuria (> 3 red blood count/ high power field) up to 48 hours postexercise	Repeat sample in 24 to 48 hours	If repeat sample abnormal: obtain urine culture, blood urea nitrogen, creatinine
Blood urea nitrogen	Up to 50% elevations with increased muscle mass	None necessary	
Creatine phosphokinase	10 to 20 times normal levels after vigorous exercise up to 3 to 5 days Up to 50% elevation with increased muscle mass	Repeat in 3 to 5 days Peak levels seen at 1 to 2 days post-exercise	Normal range: 38 to 275 U/L Consider expanded differential if levels > 5000 U/L or not normalized after 5 days
Aspartate transaminase, alanine aminotransferase	1.5 times normal levels postexercise up to 10 to 12 days Up to 50% elevation with increased muscle mass	Repeat at rested levels in 2 weeks	Normal ranges: Aspartate transaminase (5 to 40 IU/L) Alanine aminotransferase (7 to 56 IU/L) Consider work-up for hepatitis, gall stones, liver disease if abnormal

References

1. Kleinerman RA. Cancer risks following diagnostic and therapeutic radiation exposure in children. *Pediat Radiol.* 2006;36(2):121–125.
2. Valdini A, Steinhardt S, Feldman E. Usefulness of a standard battery of laboratory tests in investigating chronic fatigue in adults. *Fam Pract.* 1989;6:286–291.
3. Reid VL, Gleeson M, Williams N, et al. Clinical investigation of athletes with persistent fatigue and/or recurrent infections. *Br J Sports Med.* 2004;38:42–45.
4. Du Toit C, Locke S. The fatigued athlete: an audit of pathology test versus clinical diagnosis. *J Sci Med Sport.* 2005;8(suppl):171.
5. Brenner JS, Council on Sports Medicine and Fitness. Overuse injuries, overtraining, and burnout in child and adolescent athletes. *Pediatrics.* 2007;119:1242.
6. Ridsdale L, Evans A, Jerrett W, et al. Patients with fatigue in general practice: a prospective study. *BMJ.* 1993;307:103–106.

7. Peterson MC, Holbrook JH, Von Hales DE, et al. Contributions of the history, physical examination and laboratory investigation in making medical diagnoses. *West J Med.* 1992;156:163–165.
8. Li SF, Cassidy C, Chang C, et al. Diagnostic utility of laboratory tests in septic arthritis. *Emerg Med J.* 2007;24(2):75–77.
9. LaPorta MA, Linde HW, Bruce DL, Fitzsimons EJ. Elevation of creatine phosphokinase in young men after recreational exercise. *JAMA.* 1978;239(25):2685–2686.
10. Senert R, Kohl L, Rainone T, Scalea T. Exercise-induced rhabdomyolysis. *Ann Emerg Med.* 1994;23:1301–1306.
11. Oosterom DL. Exertion-related abnormalities in the urine. *Ned Tijdschr Geneeskd.* 2006;150(11): 606-610.
12. Fallon KE, Sivyer G, et al. The biochemistry of runners in a 1600 km ultramarathon. *Br J Sports Med.* 1999;33: 264-269.

Section III

Musculoskeletal Issues

21 How to Take a Sports Medicine History

Kelly Chain, MD and Chris Koutures, MD, FAAP

History—The Acute Injury

1. How Did the Injury Happen?

Knowing the exact mechanism of injury can be helpful to develop a differential diagnosis. Use observers, patient recall, and even video (if available).

- Was there contact or trauma, such as a fall, hit, or blow to a particular area?
- Did the patient hear any noises, such as a crack, click, or pop?
- Did the patient have any particular sensations, such as "tearing" or bones sliding out of joint?

2. What Happened Immediately After the Injury?

- Did the child continue to play, or was there removal from the activity?
- If he or she was able to continue playing, was there any change in form or level of aggressiveness?
    - What were these changes?
    - Did the child have a limp?
- If he or she was unable to return to play, what prevented his or her return?
    - Was he or she limited by pain, decreased range of motion, or stiffness?
- How did the injury initially look?
    - Was there any bruising and/or swelling?
    - If so, what was the timing of the onset of the bruising and/or swelling?
        - Did it occur immediately or did it develop gradually over time?

Immediate joint swelling within 1 hour suggests a possible intra-articular concern (fracture, ligament tear).

- Where was the pain located?
    - Identifying the precise location of the pain is important.
        - Can the child point with one finger to the exact location of the pain, or is the pain more diffuse and nonspecific?

Finger-tip or focal pain is more suggestive of serious pathology.

Koutures C, Wong V.
Pediatric Sports Medicine: Essentials for Office Evaluation (pp 139-143)

- Was the pain immediately present, or did it evolve over time?
- What actions or movements are making the pain better/worse?
- Does the pain radiate anywhere?
- How bad is the pain?
    - For older children and teens, use a 1 to 10 pain rating scale.
    - For younger children, use the happy to sad face scale.
- Is there any burning or stiffness related with the pain?

3. What Interventions Were Tried to Help Alleviate the Child's Discomfort?

- Did he or she use ice, heat, or both?
    - How often and for how long?
- Did the child take any medication?
    - If so, which medications, what were the exact doses, and how often?
- Did ice, heat, or medication help reduce the pain?
- Did the child require the use of crutches, a sling, a splint, or any other device to help protect or take weight off of the injured area?
- Since the injury occurred, has it been getting better or worse?
- Has the individual been able return to his or her sport with modified activity or was he or she able to fully participate without limitation?
- Are activities of daily living (walking up/down stairs, opening doors, lifting objects, etc) now limited due to the pain?

4. Is This a First-Time Injury Versus a Repetitive (Acute on Chronic) Injury?

- If this is a recurrent or repetitive injury, was the child at baseline function and pain free prior to the current injury, or was he or she still having symptoms and limitations from his or her previous injury?
- Was there any lingering swelling, pain, or bruising from the previous injury?

Underrehabilitated past injuries are the highest risk factor for new injuries.

History—The Chronic Injury ("Been Going on for 1 to 2 Months")

Many chronic injuries are due to repetitive stress, so questions are designed to identify activities or patterns of potential overload. Obtaining specifics on all sport participation (practices, games, private lessons, strength training, etc) and learning about recent (last 1 to 2 months) increases in game/tournament play, or participating at a "higher" level.

1. What Is the Child's Overall Sport/Activity Involvement?

- How many practices/games per week for each sport-related activity?
    - Quantify type and duration of each activity. Examples include the following:
        - How many hours per day and days per week?
        - For running, how many miles does he or she run daily/weekly?
        - For swimmers, how may yards/meters does he or she swim daily/weekly?
        - For pitchers, how many pitches does he or she pitch in one game/per week?

- Has the child recently increased his or her frequency or the intensity of his or her activity?
  - Longer practice sessions, more practices per week.
- Has he or she recently joined a more competitive team or league that requires more participation time and/or increased intensity?
- Is the child playing with older or more experienced players?
- Has the individual recently changed technique or started using any new equipment?
- Does the child play only one position or a variety of different positions?
- Have there been recent multiday tournaments or showcase events?

2. Does the Athlete Get Enough Rest?

- How many rest days per week (complete day off from all sports activities)?
- How many months in a year does he or she take off from his or her sport?

To reduce the risk of overuse injuries, sports medicine experts recommend a minimum of 1 day off per week and 2 to 3 months off from a particular sport per year.[1]

3. When Was the Onset of Pain?

- Was the pain first noticed during activity, or did the pain begin after activity?
- If the pain occurs during activity, does it occur earlier or later in the course of the activity? Does it happen every practice/game or only sporadically after certain movements or practices?
- If the pain begins after the activity is completed, how long does the pain persist (a few minutes/hours, or until the next morning)?
- Does the pain cause any modification of technique? If so, what is different?
- Does the pain limit the athlete's intensity or his or her frequency of activity?
- Is there any pain in the joints proximal and/or distal to the problem area?
- Does the pain move? If so, where?
- It is important to grade all pain symptoms on a 1 to 10 scale or a happy to sad face scale.

4. Are There Other Symptoms (Swelling, Numbness, Weakness, etc), and How Have They Progressed?

- Are the other symptoms getting better or worse?
- Do they last longer or shorter than at initial presentation?
- Have any new symptoms developed since the initial injury?

5. What Interventions Have Been Tried to Help Alleviate the Child's Pain or Other Symptoms?

- Has the athlete been forced to change his or her technique or form in any way?
- Has he or she been taking any medications?
  - If so, which medications and how often?
  - Did these provide any relief?
- Has he or she tried using ice or heat therapies?
- Has the athlete seen a medical provider? If so, what was he or she told?
- Has he or she used any braces or splints? If so, what was the result?

A comprehensive rehabilitation program needs appropriate monitoring, exercises and time. Ask about the types of exercise, length of program, and patient compliance. Often, when therapy "didn't" work, it is because the athlete did not receive proper supervision or did not allow sufficient time and effort.

- Has he or she tried physical therapy or rehabilitation exercises/stretches?
- Has the individual attempted chiropractic or acupuncture care for pain relief?

6. Is This the First Time the Athlete Has Experienced Pain or Symptoms in This Particular Area, or Is This a Repetitive/Chronic Problem?

- If this is a repetitive problem, what past diagnoses has the athlete received?
- What evaluations and work-up was done in the past?
- What imaging has been done?
  - When was the last time imaging was done, and did it show a problem?
  - Can the family bring in the past imaging for review/comparison?
- What was done for the athlete the last time he or she had this problem?
  - Did he or she receive physical therapy?
  - Was he or she given any prescriptions medications?
  - Did he or she require surgery?
- Most importantly, did any of the interventions help alleviate symptoms?
  - What worked and what did not?
- Was there complete recovery with past issues, or only partial improvement?

History—All Injuries

1. Clarify With the Athlete What Positions He or She Plays. Does He or She Have any Upcoming Goals/Major Events/ Tournaments? Where Is He or She in the Season?

- Does the child have other sports/activities/classes to be taken into consideration?

2. How Is the Athlete's Diet?

- Is he or she taking in sufficient calcium/vitamin D, calories, and iron?
- Has he or she recently been trying to gain or lose weight?
  - What has he or she been doing to accomplish this goal?

3. Are There Any Constitutional Signs/Symptoms?

- Does he or she have night pain (awakens from sleep), fevers, vomiting, diarrhea, unintentional weight gain/loss, rashes, or fatigue?

4. For Girls, a Menstrual History Is Important.

- When was her last period, and is her cycle regular?
- Is she experiencing severe cramping or does she have very heavy bleeding?
- Is she on any type of birth control?

5. Ascertain the Extent of Skeletal Maturity.

- How old is he or she, and what are his or her Tanner stages?
- If development is uncertain, a bone age x-ray can help stage development.

Skeletally immature athletes are more likely to injure growth plates than skeletally mature athletes who more commonly injure ligaments/tendons.

6. Does the Athlete Have Any Other Significant Medical or Orthopedic History?

- Is there a history of frequent injuries, sprains, fractures, etc?
- Has the athlete had any past stress fractures?

7. What Prescription and Nonprescription Medications/Supplements Has He or She Taken in the Past?

- What is he or she taking now?
- Include the dose and frequency.

Reference

1. Brenner JS, Council on Sports Medicine and Fitness. Overuse injuries, overtraining and burnout in child and adolescent athletes. *Pediatrics*. 2007;119(6):1242–1245.

22 Physical Examination Organization and Basics

Chris Koutures, MD, FAAP

Many health care providers are intimidated by performing joint examinations, "I just don't know what I'm doing, and I don't do this that often." Having an organized and consistent approach to the physical examination can improve provider and patient comfort, better ensure appropriate examination of key issues, and assist with documentation. Practice at every opportunity—even incorporate joint evaluations into younger well-child care (smaller limbs are easier to hold and perform joint-specific examinations)—and never be afraid to touch the patient!

Step 1: Preparation and Tips to Enhance Patient Comfort

- The physical examination often serves to confirm what is suspected by a thorough history. Create a focused list of potential diagnoses before starting the physical examination.
- Properly expose the area/extremity of concern.
  - It is advisable to have shorts and tank tops available to maintain patient modesty.
  - If examining the patient's lower leg and foot, remove both sets of socks and shoes.
  - Remove any braces, wraps, or dressings.
- Pull the examination table away from the wall to increase access to patient.
  - To examine paired joints, the examiner should move, not the patient.
- For paired joints, always examine the noninjured side first.
  - This allows the assessment of "normal" range of motion (ROM), strength, and joint laxity to compare with the injured side.
  - Starting the examination on the nonpainful side can reduce patient apprehension during the evaluation of the painful, injured area.
- Save the most potentially uncomfortable maneuvers for last.
  - Evoking pain may increase muscle guarding and patient apprehension and may limit the remainder of the examination.

Step 2: Observation and Visual Examination

- The physical examination begins when you enter the room.
  - Is the patient sitting or laying down on the table?
  - Is he or she using typical gestures while talking?
  - Does he or she move around comfortably about the room?
  - Is he or she moving excessively or limiting movement due to pain?
- Evaluate for swelling, bruising, or distal skin color changes.

Koutures C, Wong V.
Pediatric Sports Medicine: Essentials for Office Evaluation (pp 144-147)

Step 3: Always Involve at Least One Joint Proximal and One Joint Distal to the Area of Concern

- Referred pain from a proximal joint presenting as distal pain is common.
  - Classic example: intra-articular hip pain from slipped capital femoral epiphysis presenting as medial thigh or knee pain.
- Proximal weakness or instability can contribute to distal pain or injury.
  - Involve the neck and the periscapular region in cases of chronic shoulder or elbow pain.
  - Involve the lower back, hip, and pelvis in cases of chronic knee or lower leg pain.

Step 4: Assess for Skin Integrity and Swelling

- Diffuse joint swelling is more of a concern for intra-articular pathology than finger-tip or focal swelling.
- Use the dorsum of the hand to assess warmth of the joint.
  - Asymmetric or increased warmth suggests infection or inflammatory concerns.
- Document abrasions, lacerations, bruising, and any other alteration of the skin.
  - Any open skin around an acute injury puts the patient at a high risk for deep infection.

Step 5: Assess Range of Motion

- Use the noninjured extremity for comparison.
- Use a goniometer to measure the degrees of ROM.
- Swelling often will limit the patient's ROM.
- Increased ROM (knee/elbow hyperextension past 0 degrees) may suggest hyperlaxity of connective tissues.
- Have the patient first do active ROM.
- If limits are noted, attempt to passively move the joint through full ROM.
  - Painfully limited ROM ("block") with swelling may suggest an intra-articular injury process with loose body or displacement.

Step 6: Palpation

- Do not hesitate to consult an anatomy reference for a quick refresher. Sharing pictures and images with the patient and family often enhances understanding.
- Use methodical, organized palpation of the injured region, saving the most painful area for last.
  - Use your finger tip for best sensation.
    - Focal pain is more of a concern than diffuse pain.

Step 7: Assessing Ligamentous Integrity

- Hinged joints (knee, elbow, finger interphalangeal).
  - Ligaments are isolated when the joint is flexed to 30 degrees.
    - Example: valgus stress testing of a knee flexed to 30 degrees stresses medial collateral ligament (MCL).
  - Entire support complex (ligament, joint capsule, and muscles) are involved when the joint is at full extension (0 degrees).
    - Example: valgus stress testing of a fully extended knee stresses MCL along with posterior-medial knee complex and medial joint capsule.

TABLE 22-1. GRADING LIGAMENT SPRAINS	
GRADE	*DESCRIPTION*
Grade 1 sprain	Pain to palpation, no increased laxity versus noninjured side
Grade 2 sprain	Pain to palpation, increased laxity with firm end point
Grade 3 sprain	+/- pain to palpation, increased laxity without firm end point

TABLE 22-2. UPPER EXTREMITY DERMATOMES/MYOTOMES/REFLEXES	
NERVE	*DERMATOME/MYOTOME/REFLEX*
C5	Radial forearm/shoulder abduction/biceps brachii
C6	Thumb, index finger/wrist dorsiflexion/triceps
C7	Middle finger/wrist palmarflexion/brachioradialis
C8	Fifth finger/claw fingers
T1	Ulnar forearm/finger abduction

Rapid Assessment of Upper Motor Nerve Function

Radial nerve: "Thumbs up"
Median nerve: "OK" sign
Ulnar nerve: "Cross fingers"

  - Thus, increased laxity in full extension suggests a more complicated injury.
  - See Table 22-1 for information on grading ligament sprains.

Step 8: Joint-Specific Special Tests

- Please refer to the joint-specific chapters for information on special tests.

Step 9: Involve Assessment of the Patient's Distal Neurovascular and General Neurologic Status

- In cases of bilateral concerns, strongly consider the following central etiologies:
  - Spinal cord issues, disc herniation.
  - Autoimmune disorders, thyroid dysfunction, spondyloarthropathies.
- Capillary refill.
  - Normal is usually less than 3 seconds. Compare with the patient's noninjured side.
  - Please refer to Tables 22-2 and 22-3 for descriptions of key upper and lower extremity dermatomes, myotomes, and reflexes.

Step 10: Functional Examination

- In the setting of an acute injury, you may have to limit or defer due to patient discomfort.
- This may be performed earlier in the examination with patients who have completed/are further along in a rehabilitation program, or who desire immediate return to play and need to exhibit appropriate movement patterns and function.
- Use the hallway or a larger room/outside area if needed for appropriate space.
- Stance.
  - Is the patient balanced or putting more weight on one side?

Table 22-3. Lower Extremity Dermatomes/Myotomes/Reflexes	
NERVE	*DERMATOME/MYOTOME/REFLEX*
L4	Medial shin, foot/foot dorsiflexion/patellar tendon
L5	Mid shin/first toe dorsiflexion
S1	Lateral shin/foot plantarflexion/Achilles tendon

Table 22-4. Special Tests for Central Strength and Stability	
POSITION	*REGIONS/MUSCLES TESTED*
Duck walk—5 steps in a deep squat position (See Figure 37-3)	Stability and ROM of hips, knees, and ankle
Bridge (Figure 22-1)	Gluteal strength
Plank (Figure 22-2)	Periscapular, upper arm, and abdominal strength
Single leg squat (See Figure 17-2)	Gluteal, hip rotator, and quad strength
Lateral foot walk	Inability to walk on outside of foot = ankle instability or subtalar motion restriction

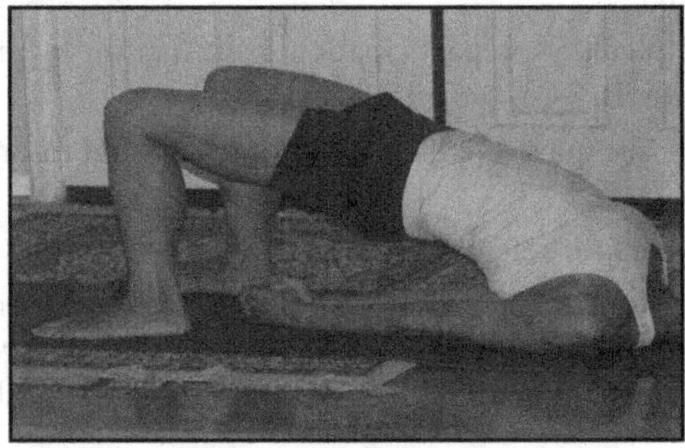

Figure 22-1. Bridge position.

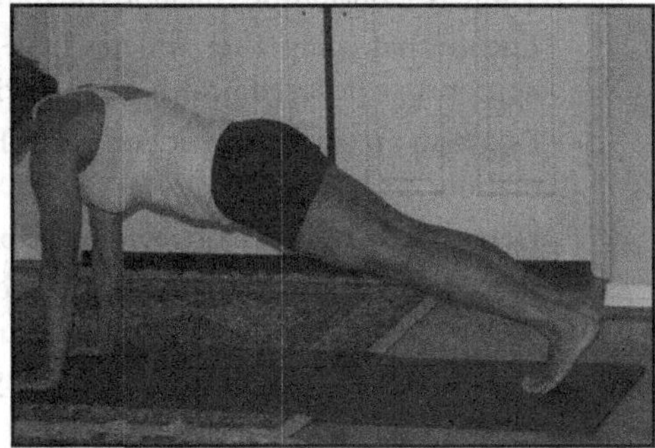

Figure 22-2. Plank position.

  - Is the patient holding one arm against his or her body?
- Gait.
  - Ask the patient to demonstrate normal walking.
  - If able, as the patient to walk on his or her toes and heels.
  - Please refer to Table 22-4 and Figures 22-1 and 22-2 for Special Tests of Central Strength and Stability.
- Running and sport-specific activities.
- If possible, have the athlete demonstrate unique movements or techniques.
  - Running in a figure of 8 pattern can assess joint stability.
  - Throwing or hitting an overhead ball or object.

23 Sideline Management Pearls

Tracy L. Zaslow, MD, FAAP, CAQSM

1. What Are the Responsibilities of a Physician on the Sidelines of a Sporting Event?

The sideline physician is responsible for optimizing medical care for all injured or ill athletes. Ideally, the sideline physician would coordinate a comprehensive medical plan to address pregame, game-day, and postgame evaluation of athletes.

- Pregame responsibilities include the following:
  - Ensure that competing athletes have completed a preparticipation examination by an appropriate licensed health care provider (MD/DO).
  - Establish an emergency action plan (EAP); see questions 11 and 12 for additional information.
  - Determine a network of health care providers for referral, as needed.
  - Prepare a sideline "medical bag." Coordinate with the on-site staff (eg, athletic trainer, athletic director) to avoid redundancy; athletic trainers and/or facilities often are equipped with automated emergency defibrillators (AEDs), spine boards, face mask remover tools, ice, and plastic bags.
- Game-day responsibilities—Help the athletes stay safe!
  - Determine the final clearance status of injured or ill athletes on game day, prior to the start of the competition.
  - Survey the playing field/court for any dangerous conditions.
  - Keep close observation from a location with an unobstructed view of the playing area; the physician does not leave the field during play.
  - If there is an emergency in the stands or an athlete needs to be transported to the hospital, consider stopping the game until the team physician returns to the sidelines.
  - Introductions of the medical team to game officials and coaches (visiting/home) prior to the game start and coordination of care with the opposing team's medical staff are important.
  - Assess and manage game-day injuries and medical problems.
  - Determine if athletes who are injured or ill during a game are cleared for same-day return to play (RTP).
  - Issue follow-up care, instructions, and anticipatory guidance for athletes who require further treatment after the competition.
  - Notify the appropriate parties about an athlete's injury or illness.

Koutures C, Wong V.
Pediatric Sports Medicine: Essentials for Office Evaluation (pp 148-155)

- Postgame responsibilities include the following:
  - Check in with both teams concerning any postgame issues.
  - If an athlete was evaluated on the field and anticipatory guidance or follow-up is recommended, this information must be communicated to the appropriate personnel (athletic trainer, coach, and/or legal guardian).

2. Are Sideline Physicians at a Sporting Event Protected From Liability by the Good Samaritan Law?

- Unfortunately, there is no absolute answer to this question.
- Every state has a "Good Samaritan" law that is designed to protect individuals from civil liability for acting negligently while providing voluntary care.[1]
- The intent of the Good Samaritan law is to encourage the provision of medical care to those in need by persons who come upon a victim by chance, thus limiting legal liability to those who provide emergency care.
- States vary on how the Good Samaritan law is applied: (1) to categories of people protected by the statute and (2) to the circumstances in which the statute is applied.
- The categories of people protected may include all personnel delivering any type of emergency care, or they may be much more restrictive, excluding physicians and sometimes even athletic trainers.
- Circumstances in which care provided is protected under Good Samaritan laws may not extend to prescheduled event coverage, even if that scheduling is done at the last minute. Additionally, Good Samaritan laws often do not apply where "volunteers" are compensated for services in some way; "compensation" may include team gear, free admission to the game, gifts, food, or intangible benefits, such as practice promotion.
- It is very important to understand that there is no national Good Samaritan law that applies to health care providers covering athletic events. Prior to covering an event as a sideline physician, check with your malpractice carrier to make sure it includes sideline coverage. The Good Samaritan laws often will not protect physicians in this setting.[2]
- While doctors should familiarize themselves with their own state laws, there are a few general rules:
  - Is the case an emergency?
  - Does the incident take place outside of the traditional health care setting?
  - Is there any previous patient-physician relationship? (This includes caring for any patients on either team in the past.)
  - Is there compensation involved?

If the answer is "yes" to the first two questions and "no" to the last two, then physicians in most states should feel fairly comfortable that the Good Samaritan laws apply.[3] If the answer is "no" to either of the first two questions and "yes" to either of the second two, then further investigation into additional malpractice coverage is recommended.

3. What "Formal Arrangements" Should Be Made Before Becoming a Sideline Physician?

- "Formal" arrangements can range from the acceptance of the sideline responsibilities via a quick e-mail or phone call to an elaborate written contract. This wide range depends on the type of event, the experience of the physician, and the level of pregame planning required by the sideline physician (eg, as medical director of a marathon, the sideline physician must coordinate all medical staff and supplies versus a physician covering a single tennis tournament or high school football game).

- It is important to consider malpractice/Good Samaritan coverage in advance to avoid any surprises. The details that may be included are time/date/length/type of event requiring coverage, physician responsibilities, malpractice/Good Samaritan coverage, and support staff that is available.

4. Should the Sideline Physician Have the Final Say in Return-to-Play Decisions and Disposition of an Injured or Ill Athlete?

Absolutely! To prevent any confusion during an athletic event, the sideline physician should discuss these issues in advance with the athletic director, athletic trainer, and coaches. As a sideline physician, you are responsible for all medical issues (injury or illness) that occur during an athletic event and thus must have the "final say" without argument regarding the RTP and disposition of an athlete.

5. What Injury Scenarios Should Be Routinely Practiced by the On-Field First Responders?

Catastrophic injuries are uncommon in sports, but adequate preparation is the secret to successful, well-coordinated emergency care. The emergency response team must be ready for the worst-case scenario, and the best way to be ready is to practice multiple scenarios to clarify roles, establish protocols, and familiarize the team with the equipment/resources available. Important scenarios to practice include head/neck injury and sudden collapse.

Head/Neck Injury

- Consideration of care for both the conscious and unconscious athlete should be practiced with attention to cervical spine immobilization.
- Review the basics: airway, breathing, and circulation.
- Discuss the importance of not removing the helmet from players who wear helmets and pads.
- Practice the focused neurologic examination.
- Plan protocols for transporting athletes and/or performing cardiopulmonary resuscitation (CPR) to emphasize that these are the only two indications to move the athlete.
- Review the log roll protocol for placing an athlete on a long spine board.
  - Requires four or more qualified responders each with a specific role.
    - One person maintains manual control of the cervical spine.
    - Two people are positioned on the same side of the torso to turn the patient toward them while preventing any segment from rotation, flexion, extension, or lateral bending.
    - The fourth person is responsible for sliding the long spine board behind the athlete.
  - Neutral anatomic alignment of the entire vertebral column must be maintained during any turning or other movement of the athlete.
- Review the availability of all equipment that may be needed for the transportation of the unconscious athlete, such as a spine board, facemask removal tools (bolt cutters/screw driver/Trainer's Angel), rigid cervical collar, and telephone to activate the emergency response team.
- Consider additional clinical questions during scenarios regard management with observation versus further work-up and potential for RTP.

Sudden Collapse

- Educate all first responders on how to palpate a pulse; confirming pulselessness can be difficult for inexperienced rescuers.
- Practice performing CPR and using the AED.
- Review where the AED is stored and how it will be accessed in an emergency.

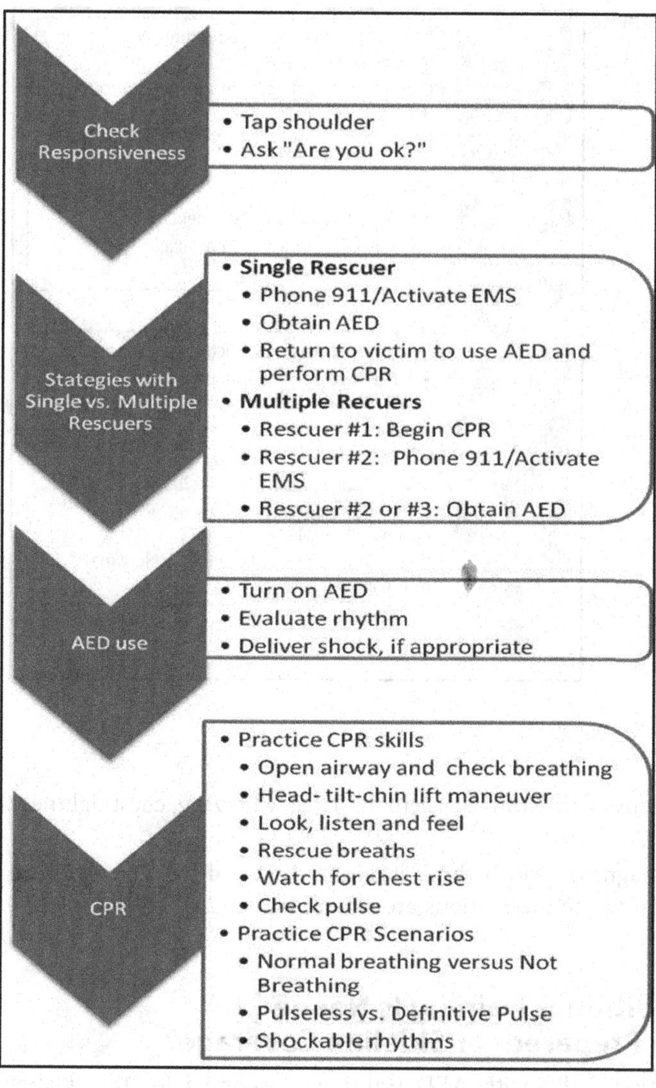

Figure 23-1. Practice strategies for an athlete with witnessed collapse.

- Discuss the activation of the Emergency Medical System. Figure 23-1,[4,5] which demonstrates an algorithm that can be used when an athlete suddenly collapses.

Heat Stroke

- Review the signs and symptoms of heat stroke (eg, elevated body temperature [> 104°F], nausea, vomiting, tachypnea, headache, muscle cramps/weakness, confusion, loss of consciousness).
- Understand how to measure rectal temperature.
- Review the concepts of rapid cooling: immersion in cold/ice water immediately; otherwise, water, fans, shade, wet towels, and ice bags may be used to lower core temperature. Additionally, it is important to review temperature-monitoring protocols to avoid excessive cooling.
- Rehearse the actual placement of an athlete in an immersion bath, being sure to monitor the person during cooling and the removal from the bath; due to the large size of some of the affected athletes, this can be significantly challenging in an emergency situation.
- Discuss the protocol for transport, with the understanding that cooling must occur first, and then transport.

Figure 23-2. Practice strategies for an athlete with asthma exacerbation.

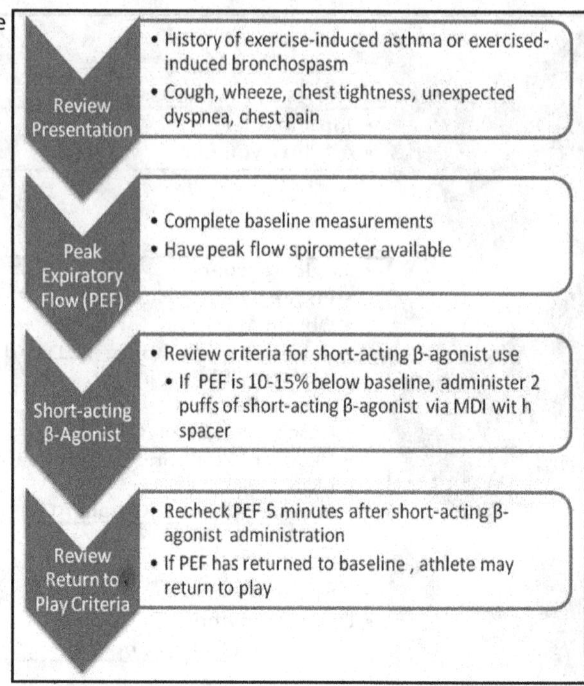

Asthma Exacerbation

- Review the signs and symptoms of an asthma exacerbation. (eg, wheezing, chest tightness, cough, shortness of breath).
- For athletes who have been diagnosed with asthma, it is important to discuss their history, medications, and the location where medications are stored. Figure 23-2 shows an algorithm to use as a review guide.[6]

6. What Additional Training Is Needed to Be Adequately Prepared for Sideline Coverage?

- Cardiopulmonary resuscitation—CPR with AED training is essential for the sideline physician and the entire team of first responders. Because most sideline physicians spend the majority of their time in outpatient clinic settings, CPR and emergency response are not part of the daily routine, and therefore updating certification every 2 years is recommended. Lastly, CPR/AED training reviews the different techniques that are appropriate for each age group; emergency treatment of the child is different than that for an adult.
- Additional advanced life support—Physicians may also consider Pediatric Advanced Life Support and Adult Cardiac Life Support. Topics included in the training are the ability to manage the patient's airway, initiate intravenous access, read and interpret electrocardiograms, and use emergency pharmacologic treatments. This further training can only help to hone these emergency response skills and confidence in an emergency situation. If there is an advanced Emergency Medical Technician (EMT) team (see question 11) onsite for the sporting event, they can provide expertise as well.
- "Team Physician Courses"—These are excellent ways to acquire further expertise in sideline coverage. Courses will often review the care of the "downed" athlete, cervical spine stabilization, immediate fracture care, and the approach to sudden collapse, in addition to providing tools on how to coordinate and prepare an emergency response team. Courses are offered through the American Medical Society for Sports Medicine and the American College of Sports Medicine.

- Other sources of sideline physician education—These other sources are sport specific (eg, National Football League Team Physician's Society) and level specific (eg, United States Olympic Committee), and include local medical society meetings (eg, chapter meetings of the American Academy of Pediatrics) and professional journals and other electronic media sources.

7. Should an Unconscious Football Player's Helmet Be Removed on the Field so a Better Physical Evaluation Can Be Performed?

- No! The removal of the football player's helmet will allow the cervical spine to hyperextend due to the pads worn by the player.
- If there is any potential cervical-spine injury, all efforts must be focused on maintaining stabilization of the cervical spine to prevent potential complication. The patient should be positioned supine in neutral alignment with no rotation or bending of the spinal column by manual control of the cervical spine. One person should be assigned full responsibility of maintaining neutral alignment until the athlete is secured to a long spine board with a helmet and pads in place. When the patient must be moved, a coordinated log roll must be performed (see question 5 head/neck injury, log rolling protocol). Neurologic function must be assessed before and after any position change.
- Until radiographs/computed tomography scans are completed to clear the cervical spine, the helmet and pads must remain in place.

8. What Is Commotio Cordis, and What Is the Management of This Condition?

- Commotio cordis is defined as a blunt, nonpenetrating trauma to the chest that results in an irregular heart rhythm (usually ventricular fibrillation) and often leads to sudden death. The term is derived from Latin, meaning "agitation of the heart." It is most common in children younger than 15 years of age.[7]
- Commotio cordis results from blows to the chest by projectiles (eg, baseballs, softballs, lacrosse balls, hockey pucks) or blunt body trauma with other athletes. The impact must occur directly over the heart (at or near the center of the cardiac silhouette) within a 10- to 20-msec window during the upstroke of the T wave. This window is an electrically vulnerable period when inhomogeneous dispersion of repolarization is the greatest, creating a susceptible myocardial substrate for provoked ventricular fibrillation.
- Other factors that increase risk of commotio cordis include the hardness, size, and shape of the object causing the blow; hard, small, sphere-shaped objects are the most dangerous. Additionally, the thin compliant chest wall of a young athlete is less capable of blunting the arrhythmogenic consequences of precordial blows.[8,9]
- Commotio cordis presents clinically as instantaneous cardiovascular collapse, but 20% of victims do remain physically active for a few seconds after the blow. Survival rates are rising and have increased to 35%, whereas for the preceding 10 years survival rates hovered around 15%.[7] These improvements in survival rates are related to increased public awareness, increased availability of AEDs, and earlier activation of emergency care. Prompt defibrillation is the key to survival! Knowing the exact location of the AED and how to operate it are essential to providing the optimal care for commotio cordis.
- Since survival rates are so low, can commotio cordis be prevented? Yes, just avoid precordial blows. While theoretically a great idea, eliminating all precordial blows is an unrealistic goal. To minimize the risk, coaching techniques should be improved to encourage safety. For example, teaching batters how to turn away from errant pitches or coaching hockey/lacrosse players to avoid using their chest to block a ball/puck. Also, equipment designed for safety should be used (eg, safety baseball that is engineered completely from rubber without the hard core of standard baseballs).

- Equipment such as chest protectors/vests have not been shown to be effective against commotio cordis, but they do reduce the risk of blunt bodily injury.[8-11] A well-organized EAP with accessible AEDs is the best way to maximize survival.

9. What Is the Physician's Role Compared With the Certified Athletic Trainer or Other First Responders, Such as Emergency Medical Services?

- The certified athletic trainer (ATC) and other first responders are respected members of the medical team.
- The physician has the final word when it comes to medical management and RTP decisions.
- Before the game begins, the medical team should establish the accepted approach to athlete care.
- If there is an injury on the field, the ATC will be the first to evaluate the player while the physician observes from the sidelines. If there is any concern, the trainer will flag the physician to come onto the field for an assessment. Other medical teams prefer to have the whole team respond as one.
- It is important to discuss everyone's roles prior to the start of the game to prevent any confusion or delay in care when a medical emergency arises.

10. What Are the Different Levels of Emergency Medical Technicians/Ambulances That Are Available?

- A basic ambulance service is staffed with entry-level emergency responders who are trained to do noninvasive care.[12]
- Intermediate levels of EMT training can perform more invasive procedures such as intravenous therapy and cardiac monitoring. This level of care is likely adequate for most injured/ill athletes.[12]
- The most advanced level of emergency care is provided by paramedics. Paramedics are trained to perform high-level medical procedures, including fluid resuscitation, pharmaceutical administration, obtaining intravenous access, cardiac monitoring (continuous and 12-lead), neurologic stabilization, and monitoring and other advanced procedures.[12]

11. Why Is an Emergency Action Plan Important? Who Is Responsible for Making an Emergency Action Plan? What Items Should Be Included?

- The purpose of an EAP is to provide instructions to members of the sports medicine team in the event of a medical emergency regarding student athletes. An emergency is defined as a sudden life-threatening injury or illness that requires immediate medical attention. An EAP helps to ensure that expedient action will be taken in the case of emergency to provide the best possible treatment.
- Ideally, a land line is the preferred method for activating Emergency Medical Services (EMS), as cell phones often contact Highway Patrol in the area code of the cell phone and not necessarily in the area code of the incident.
- The sports medicine team, which includes the physician, athletic director, athletic trainer, and coaches, all must understand the EAP, but usually the physician is the one who develops the EAP in collaboration with the team. Items to address include who will provide the care, emergency equipment availability and its specific location, activation of EMS, directions to the emergency site, list of emergency contacts, and step-by-step instructions for emergency care.

- Nonmedical personnel can be utilized to ensure that gates are opened and can help direct EMS to the appropriate site of the incident.
- Determining a protocol regarding first responders is essential. Acute care in an emergency should be directed by the most qualified individual on the scene; those with lesser credentials are to yield leadership to those with the higher level of training, but they should be ready to take direction to provide care as needed.
- Ideally, the emergency equipment includes an anaphylaxis kit/Epi-pen, long spine board, medication kit (including advanced medications and oxygen), splints, and an AED. This equipment must be available in known and accessible locations. With an EAP, the goal is to prevent access problems, such as having the AED locked in a cabinet to which no emergency responders have the key.
- All items/equipment used during the EAP should be stored in an area that is easy to access and the whole EAP team should be informed of the location.
- The certified athletic trainer usually possesses the main equipment of the EAP and the doctor maintains the medical bag item. The physician and certified athletic trainer should communicate in advance to ensure all items are provided and determine who will be responsible for each item.

12. Does an Emergency Action Plan Include a Plan for a Spectator Who Has a Medical Issue? Who Is Responsible for Caring for a Spectator With a Medical Problem?

- EAPs may or may not include spectators who have medical issues during sporting events. Because of this variability, it is essential that this issue is discussed prior to the event. If the sideline physician is responsible for spectator medical emergencies, all involved parties should consider stopping the game if the physician must leave the sideline to address an emergency. If the sideline physician is not responsible, then other personnel must be assigned to cover any spectator emergencies; usually an EMT team is assigned to this responsibility.

References

1. Velasquez ex rel Velasquez v Jimenez, 798 A2d 51, 57 (NJ 2002). In: Quandt EF, Mitten MJ, Black JS. *Legal Liability in Covering Athletic Events*. Sports Health. 2009;1(1):84-90
2. Quandt EF, Mitten MJ, Black JS. Legal liability in covering athletic events. *Sports Health*. 2009;1(1):84-90.
3. Albert T. Good Samaritan law shields California doctor from liability. American Medical News Web site. www.ama-assn.org/amednews/2005/03/14/prca0314.htm. Published March 14, 2005. Accessed February 9, 2012.
4. Harmon KG, Drezner JA. Update of sideline and event preparation for management of sudden cardiac arrest in athletes. *Curr Sports Med Rep*. 2007;6:170-176.
5. Roberts, Mustafa M, Penrod M, Bills DN. Event and sideline management of sudden cardiac death. *Curr Sports Med Rep*. 2002;1:141-148.
6. Allen TW. Sideline management of asthma. Current Sports Medicine Reports. 2005;4:301-304.
7. Maron BJ, Estes NA. Commotio cordis. *N Engl J Med*. 2010;362;10:917-927.
8. Maron BJ, Poliac L, Kaplan JA, Mueller FO. Blunt impact to the chest leading to sudden death from cardiac arrest during sports activities. *N Eng J Med*. 1995;333:337-342.
9. Maron BJ, Gohmna TE, Kyle SB, Estes NAM III, Link MS. Clinical profile and spectrum of commotio cordis. *JAMA*. 2002;287:1142-1146.
10. Maron BJ, Doerer JJ, Haas TS, Estes NAM III, Hodges JS, Link MS. Commotio cordis and the epidemiology of sudden death in competitive lacrosse. *Pediatrics*. 2009;124:966-971.
11. Doerer JJ, Haas TS, Estes NAM III, Link MS, Maron BJ. Evaluation of chest barriers for protection against sudden death due to commotio cordis. *Am J Cardiol*. 2007;99:857-859.
12. The National Highway Traffic Safety Administration. National EMS Scope of Practice Model. National Registry of Emergency Medical Technicians Web site. www.nremt.org/nremt/downloads/Scope%20of%20Practice.pdf. Published February 2007. Accessed February 14, 2012.

24

General Response to the Acute Injury

Anthony Saglimbeni, MD and Neesheet Parikh, DO

1. What Are the Components of the PRICE Mnemonic for the Initial Management of an Acute Musculoskeletal Injury?

- P-Protection—Helps to prevent further injury and increases comfort, and can include crutches, braces, splints, and/or slings.
- R-Rest—Varies from partial to absolute rest, depending on the injury type and severity. Rest also benefits by not increasing the injury.
- I-Ice—Helps to decrease pain and inflammation. Use ice for a maximum of 20 minutes, every hour after initial injury; do not place ice directly on the skin.
- C-Compression—Gentle, consistent pressure helps to reduce inflammation.
- E-Elevation—Elevate the affected area at or above the level of the heart to increase venous return and thereby decrease swelling.

2. What Situations Might Respond Best to the Use of Ice or Cold, and Which Would Respond Best to the Use of Heat?

Ice is typically used to decrease pain and inflammation by reducing tissue swelling, metabolic needs of injured tissue, and firing of pain receptors. Ice is best used after an acute injury and after an activity is completed. Using ice prior to activity may decrease flexibility as well as function.

Heat is used to maximize tissue healing by assisting with the removal of oxidants and other harmful injury byproducts as well as increasing the delivery of nutrients and oxygen to injured areas through increased blood flow. Table 24-1 provides information on when to use ice and when to use heat.

3. What Are the Pros and Cons of Using Nonsteroidal Anti-Inflammatory Drugs and Acetaminophen in Managing an Acute Injury?

Acetaminophen

- Pros
  - Pain relief
  - No adverse effect on kidney
  - No gastrointestinal bleed risk

Koutures C, Wong V.
Pediatric Sports Medicine: Essentials for Office Evaluation (pp 156-160)

Table 24-1. When to Use Ice Versus Heat	
ICE	*HEAT*
• Joint pain • Joint sprain • Fractures • Tendon rupture • Muscle strains (acute)	• Muscle strains (subacute or chronic) • Chronic joint pain • Muscle spasm • Joint stiffness

- Cons
  - Liver toxicity at high doses
  - No anti-inflammatory effect
  - Found in other pain relievers, which can cause overdose

NSAIDs

- Pros
  - Anti-inflammatory
  - Pain relief
  - Reduces swelling
- Cons
  - May decrease fracture healing
  - Can affect kidney function
  - Gastrointestinal bleed potential

4. Are There Any Situations Where a Steroid Injection May Be Considered in the School-Aged Athlete?

It is very unlikely that a school-aged athlete may need an anti-inflammatory steroid injection, but there may be special circumstances that may warrant consideration of this treatment, such as a high level of competition (eg, elite championship game, Olympics, world championships).

In cases where steroid injection is considered in the school-aged athlete, the usual adult risk factors of recurrent and prolonged use are more critical due to the younger age of the child and more potential opportunity for future need of steroid injection. Furthermore, as with adults, the steroid injection is usually just a temporizing measure to eliminate or reduce inflammation, and may not be curative. This should be emphasized to the legal guardian when using a steroid injection in school-aged athletes.

5. While Performing the Phone Triage of an Acute Injury, Which Descriptions Require Emergent or Urgent Care Evaluations Versus Next-Day Office Evaluations?

While questioning the athlete or parent, keep in mind the mechanism of injury, location and severity of the injury, comfort of the athlete and family members, and the physician's comfort in relation to the patient.

When in doubt, send the patient to the emergency department or urgent care facility.

- Questions should lead to screening for fractures, dislocations, sprains, nerve injury, vascular injury, head injury, and neck injury.
- For orthopedic injuries, obvious deformity, significant discoloration, and extreme pain or swelling are indications to seek early assessment.

Table 24-2. Buzzwords to Send the Patient to Emergency or Urgent Care	
• Loss of consciousness	• Visual disturbance
• Bilateral numbness or tingling after trauma or fall	• Small projectile to eye
• Worsening headache after head injury	• Dislocation
• Unable to bear weight on injured extremity	• Significant caller concern
• Open wound	• Midline neck pain

Some red flags that should alert the health care provider that the patient should be sent for emergency or urgent care include loss of consciousness, visual disturbance, and an open wound (Table 24-2).

6. What Are Some Simple Office-Based Criteria That Can Be Used to Determine if an Athlete Can Return to Play Immediately or Soon After an Acute Injury?

This is often one of the most difficult decisions a sports medicine physician has to make. There should be a multifactorial approach to deciding whether an athlete can return to play (RTP) or should sit out, which may include the following factors:

- Type of injury
- Level of competition
- Future goals of the athlete

In general, an athlete may RTP when he or she is able to progress to the functional requirements of the sport without any evidence of pain or instability and the risk of further injury is minimal.

Functional testing should be completed prior to RTP. This may be done on the sideline, in the training room, or in the office. Things to look for include the following:

- Swelling
- Limping
- Guarding
- Tenderness to palpation
- Abnormal function of the affected area
    - Cannot jump, reduced handgrip, visible change in throwing mechanics

7. Does Every Sports-Related Injury Require X-rays? If Not, What Are Some Good Criteria to Guide the Physician When Deciding Who Should Get X-rays?

Not every sports-related injury requires x-rays. Criteria such as the Ottawa ankle rules (see Chapter 40, question 4) are a good guide in deciding who needs ankle x-rays. Another helpful tool may be the finding of focal pain (finger tip) with palpation or when vibrating bone prominences with a tuning fork. When deciding if an athlete can go back to play quickly after an injury, immediate x-rays may be helpful.

8. What Situations Require Immobilization or Crutches, and for How Long?

In general, crutches should be used if weight bearing causes significant pain, abnormal gait, a sense of instability, or if there is a risk of further injury. Immobilization, splinting, or casting should be considered if a fracture is suspected or if there is significant pain, especially while

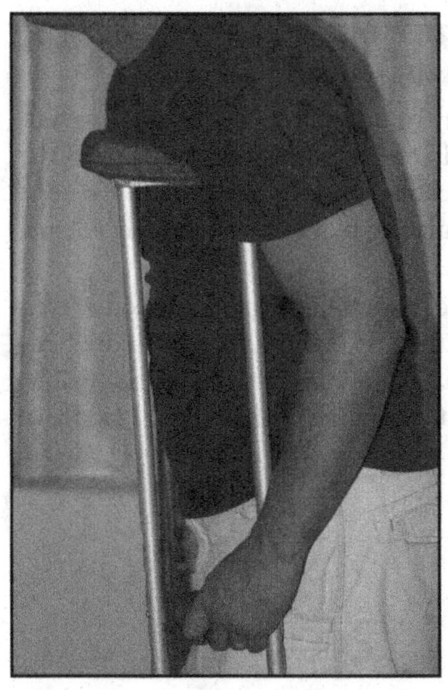

Figure 24-1. Crutch fit with 30 degrees of elbow flexion.

awaiting specialty consultation. Children often need to be placed on crutches or have injuries immobilized to slow them down and reduce the temptation to use the injured area. Thankfully, children handle immobilization better than adults, with less risk for joint stiffness and muscle atrophy, so never hesitate to protect a child from himself or herself or from peer pressures. The length of immobilization is dependent on the type of injury and whether or not surgery is required. Typically, a fracture should be immobilized for 4 to 6 weeks.

9. What Are Some Basic Tips for Proper Fit and Safe Use of Crutches?

- Appropriate crutch height should be assessed by placing the tip of the crutch about 6 inches from the outer margin of the foot and 2 inches in front of the foot.
- The top of the crutch should then be approximately 1 to 2 inches below the anterior fold of the axilla to prevent injury of the brachial plexus.
- The hand support should be placed where the hand would naturally fall when the elbow is at 30 degrees of flexion (Figure 24-1).

10. What Are Some Basic Materials and Methods to Immobilize an Acute Injury?

- Spine board
- Soft or hard cervical spine immobilizer
- Cardboard splints and tape/wrap
- Ready-made plaster or fiberglass
- Portable malleable aluminum padded large splints to immobilize extremities
- Compression elastic bandages and fasteners
- Shoulder sling
- Figure 8 brace
- Malleable aluminum padded small splints to immobilize digits

11. Can Stretching or Massage Help an Athlete Return Quicker From an Injury?

Yes, stretching or massage can help athletes return quicker from injury by helping relieve tension, desensitizing trigger points, and reducing swelling and soreness. Massage can lead to the vasodilatation of extremities, reduce or treat muscle spasms, reduce swelling, and reduce soreness. It can be especially useful after sprains or contusions by stimulating blood flow, reducing edema, breaking apart undesired fibrosis, and relaxing muscle spasm.

Although evidence that stretching prevents injury is limited, stretching is generally considered to enhance flexibility and therefore improve performance. Current thought suggests more benefit to stretching after rather than before activity as warm muscles are likely to be more flexible. There is also speculation that injury prevention is a benefit of stretching, although real evidence is lacking.

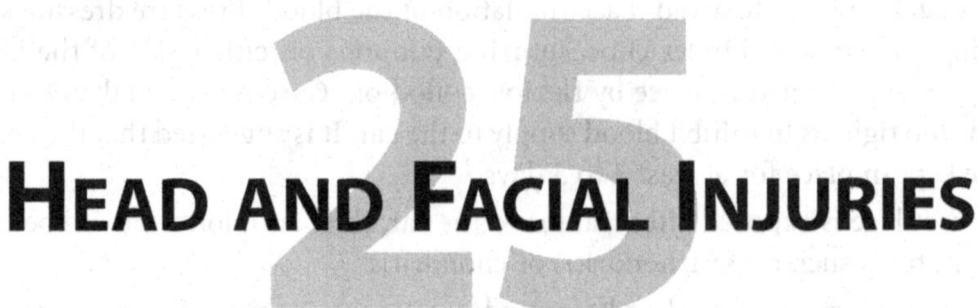

25 Head and Facial Injuries

Mary M. Hung, DO, MS and Valarie Wong, MD, FAAP

1. When Should a Clinician Worry About an Intracranial Bleed in an Athlete?

- The sports with the highest incidences of intracranial bleeds are football, boxing, ice hockey, rugby, lacrosse, martial arts, gymnastics, skiing, soccer, and pole vaulting (track).
- Signs and symptoms that may indicate the presence of an intracranial bleed include the following: decreasing level of consciousness, seizure activity, progressively worsening headache, multiple episodes of emesis, dizziness/ataxia, significant deviation from baseline activity, focal neurologic deficits, and altered mental status.
- Concerning signs on physical examination that may indicate an intracranial bleed are the following: hemotympanum, clear rhinorrhea or otorrhea that is suggestive of cerebrospinal fluid (CSF), raccoon eyes, Battle's sign, and palpable skull fracture. When any of these symptoms are present, the athlete must be sent to the emergency department for a head computed tomography (CT) scan without contrast.[1]
- Some of these signs and symptoms may also be present when an athlete has a concussion. Please refer to Chapter 26, which discusses concussions, for more detailed information.

2. What Is a Cauliflower Ear, and How Should It Be Managed?

- Cauliflower ear is a complication of an auricular hematoma that occurs if it is left untreated. When the ear experiences blunt trauma, there is a disruption of the perichondrium, shearing the blood vessels in the area and causing the accumulation of blood in the subperichondrial space of the pinna. If the resultant hematoma is not evacuated in a timely manner, then neocartilage and fibrous tissue start forming where the hematoma has accumulated, resulting in a permanent deformity of the pinna.[2]
- The sports that have a high incidence of trauma to the ears are wrestling, rugby, water polo, mixed martial arts, and boxing.
- When trauma to the pinna occurs, immediately apply direct pressure to the area. The direct pressure will help to minimize the bleeding into the subperichondrial space of the pinna. Next, the application of an ice pack will help to reduce any swelling that may occur.
- The hematoma does not occur immediately after trauma. It takes some time for the hematoma to form. A hematoma may form anywhere from 24 to 48 hours so it may be evacuated anytime during this time frame. A large bore needle or an incision can be made into the subperichondrial space of the pinna to evacuate the hematoma. Pressure must be

Koutures C, Wong V.
Pediatric Sports Medicine: Essentials for Office Evaluation (pp 161-167)

immediately applied to avoid reaccumulation of the blood. Pressure dressings can include clipping the ear with binder clips, suturing tampons on either side of the hematoma, or using gauze pads held in place by flexible collodion. Care must be taken to not compress the ear too tight as to inhibit blood supply to the ear. It is suggested that the pressure dressing be kept in place for at least 3 to 5 days.[2]

- If the cartilage is exposed after trauma to the ear, then antibiotics should be used to avoid complications such as perichondritis or chondritis.
- If the cauliflower ear has already formed, treatment consists of surgical resection of the fibrous tissue and neocartilage, and subsequent recontouring of the ear.
- If the accumulation of blood reaches the inner ear canal, then hearing may be impaired. Therefore, in this case, urgent evacuation is necessary.
- To prevent cauliflower ear, an athlete may wear protective head gear that covers the ears or custom ear molds. It is important that the protective gear fits properly because the equipment can cause hematomas if it is not fitted appropriately.

3. Which Sports Carry a Risk of Blunt Orbital Trauma? How Can Orbital Trauma Be Recognized on the Sidelines?

- Any sport that involves small, high-velocity objects (eg, baseballs, racquet balls), any contact sport such as football, any sport that uses equipment such as sticks or bats, or any sport that involves the intentional injury to the head such as boxing or full-contact martial arts carries a risk of blunt orbital trauma.
- The signs and symptoms of orbital trauma that may be seen on the sidelines are visual changes such as diplopia or visual loss, pain or paresthesia, proptosis of the eye, rupture of the globe, or unequal pupils. Table 25-1 discusses other signs of orbital trauma and their recommended management plan.[3]

4. What Are the Symptoms of and Management Options for Retinal Detachments?

- **This is a medical emergency!** Athletes with retinal detachments complain of seeing floaters, flashing lights, blurry vision, or dark shadows in the corner of their vision (dark curtain coming over the eye). **Retinal detachments are painless.** If a patient has visual loss or a decrease in monocular vision, urgent referral to an ophthalmologist is necessary.
- Treatment/management—The athlete must be examined within 24 hours by an ophthalmologist. The examination usually will also include an evaluation of visual acuity and any visual field deficits. A dilated retinal examination is recommended. Athletes should not return to play for at least 1 month after experiencing a retinal detachment. The actual time away from sports will depend on the extent of the detachment. The treatment is surgical repair of the detached retina by a retinal specialist.[4]

5. What Type of Equipment Is Recommended to Protect the Eye During Sports?

- See Chapter 4, question 11, for information on eye protection.

6. What Are Some Issues That May Be Associated With Nasal Bridge Fractures?

- Complications associated with nasal bridge fractures are a septal hematoma and nasal airway obstruction. It is essential to examine the athlete's nose with an otoscope to see if there is a hematoma. **A septal hematoma needs emergent surgical drainage, packing,**

Table 25-1. Types of Orbital Injuries and Their Management	
TYPE OF INJURY	*SYMPTOMS/MANAGEMENT*
Eyelid edema and ecchymosis	• Self-limiting • Treatment includes ice and analgesics • Symptoms: swelling and bruising of the eyelid
Periorbital ecchymosis	• Prompt eye examination for possible fractures, intraocular hemorrhage, or globe rupture • If any of the above are present, referral to an ophthalmologist is necessary • Symptoms: bruising around the eye
Eyelid lacerations	• Primary care physician can close simple lacerations • If lid margin or canaliculus is involved, referral to an ophthalmologist is recommended • If the canaliculus is involved, intubation of the nasolacrimal duct is required in addition to the laceration repair • Involvement of the eyelid margin requires careful repair to prevent notching and lid misalignment • If fat is visualized in the laceration, most likely there is damage to the orbicularis oculi, levator muscle (elevates the eyelid), or the orbital septum; referral to an ophthalmologist is a must for repair to prevent ptosis
Corneal abrasions	• Symptoms include photophobia, tearing, blurry vision, pain, and a gritty feeling when the eyelid closes • To diagnose, instill fluorescein dye in the affected eye and use a Wood's lamp or a cobalt-blue filtered light; the abrasion should light up or glow • Apply topical antibiotic ointment • Re-evaluate in 24 hours
Foreign body	• Symptoms include inflammation, discomfort, and increased tearing • Detected with good lighting and a magnifying glass or an ophthalmoscope • If the object is deep and metallic, a slit lamp eye examination is sometimes necessary • If the object is not found and there is high suspicion for a foreign body, radiographic imaging may be needed for possible intraorbital foreign body • Removal of the foreign object can be as easy as irrigating the eye or by using a moistened end of a cotton swab • If it is embedded in the eye or in the cornea, an ophthalmologist should remove it • If the object is metallic, prompt removal is necessary to prevent rust formation in the cornea; this requires an ophthalmologist follow-up in 1 to 2 days of removal for further treatment, if warranted

(continued)

Table 25-1 (continued). Types of Orbital Injuries and Their Management	
TYPE OF INJURY	*SYMPTOMS/MANAGEMENT*
Hyphema	• Definition: blood in the anterior chamber of the eye secondary to a blunt or perforating trauma • Symptoms include acute loss of vision and pain, which can cause permanent loss of vision • Management involves shielding the eye, bed rest, elevating the head >30 degrees, applying a cycloplegic agent, and the use of steroids (topical or oral) • Avoid using nonsteroidal anti-inflammatory drugs and aspirin • If there is evidence of increased intraocular pressure that is not controlled with medications, then the clot must be removed to prevent vision loss • These patients need to be followed up on a regular basis due to the high risk of developing glaucoma in the future
Adapted from Rodriguez JO, Lavina AM, Agarwal A. Prevention and treatment of common eye injuries in sports. *Am Fam Physician.* 2003;67(7):1481-1488.	

and antibiotic coverage from an otolaryngologist. The presence of a septal hematoma may increase the risk of developing a brain abscess, a subarachnoid empyema, subsequent meningitis, a cavernous sinus thrombosis, a lateral sinus thrombosis, or a naso-oral fistula. A septal hematoma that is not diagnosed can cause septal cartilage necrosis and possible midface growth retardation.

- A CT scan of the maxillofacial region may be more helpful in terms of diagnosing a nasal bridge fracture. This study can be quite useful if associated facial fractures are suspected.
- An athlete who has some compromise to his or her nasal airway can be managed in the emergency department. If there are associated complications such as nasal deformities or nasal septum deviation, this can also be referred nonemergently to an otolaryngologist or a plastic surgeon.[5]

7. What Type of Imaging Is Best for Identifying Facial Fractures?

- CT with three-dimensional reconstruction imaging is diagnostic and most accurate in detailing and localizing facial fractures.

8. What Are Some Tips for Assessing Head and Facial Injuries?

- The first priority when a head or facial injury is suspected is to assess the athlete's airway, breathing, and circulation (ABC). If his or her ABC's are stable, then look for signs and symptoms of fractures as described in question 6 and in Table 25-2.[6]

9. What Is a "Blow-Out Fracture," and What Clinical Findings Would Suggest It?

- A blow-out fracture is the result of blunt trauma to the orbit, causing compression of the globe and increased intraorbital pressure, which results in buckling inferiorly of the infraorbital floor. As a result, there is entrapment of muscle, nerves, and tissues. When

TABLE 25-2. HELPFUL QUESTIONS FOR DIAGNOSING SUSPECTED FRACTURES		
QUESTION	*ANSWER*	*SUSPECTED DIAGNOSIS*
Do you have vision changes?	Yes, binocular diplopia	Periorbital or internal fractures Nonspecific finding
	Yes, monocular diplopia	Globe injury
Do you feel numbness anywhere on your face?	Yes	Bony foramina fractures that contain branches of the trigeminal nerve
Does your bite feel different?	Yes, may feel misaligned or have premature contact with their teeth	Mandibular or maxillary fractures
Do you feel pain in a certain part of your face? (There may be areas that are not visually obvious but yet still painful, giving rise to better localization)	Yes, tenderness preauricularally upon moving the mandible	Condylar process fracture
	Yes, cheek pain upon opening the mouth	Zygomatic or maxillary complex fracture
	Yes, angle of the mandible pain	Fracture of the angle of the mandible
Adapted from Zimmermann CE, Troulis MJ, Kaban LB. Pediatric facial fractures: recent advances in prevention, diagnosis and management. *Int J Oral Maxillofac Surg.* 2006;35(1):2-13.		

the orbital floor is displaced superiorly, it is called a "blow-in" fracture. Objects that cause "blow-out" fractures are usually larger than the diameter of the opening of the orbit.

- A "white-eyed" blow-out fracture is an orbital fracture that causes entrapment and diplopia with a benign presentation. Most patients experience nausea and have defects in superior and inferior gaze, but have few external signs of trauma. These are commonly misdiagnosed.
- The signs and symptoms classically seen in blow-out fractures are similar to that discussed previously regarding blunt orbital trama in addition to:
  - Enophthalmos, orbital dystopia, hypesthesia usually along the distribution of the maxillary branch of the trigeminal nerve, obstruction of the lacrimal duct, retinal hemorrhage, blindness, optic neuropathy, epistaxis, subconjunctival hemorrhage, blepharoptosis, orbital emphysema, ophthalmoplegia, CSF rhinorrhea.
- If a health care provider suspects that a blunt trauma to the orbital region has occurred, a CT scan of the patient's orbit with coronal cuts should be ordered to best visualize the location and size of any fractures. If the physical examination exhibits no restrictions in extraocular movements, the orbit is not malaligned, and the CT scan shows an isolated orbital fracture, then the patient can be observed with regular follow-up.
- Antibiotics can be given prophylactically to decrease the incidence of infection. Corticosteroids can also be prescribed to minimize swelling and delay fibrosis progression. All patients should be evaluated when edema has resolved to assess for persistent diplopia, enophthalmos, and limitations of ocular movements.
- Surgical intervention is required within 3 to 5 days of injury if one or more of the following are present: large orbital floor fracture involving more than 50% of the orbital floor, muscle entrapment, significant initial enophthalmos of more than 2 mm, or significant displacement of the bones on radiographic imaging.[7]

10. What Is the Best Way to Manage Dental Trauma? How Can Dental Trauma Be Prevented?

- An initial assessment of the teeth can be performed by percussion of the teeth for pain or mobility and asking about the sensitivity of the teeth to heat and cold. Also, a brief examination of the periodontium and other surrounding structures should be undertaken. A prompt referral to a dentist is usually warranted so that proper x-rays of the mouth can be taken to thoroughly assess the extent of the patient's injury to the teeth.
- If the injured tooth is primary dentition and is found to be causing injury to the underlying permanent dentition, it needs to be extracted. Possible consequences of permanent dentition injury include hypoplasia of the enamel, hypocalcification, crown or root dilacerations, or eruption complications. If the child's enamel calcification has not yet been completed, there is a greater risk of permanent dentition complications.
- Trauma to the permanent dentition is usually associated with pulp and periodontal ligament complications. Prognosis mainly depends on timely assessment and treatment by a dentist as soon as the trauma occurs. Prevention includes proper protective gear such as helmets, mouthguards, and face masks.
- If a tooth becomes avulsed, it will begin to degrade after 15 minutes. After 60 minutes, the probability of saving the tooth is very low.
- The best way to store and transport an avulsed tooth is to place it back in its original position in the mouth or underneath the tongue. The next best way to store a tooth is an over-the-counter solution called "Save-A-Tooth." The solution prevents the tooth from dehydrating. The avulsed tooth can be kept in the solution for up to 24 hours.
- Other storage or transport media include cold cow's milk or cold isotonic solution.
- If the avulsed tooth lands in dirt, handle the crown only (being careful not to touch the root), irrigate the tooth thoroughly but gently with clean water (do not scrub it) to remove any debris before it is placed back into the mouth or a transport solution. Once the athlete is stabilized, it is important to refer him or her to a dentist for placement of a splint to keep the avulsed tooth in place. If it is a primary tooth, it may be left out, but the athlete still needs to see a dentist for possible injury to the permanent teeth that have not yet erupted.[8,9]

11. When Should Mouthguards Be Recommended, and What Are the Differences Between Off-the-Shelf Mouthguards and Custom Mouthguards?

- Mouthguards are recommended for any athlete who plays any contact or collision sport. The only sports whose players are required by the National Federation of State High School Associations to wear mouthguards are football, ice hockey, lacrosse, and field hockey.
- There are three different types of mouthguards: custom-made, mouth-formed, and stock mouthguards.
  - Custom-made mouthguards are made by the dentist from a mold of the athlete's teeth. The American Society for Testing and Materials suggests that maximal protection is reached if the mouthguard covers all teeth in one "arch."[9] The Academy for Sports Dentistry highly recommends this type of mouthguard for the most protection. It is usually the most comfortable and best fitting of all the mouthguards to wear.[9]
  - Mouth-formed ("boil-and-bite") mouthguards can be bought at commercial department stores or sporting goods stores. The athlete places the product in boiling water, and then it is pressed against the teeth and tongue to make the impression. This type is the most popular among athletes, but it is variable in its protective effectiveness and sometimes is uncomfortable to wear.

- Stock mouthguards can also be bought at commercial department stores, over-the-counter, or sporting goods stores. It is premade, with no custom impression made from the athlete's teeth. In order for it to be effective, the athlete must bite down on the mouthguard to stay in place. Sometimes it can be difficult for the athlete to breathe and talk while wearing the mouthguard during a sporting event. It is considered to be the least protective out of the three mouthguards, but it is the most affordable. Stock mouthguards may be the only option for athletes who have braces or certain dental appliances.[9]

References

1. Kuppermann N, Holmes JF, Dayan PS, et al. Identification of children at very low risk of clinically-important brain injuries after head trauma: a prospective cohort study. *Lancet.* 2009;374(9696):1160-1170.
2. Giles WC, Iverson KC, King JD, Hill FC, Woody EA, Bouknight AL. Incision and drainage followed by mattress suture repair of auricular hematoma. *Laryngoscope.* 2007;117(12):2097-2099.
3. Rodriguez JO, Lavina AM, Agarwal A. Prevention and treatment of common eye injuries in sports. *Am Fam Physician.* 2003;67(7):1481-1488.
4. Sarrazin L, Averbukh E, Halpert M, Hemo I, Rumelt S. Traumatic pediatric retinal detachment: a comparison between open and closed globe injuries. *Am J Ophthalmol.* 2004;137(6):1042-1049.
5. Desrosiers AE III, SR Thaller. Pediatric nasal fractures: evaluation and management. *J Craniofac Surg.* 2011;22(4):1327-1329.
6. Zimmermann CE, Troulis MJ, Kaban LB. Pediatric facial fractures: recent advances in prevention, diagnosis and management. *Int J Oral Maxillofac Surg.* 2006;35(1):2-13.
7. Petrigliano FA, RJ Williams III. Orbital fractures in sport: a review. *Sports Med.* 2003;33(4):317-322.
8. Guideline on management of acute dental trauma. *Pediatr Dent.* 2008;30(7 Suppl):175-183.
9. Policy on prevention of sports-related orofacial injuries. *Pediatr Dent.* 2008;30(7 Suppl):58-60.

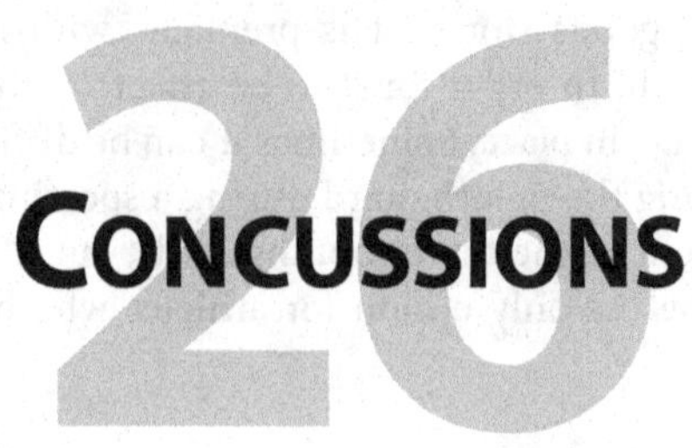

Concussions

Phuong N. Huynh, MD and Amanda Weiss Kelly, MD

1. Is Loss of Consciousness Required for Diagnosing Sports-Related Concussions?

No. According to the 4th Consensus Statement on Concussion in Sport (Zurich Guidelines), a concussion is "a complex pathophysiological process affecting the brain, induced by traumatic biomechanical forces."[1] Historically, loss of consciousness (LOC) was used as a marker of severity and applied to multiple grading scales to help determine return to play (RTP)/management. However, LOC does not correlate with severity and is not required for the diagnosis of a concussion. Less than 10% of concussions involve LOC.[2,3]

2. What Signs or Symptoms May Suggest a Concussion?

Signs and symptoms of a concussion can gradually appear over time and can take hours to days to reach full intensity.[1,4,5] A child with a suspected concussion should be monitored closely after injury for worsening signs and symptoms (Table 26-1).[1,5] There are also symptoms that would be more concerning for neurologic conditions other than concussions, such as intracranial hemorrhage (Table 26-2).[5] A commonly used tool to evaluate the symptoms of a concussion is the Sport Concussion Assessment Tool 3 (SCAT3), which can be accessed at http://bjsm.bmj.com/content/47/5/259.full.pdf. The 4th Consensus Statement incorporates a Child-SCAT3 for evaluation of children aged 5 to 12 years, and can be accessed at http://bjsm.bmj.com/content/47/5/263.full.pdf.

Postural balance has been assessed with the Balance Error Scoring System test (BESS), and a modified version is part of the SCAT3 evaluation. It consists of counting balance errors with the athlete in three stances: double leg, single leg, and tandem on a firm and foam/unsteady surface (Figure 26-1).[1] Since balance can be affected by physical activity/fatigue, it is best to use this test 20 minutes after exertion.[6] The Child-SCAT3 has a modified BESS test, which only incorporates the double leg and tandem stances.

Cognitive deficits can be measured with neurocognitive testing. A sideline assessment tool for quick screening, also included in the SCAT3, is the Standardized Assessment of Concussion (SAC) that evaluates orientation, immediate and delayed recall, and concentration.[1] A preinjury SAC can serve as a baseline test for comparison after a head injury. Computerized and traditional pen and paper neuropsychologic testing allows for the evaluation of reaction time changes, memory, and concentration.[7]

3. Do Evidence-Based Grading Systems Exist for Classifying Concussions?

No. There are numerous grading systems published to classify concussions; however, none of them are evidence-based and instead depend mainly on expert opinion. The most recent Zurich

Koutures C, Wong V.
Pediatric Sports Medicine: Essentials for Office Evaluation (pp 168-174)

Table 26-1. Concussion Symptoms Assessed in the Sport Concussion Assessment Tool 3 and Acute Concussion Evaluation

SYMPTOMS			*SCAT3 ONLY*[1]	*ACE ONLY*[5]
Headache	Sensitivity to light	Drowsiness	Pressure in head	Numbness/tingling
Nausea/vomiting	Sensitivity to noise	Trouble falling asleep	Neck pain	Sleeping more than usual
Dizziness	Feeling slowed down	More emotional	"Don't feel right"	Sleeping less than usual
Blurred vision/visual problems	Feeling "in a fog"/mentally foggy	Irritability	Confusion	
Balance problems	Difficulty concentrating	Sadness		
Fatigue/low energy	Difficulty remembering	Nervous/anxious		

Adapted from US Department of Health and Human Services, Centers for Disease Control and Prevention. Head's up: facts for physicians about mild traumatic brain injury (MTBI). www.cdc.gov/concussion/headsup/pdf/Facts_for_Physicians_booklet-a.pdf. Accessed February 27, 2012.

Table 26-2. Signs and Symptoms for Emergency Department Referral

- Seizures
- Focal neurologic deficits
- Obtunded or somnolent
- Persistent vomiting
- Speech problems
- Behavioral and/or emotional changes
- Loss of consciousness for > 30 seconds
- Disorientation
- Neck pain
- Significant worsening or severe headaches

Adapted from the US Department of Health and Human Services, Centers for Disease Control and Prevention. Head's up: facts for physicians about mild traumatic brain injury (MTBI). www.cdc.gov/concussion/headsup/pdf/Facts_for_Physicians_booklet-a.pdf. Accessed February 27, 2012.

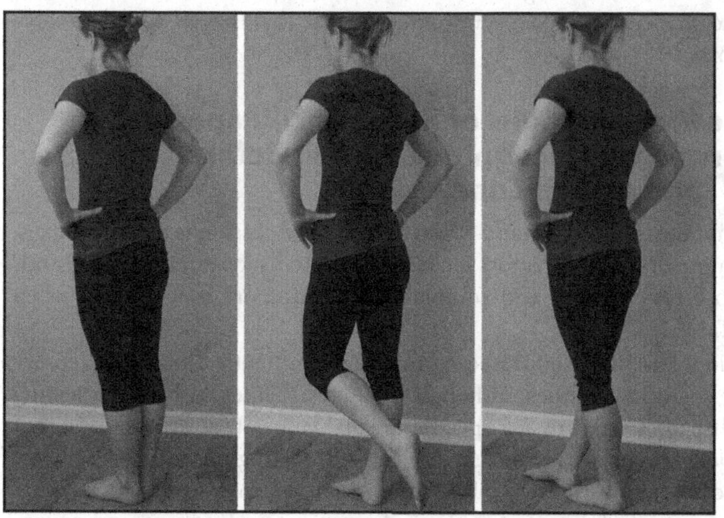

Figure 26-1. Balance Error Scoring System testing stances. From left to right: double leg, single leg, and tandem.

Table 26-3. The Pros and Cons of Neurocognitive Testing by Paper/Pencil and Computer[7]

	PAPER/PENCIL	*COMPUTER*
Pros	• Can detect difference between preexisting conditions (learning disability, attention deficit hyperactivity disorder, headaches) and concussion • Allows for more specific modifications in the classroom	• Multiple forms decrease practice effect • More precise reaction time • Quick • Many athletes can test at same time • Easier to obtain baseline tests
Cons	• Practice effect • Time • Access to neuropsychologist	• Hard to control surrounding environment • Difficult to interpret if athlete has underlying conditions (learning disability, attention deficit hyperactivity disorder)

Guidelines recommend individualized management of all concussions, since no classification system accurately predicts the time to recovery.[1,3]

4. What Are the Current Thoughts About "Second Impact Syndrome"? Does It Exist, and What Is the Proposed Pathophysiology Behind It?

Second impact syndrome is defined as cerebral edema occurring "when an athlete who sustains a head injury—often a concussion—sustains a second head injury before symptoms associated with the first have cleared."[2] There are some who do not believe that it exists as a separate entity. McCrory et al point out a process called *malignant brain edema syndrome*, which is characterized by cerebral swelling due to trauma and can occur after a single traumatic event.[8,9] They believe that many of the reported cases of second impact syndrome either occur without a second hit or are related to intracranial hemorrhage. Others, like Cantu, believe that a concussion leads to the loss of cerebral blood flow autoregulation, making the brain more vulnerable to cerebral swelling.[2] When a second head injury occurs prior to resolution of symptoms from the initial injury, it leads to increased cerebral blood flow, causing increased intracranial pressure, cerebral edema, and possibly herniation and death. Second impact syndrome is so rare that the only data available in humans are from case reports.[2,8-10]

5. What Are the Pros and Cons of Both Pencil/Paper and Computerized Neurocognitive Testing Before and After a Concussion?

Neurocognitive testing is not meant to be a stand-alone test, as a concussion is a clinical diagnosis made with the consideration of multiple factors including symptoms, postural balance, and/or neurocognitive testing. Both pencil/paper and computerized testing are best utilized when there is a baseline available (Table 26-3).[1,3,7]

In the school-age population, baselines should be repeated intermittently since children are still growing and developing cognitive abilities, although the optimal interval between testing baselines has not been established. There are age-specific normal values that can be used, but individual baselines are the best for comparison. Neuropsychologic testing may be normal even when the child is symptomatic, so diagnostic and RTP decisions should be made only after taking into consideration the patient's report of symptoms, physical examination findings, and neuropsychologic testing data.[1,3]

Table 26-4. Sample Return-to-Play Progression	
ATHLETE MUST BE SYMPTOM-FREE PRIOR TO STARTING A RETURN-TO-PLAY PROGRESSION	
Day 1	Light aerobic exercise • Elliptical trainer • Stationary bike • Light jogging
Day 2	Sport-specific exercise at higher aerobic intensity • Running • Skating
Day 3	Noncontact training drills • Ball skills/control • Running routes • Shooting drills • Light resistance training
MEDICAL CLEARANCE SHOULD BE OBTAINED PRIOR TO STARTING DAY 4 OF PROGRESSION	
Day 4	Full contact training/practice
Day 5	Full game or competition
Adapted from McCrory P, Meeuwisse W, Aubry M, et al. Consensus statement on concussion in sport: the 4th international conference on concussion in sport held in Zurich, November 2012. *Br J Sports Med.* 2013;47:250–258.	

6. Once an Athlete Suffers a Concussion, What Are the Suggested Criteria to Allow a Return to Play?

Research from 2004 shows that mild or "ding" concussions can have cognitive sequelae that were previously not recognized.[11] This has led to a more conservative approach to RTP that prevents the young athlete from returning to a game on the same day that he or she sustained the injury. The athlete needs to be completely symptom free, off of any medications used to treat the signs/symptoms of a concussion, and tolerating normal cognitive activity for at least 24 hours prior to beginning a RTP progression. School performance and computerized neuropsychologic testing can be used to determine a return-to-baseline cognitive function. Other considerations, such as duration of symptoms, history of prior concussions, and severity of symptoms, may contribute to RTP decisions.

The Zurich Guidelines propose a stepwise RTP (Table 26-4).[1] There should be at least 24 hours between each step and if there is any return of symptoms, the athlete needs to go back to the prior, symptom-free phase.[3] This progression may also be extended for younger athletes since their brains are more vulnerable to the effects of head injury.[7] It is helpful to educate the athlete regarding this progression so that proper expectations are set from the beginning of management.

Neuropsychologic deficits may persist even when the athlete reports being symptom free. One group demonstrated that some high school athletes did not return to baseline on computerized testing at 36 hours after injury even though they were asymptomatic. Return to baseline was noted an average of 6 days after injury/symptom resolution.[11] This makes a case for being even more conservative in RTP decisions and making all RTP decision making on an individualized basis, as recommended by the Zurich Guidelines. This may mean a longer symptom-free time prior to progression or progression spaced over multiple days instead of 24 hours.[3]

Table 26-5. Symptom-Based Postconcussion School Modifications[5]	
SYMPTOM/DEFICIT	*ACCOMMODATIONS*
Any symptoms	• If patient has worsening symptoms, breaks in the nurse's office or early school dismissal • Limit general workload • Frequent breaks when doing homework • No physical activity, including gym class
Light sensitivity	• Decrease computer use • Sunglasses in the classroom
Noise sensitivity	• Early class dismissal for transport in quiet hallways • Lunch in a classroom or library • Avoid team practice • Ear plugs
Decreased processing speed	• Extra time for tests • Extra time for homework
Impaired memory	• No testing • Limit new concepts

7. What Modifications Might Be Needed to Assist in the Return to the Classroom?

Since concussions can be exacerbated by cognitive activity and physical activity, it is very important to limit cognitive stimulation in addition to physical activity. A child should stay home from school until his or her symptoms improve. Decreasing recreational reading, access to computers, texting, and video games are also recommended during the symptomatic time period. Once the child returns to school, special accommodations (Table 26-5) should be in place to decrease unnecessary stimulation.[5]

Return to school should be a progression.

- Start with half-day attendance, and progress to full days as tolerated.
- Defer testing until the student is tolerating full days at school and homework.
- Limit situations where the student could suffer another blow to the head.
- If prolonged symptoms occur or the student has an underlying learning disability or attention deficit/hyperactivity disorder, formal neurocognitive testing may be helpful in making specific modifications, such as allowing extra time for tests in children with documented processing speed deficits.

8. How Many Concussions Are Too Many?

There is no evidence-based answer to this question, and management should be individualized.[12] Any potential number of concussions could possibly lead to permanent sequelae of repetitive brain trauma, such as persistent cognitive deficits or the extreme case of chronic traumatic encephalopathy (CTE), which was initially described in boxers and coined *dementia pugilistica*. However, multiple sports have been implicated, including football and wrestling. CTE presents later in life with cognitive deficits, emotional lability, and movement disorders. Autopsies have shown histopathological changes consistent with CTE.[13,14] There are no evidence-based links to a certain number or magnitude of concussion and the risk of CTE that help guide RTP decisions.

Historically, the limit of three concussions was proposed for retirement from sports. Given the variable responses to head trauma, it is hard to specify a number, since one concussion could be enough to retire an athlete if symptoms do not resolve or the athlete does not return to his or her

Table 26-6. Risk Factors for a Concussion and Postconcussion Syndrome/Prolonged Symptoms	
Concussion[3,12]	*Postconcussion Syndrome/Prolonged Symptoms*[15]
• Female > male • History of prior concussion • Males—Football • Females—Soccer, basketball	• Female > male • +/– history of prior concussion • Light and noise sensitivity • Amnesia • Migraines • Cognitive deficits • Mental health diagnosis

baseline level of cognitive functioning. Other athletes are asymptomatic with normal neurocognitive testing after more than three concussions. Neurocognitive testing and school performance can determine his or her current cognitive function.[12] The athlete and family should be involved in the discussion so that they are aware of the possible long-term consequences. Ultimately, athletes who experience a decreased threshold for concussion, take an extended time period to return to normal function after concussion, or continue to have persistent symptoms may need to consider retirement from contact and collision sports.[12]

9. Which Athletes and Sports/Activities Are at Higher Risk for a Concussion?

Table 26-6 provides information on particular risk factors for suffering a concussion and also for higher possibility of postconcussion syndrome/prolonged symptoms after a concussion.[3,12,15]

10. Can Mouthguards, Helmets, and Protective Headbands Prevent Concussions?

There are no definitive data that support the use of protective equipment such as mouthguards, helmets, and headbands to prevent a concussion. Mouthguards prevent dental injury, so there is still a place for their use. Helmets decrease the chance of skull fracture and intracranial hemorrhage. There are a few studies showing support for decreased concussions with helmet use, but due to design flaws in the studies, it is difficult to make conclusions regarding the effectiveness of helmets in decreasing concussions. There is no evidence for the use of headbands in soccer to prevent a concussion.[16]

11. How Should a Helmet Be Properly Fitted?

A helmet size should be chosen based on manufacturer specifications. Once a helmet is chosen, the front of the helmet should end three-quarters to one inch above the brow line. When the helmet is on with the air cells inflated (if present), it should not move when the facemask is pulled to the side against the athlete's resistance. Chinstraps should not be necessary to keep it on, but they should still be appropriately fastened before play.[17] See Chapter 11, question 3, for more discussion on helmets.

12. Does Neck Strengthening Prevent Concussions?

Research has yet to prove that neck strengthening prevents concussions. The theory behind strengthening cervical musculature in preventing concussions is that contracting the cervical musculature will better support the head/neck, limiting impact to the head.[18] However, video analysis of concussion injuries reviewed in Australian football, soccer, and rugby has found that the vast majority of concussive impacts are accidental and that athletes are unable to tense the neck to embrace sudden impact.[19]

There is still much debate over which of these biomechanical forces (linear/translational versus rotational acceleration, changes in velocity, impact speed, head displacement) are the most important in terms of being responsible for causing the clinical changes seen with concussions.[20] According to the first study that looked at static neck strength and head impact biomechanics in youth ice hockey players,[18] the data collected did not support that increased baseline cervical neck strength alone was enough to reduce head accelerations in head impact injuries. Another small study looked at 16 college-aged male athletes to examine the effects of cervical resistance training on kinematic responses in standard football tackling and on sternocleidomastoid and upper trapezius muscle activity using an electromyogram[21]; it failed to show an enhancement in dynamic stabilization of the head and neck during a standard football tackle.

References

1. McCrory P, Meeuwisse W, Aubry M, et al. Consensus statement on concussion in sport: the 4th international conference on concussion in sport held in Zurich, November 2012. *Br J Sports Med.* 2013;47:250–258.
2. Cantu RC. Second-impact syndrome. *Clin Sports Med.* 1998;17(1):37-44.
3. Halstead ME, Walter KD. Sport-related concussion in children and adolescents. *Pediatrics.* 2010;126(3):597.
4. Guskiewicz KM, Bruce SL, Cantu RC, et al. National athletic trainers' association position statement: management of sport-related concussion. *J Athl Train.* 2004;39(3):280.
5. US Department of Health and Human Services. Head's up: facts for physicians about mild traumatic brain injury (MTBI). www.cdc.gov/concussion/headsup/pdf/Facts_for_Physicians_booklet-a.pdf. Accessed February 27, 2012.
6. Susco TM, McLeod TCV, Gansneder BM, Shultz SJ. Balance recovers within 20 minutes after exertion as measured by the balance error scoring system. *J Athl Train.* 2004;39(3):241.
7. Putukian M. Repeat mild traumatic brain injury: how to adjust return to play guidelines. *Curr Sports Med Rep.* 2006;5(1):15.
8. McCrory P, Davis G, Makdissi M. Second impact syndrome or cerebral swelling after sporting head injury. *Curr Sports Med Rep.* 2012;11(1):21.
9. McCrory P. Does second impact syndrome exist? *Clin J Sport Med.* 2001;11(3):144.
10. Wetjen NM, Pichelmann MA, Atkinson JL. Second impact syndrome: concussion and second injury brain complications. *J Am Coll Surg.* 2010;211(4):553-557.
11. Lovell MR, Collins MW, Iverson GL, Johnston KM, Bradley JP. Grade 1 or "ding" concussions in high school athletes. *Am J Sports Med.* 2004;32(1):47.
12. Maroon JC, Lovell MR, Norwig J, Podell K, Powell JW, Hartl R. Cerebral concussion in athletes: evaluation and neuropsychological testing. *Neurosurgery.* 2000;47(3):659.
13. Sedney CL, Orphanos J, Bailes JE. When to consider retiring an athlete after sports-related concussion. *Clin Sports Med.* 2011;30(1):189-200.
14. Gavett BE, Stern RA, McKee AC. Chronic traumatic encephalopathy: a potential late effect of sport-related concussive and subconcussive head trauma. *Clin Sports Med.* 2011;30(1):179-188, xi.
15. Jotwani V, Harmon KG. Postconcussion syndrome in athletes. *Curr Sports Med Rep.* 2010;9(1):21.
16. Daneshvar DH, Baugh CM, Nowinski CJ, McKee AC, Stern RA, Cantu RC. Helmets and mouth guards: the role of personal equipment in preventing sport-related concussions. *Clin Sports Med.* 2011;30(1):145-163.
17. National Collegiate Athletic Association. 2011-2012 NCAA sports medicine handbook. www.ncaapublications.com/p-4203-2011-2012-sports-medicine-handbook.aspx. Accessed November 29, 2011.
18. Mihalik JP, Guskiewicz KM, Marshall SW, Greenwald RM, Blackburn JT, Cantu RC. Does cervical muscle strength in youth ice hockey players affect head impact biomechanics? *Clin J Sport Med.* 2011;21(5):416.
19. McCrory P, Turner M, McIntosh A. Preventing injuries to the head and cervical spine. In: Bahr R, Engebretsen L, eds. *Handbook of Sports Medicine and Science: Sports Injury Prevention.* Vol 13. Hoboken, NJ: Blackwell Pub; 2009:175-186.
20. Demorest RA. The future of preventing concussion in children and adolescents. In: Apps JN, Walter KD, eds. *Pediatric and Adolescent Concussion.* New York, NY: Springer; 2012:177-194.
21. Lisman PJ, Signorile JF, Del Rossi G, et al. Cervical strength training does not enhance dynamic stabilization of head and neck during football tackling: 2589. *Med Sci Sport Exercise.* 2010;42(5):679.

Acknowledgment

We would like to thank Jane Chung, MD for her contribution to question twelve of this chapter.

27 Neck Pain and Cervical Spine Issues

Kentaro Onishi, DO and David Kruse, MD

1. The Cervical Spine Has a Natural Lordosis. What Does This Mean, and Why Is This Important in Preventing Cervical Spine Injuries? What Is Spear Tackling in Football, and Why Is It Strongly Discouraged?

- With the invention of the helmet, the incidence of brain hemorrhage has decreased in football, although some reports have described a paradoxical increase of traumatic cervical injuries over recent years.[1] The sports that are associated with high incidences of cervical injuries are football, rugby, ice hockey, and wrestling.[2]
- The 4 types of injuries commonly sustained by the cervical spine are as follows:
  - Soft-tissue injuries (cervical muscle strain, ligamentous sprain)
  - Bony injuries (cervical vertebral fractures/dislocation)
  - Peripheral nerve injuries
  - Spinal cord injuries
- It is reported at least 10% to 15% of football players sustain some type of cervical spine injuries during their athletic career.[2]
- The cervical spine maintains its protective, natural lordotic curvature via a complex interaction with multiple soft-tissue structures. When maintained, cervical lordosis allows the dissipation or transmission of forces to these structures upon impact. When this curvature is lost and assumes a straight or kyphotic alignment, the cervical spine loses its ability to withstand these forces and becomes more prone to injury.[3]

In football, spear tackling has been banned and discouraged. Correct tackling technique in football involves the contact of well-padded shoulders with the head up (Figure 27-1). However, in a spear tackle, athletes use the crown of the helmet as the point of initial contact (Figure 27-2). The cervical spine of the tackler assumes a flexed position of about 30 degrees when performing a spear tackle. Such flexion at the neck results in the loss of natural protective lordosis of the cervical spine, and less ability to dissipate the axial loading force. The spine is then prone to fracture and/or dislocation of the cervical vertebrae with possible spinal cord injury. This is the reason why spear tackling has been banned in American football, and players are told to "see what you hit."

2. What Are Some Key Examination Tips in the Event of an Acute Cervical Spine Injury?

- When evaluating an athlete with suspected neck injury on the field, the goal of the evaluation is to determine whether the player has sustained a spinal cord injury or an unstable spinal column fracture. When these conditions are suspected, appropriate field

Koutures C, Wong V.
Pediatric Sports Medicine: Essentials for Office Evaluation (pp 175-182)

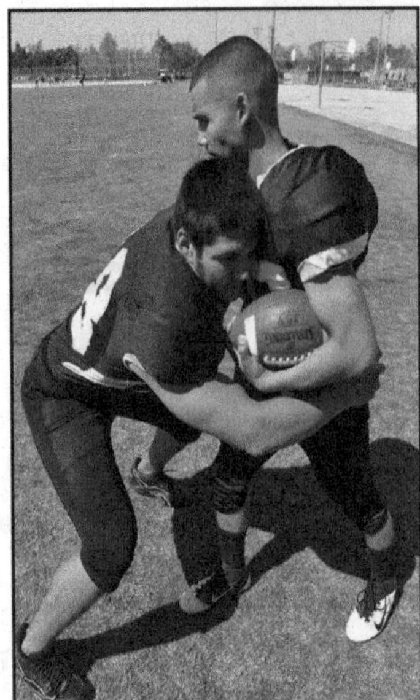

Figure 27-1. Proper tackling technique. Contact with the shoulder pads with the head up. (Reprinted with permission of Dr. David W. Kruse and the Godinez Fundamental High School Football Team.)

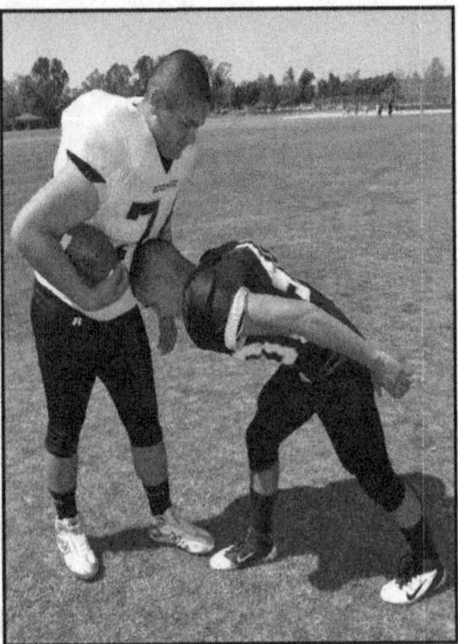

Figure 27-2. Spear tackling. Tackler leading with the crown of his head in a down position. (Reprinted with permission of Dr. David W. Kruse and the Godinez Fundamental High School Football Team.)

management of an unstable cervical spine injury should be performed and emergency medical services (EMS) should be activated for transfer to the nearest hospital. Both of these conditions require appropriate imaging and subsequent stabilization of the spine to minimize potentially permanent neurologic sequelae.

- When neck injuries occur, sport medicine physicians are expected to be equipped with a methodological approach, such as the approach outlined below, when evaluating these athletes:
  - Step 1: focused history—Should include questions regarding neck pain (location, radiation, quality, severity, and history of experiencing such pain) and neurologic symptoms (numbness, tingling, or weakness in the arms or legs).
  - Step 2: physical examination—Includes mental status and musculoskeletal examinations.
    - Mental status examination—A cognitive assessment should be performed throughout the evaluation. Concurrent neck and head injuries are common. If the athlete becomes unconscious or is unable to communicate, an unstable neck injury must be assumed.
    - Musculoskeletal examination—Includes (1) the inspection for obvious deformity; (2) palpation over spinous and transverse processes as well as over paravertebral musculatures to look for spasms; and (3) active range of motion (AROM) of the neck as tolerated. Passive range of motion (PROM) is not recommended.
- Appropriate helmet and facemask management is essential. The Inter-Association Task Force for Appropriate Care of the Spine-Injured Athlete established guidelines for prehospital helmet removal. The helmet should be removed if the helmet and other equipment (such as straps and shoulder pads) will fail to hold the head securely during transport to the hospital and adequate airway access and control are difficult (with or without removing the facemask).[4]
- It should be noted that football helmets usually provide neutral spine alignment when they are in place with shoulder pads. Consequently, the Task Force has recommended

TABLE 27-1. NEXUS CRITERIA
ORDER 3-VIEW X-RAY IF ANY OF THE FOLLOWING IS PRESENT:
• Posterior midline cervical spine tenderness • Evidence of intoxication • Altered level of alertness • Focal neurologic deficit • Painful distracting injuries
Abbreviation: NEXUS, National Emergency X-radiography Utilization Study.

against the removal of the helmet in the absence of the two previously noted conditions. In contrast, a motorcycle helmet is usually loosely fit and should be removed to provide secure immobilization of the neck before transportation.[4] As for the management of the facemask, it should be removed at the earliest possible time to enable improved access to the airway.[5]

If the decision is made to remove the face mask/helmet, it is a multistep process to successfully remove the equipment without neck motion. This process requires at least two trained health care providers, but four providers is preferred.

3. What Are the Key Imaging Studies for Cervical Spine Injuries?

- During the evaluation of a sports-related cervical spine injury, three types of imaging should be considered: (1) plain radiograph/x-ray; (2) computed tomography (CT) scan; and (3) magnetic resonance imaging (MRI). Criteria set forth to determine the need for plain radiographs is provided by the National Emergency X-radiography Utilization Study (NEXUS) criteria (Table 27-1).[6]
- If any one of the five NEXUS criteria is present, x-rays need to be obtained. If none of NEXUS criteria are present, then have the athlete actively rotate his or her head. If the athlete is unable to do so, then plain radiographs are indicated. Three views (anteroposterior [AP], lateral, and odontoid views) are often sufficient to properly evaluate the cervical spine. The second type of imaging is CT. There is a true risk for false-negative findings on x-ray evaluation in the setting of cervical spine fractures, especially at the transition zone between C7 and T1. If the risk for fracture is deemed high, then CT scan is often used. Lastly, MRI serves to best evaluate damage to the spinal cord or other neural tissues, which might be important in the nonacute setting to predict the extent of the injury.

4. What Is a Cervical Strain/Sprain, and How Is It Managed?

- One of most common sports-related cervical injuries is acute cervical strain/sprain. A strain is muscle-tendon injury. Athletes with cervical strain will report localized tenderness without any neurologic deficits. On examination, there may be limited ROM due to pain and tenderness on palpation over soft tissues. This should be treated symptomatically with conservative management using basic pain modalities such as alternating ice and heat, massage, stretching, and strengthening. Oral anti-inflammatory medication can also be effective. The athlete can return to play when full pain-free ROM is obtained.
- A cervical sprain is a ligamentous injury. Cervical sprains are usually regarded as benign in nature as compared with unstable fractures or spinal cord injury, but they still can result

in significant time loss from play for the athlete. Cervical sprains can be divided into the following categories:

- Grade 1—Mild; results in no macroscopic tear of the tissue. Management is based on pain relief similar to cervical strain, and return to play is based on pain control and full pain-free ROM.
- Grade 2—Moderate; results in a partial tear of the ligament but no significant instability. Management is again based on resolution of pain and swelling with gradual return of ROM and strength; recovery will take longer.
- Grade 3—Severe; results in a complete tear of the structure with significant joint instability. If instability is suspected, then lateral flexion and extension x-ray evaluation is indicated. Specialty referral should be considered if there is evidence of an unstable injury. Radiographic evaluation of the extent of the sprain can be done using either MRI or musculoskeletal ultrasonography. Return to play is more conservative using similar parameters of pain-free ROM and symptom resolution, and after return of a stable examination. For significant unstable injuries, it would be reasonable to consider retirement from contact sports.

5. What Is a Burner/Stinger? If an Athlete Has Recurrent Stingers, What Other Issues Should Also Be Considered? Is There Such a Thing as "Bilateral" Stingers?

- In football, transient cervical radiculopathies or brachial plexopathies are common and are colloquially known as a "stinger" or a "burner." It is often a result of a direct blow to the neck area, causing a stretch or compression injury of the cervical spine nerve roots or the brachial plexus. These athletes often report transient, shock-like pain at the time of impact followed by some type of regional or localized neurologic deficit often in a C5 or C6 distribution. As a result of the anatomical location of injury, these peripheral neuropathies are unilateral and usually recover within minutes to hours. When these peripheral neuropathies are severe, it may result in architectural nerve injury that may take weeks or even longer to heal.
- When a stinger occurs, the physical examination should include the following:
  - Cervical spine ROM and palpation (see question 2 in this chapter)—Should be benign.
  - Upper extremity neurologic examination—Test for deficits in strength and sensation in all distributions, most commonly C5 and C6. See Chapter 22, step 4, for information on myotomes and dermatomes of the upper extremity.
- X-ray analysis is usually normal. If symptoms are bilateral, then cervical spine precautions should be implemented and the athlete sent to the emergency department for cervical spine x-ray or CT scan. If unilateral, neurologic deficits persist 3 to 4 weeks after injury, then further work-up with an electromyogram and/or MRI should be done to evaluate for more significant nerve injury.
- Traditionally, bilateral neurologic loss implies spinal cord injury. There is an entity known as cervical cord neuropraxia (also referred to as transient quadriparesis) that results in transient sensory or motor paralysis in all four extremities with a quick return of lost function (in minutes to hours). If suspected, cervical spine precautions should still be implemented and the athlete should be transported to the emergency department for further evaluation.

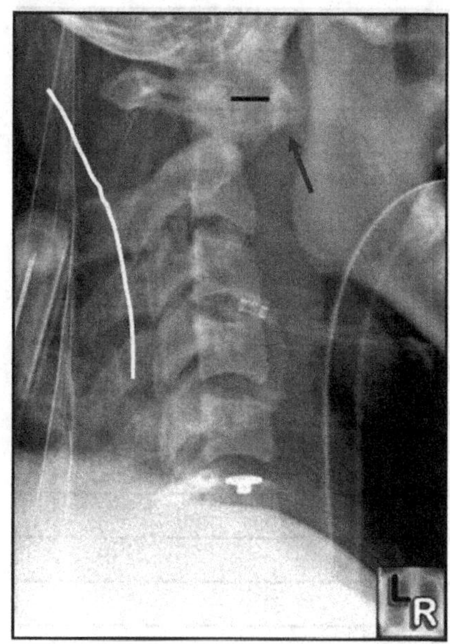

Figure 27-3. Lateral view of an atlantoaxial dislocation due to instability. Notice the imaginary line (spinolaminar line) drawn on the left side of the image and the anterior displacement of C1 to the right of the image, compromising available space for the spinal cord to pass through. (Reprinted with permission from learningradiology.com and its author, Dr. William Herring, MD, FACR.)

6. How Is a Cervical Vertebral Fracture Identified/Suspected on the Field, and What Is the Initial Management?

- On the sideline, a systematic approach following the NEXUS criteria is the best method to rule out fractures of the cervical spine (see Table 27-1; also refer to question 2, step 2). When the patient is able to perform active ROM without pain, the athlete can be safely precluded from need for transfer. However, if the athlete meets one of these criteria or is unable to move through full ROM without pain, then a fracture should be suspected and emergency protocols with cervical spine immobilization should be instituted.
- Initial on-field management should rely on standard emergency medical responses including the following:
    - Initial advanced cardiovascular life support evaluation for airway management and the activation of EMS system.
    - Stabilization of the head—Performed by a designated individual who cradles the player's helmet/head with his or her hands/arms.
    - The sports helmet should remain on if there is no airway compromise, but the facemask can be removed.
    - Once EMS support arrives, transfer to a stabilization board should be performed.
    - Refer to Chapter 23, question 5, for additional information on how to manage head/neck injuries.

7. What Are Some of the Neck Issues That an Athlete With Trisomy 21 May Have, and Why?

Trisomy 21 (Down syndrome) affects the integrity of the cervical spine via two main conditions—(1) atlantoaxial instability (AAI) and (2) congenital vertebral malformations of the cervical spine. An athlete with Trisomy 21 and AAI has innately loose transverse ligaments of the atlas (C1), which allows posterior displacement of the odontoid process (C2), potentially leading to spinal cord stenosis (Figure 27-3).

Table 27-2. Description of Klippel-Feil Syndrome Types	
TYPE	*DESCRIPTION*
Type I	Presence of single level fusion in cervical spine
Type II	Presence of multiple, noncontiguous-fused segments below level of C2 with cervico-occipital synostosis
Type III	Presence of multiple, contiguous-fused segments with nonfused segments in between fused segments

Table 27-3. Absolute Contraindications to Contact Sports Participation in Patients With Klippel-Feil Syndrome
Presence of cervico-occipital anomalies
C2 involvement
Presence of disc disease or degenerative disease
Fusion of more than 3 vertebral segments

- During the initial sports physicals for children with Trisomy 21, the clinician is expected to perform a very detailed history and neurologic examination to see if the patient exhibits signs and symptoms consistent with spinal cord injury. The American Academy of Pediatrics (AAP) Council on Sports Medicine and Fitness and the AAP Committee on Genetics both state that symptoms consistent with spinal cord injury are the best predictor of AAI.[7,8] Symptoms clinicians should be looking for include the following:
  - Numbness, tingling, weakness in the limbs, increased reflexes, or emergence of pathologic reflexes such as Babinski, Hoffman, and ankle clonus.
  - Bowel and bladder accidents or the loss of bowel and bladder control.
- Initial imaging should include flexion and extension views of the cervical spine. Should one detect radiographic evidence of AAI in the absence of clinical symptoms, then annual x-rays of the cervical spine are recommended.[7]
- General guidelines for clearance for return to sports are still lacking in these patients. Most authorities in pediatric sports medicine recommend against the participation in contact sports if the atlantodens interval is greater than 4.5 mm.[7] The Special Olympics requires patients with Trisomy 21 who are participating in higher-risk activities to have cervical spine x-ray screenings (see Chapter 18, question 3, for more details).[7]
- C1 hypoplasia places children with Trisomy 21 at higher risk for cervical spinal cord injury and myelopathy due to a smaller canal space available for the cord to pass through at the C1 level.

8. What Are the Cervical Concerns of an Athlete With Klippel-Feil Syndrome, and Can He or She Participate in Sports? Can a Child With Agenesis or Hypoplasia of the Odontoid Participate in Sports? Can a Child With a Chiari Malformation Participate in Sports?

- Klippel-Feil syndrome (KFS) is a multisystem disease that includes the congenital fusion of the cervical spine. In 2006, Samartzis et al proposed three classes of cervical spine deformities to characterize patients with KFS (Table 27-2).[9] Patients with KFS types II and III are at high risk for developing myelopathy or radiculopathy with minor trauma. Also, the risk of myelopathy increases if the level of cervical fusion is between C1 and C3.

Table 27-4. Contraindications to Contact Sports Participation in Patients With Chiari Malformation Type I	
ABSOLUTE CONTRAINDICATION	If Chiari malformation type I is radiographically confirmed, AND any of the following: • Syringomyelia is seen • Obliteration of subarachnoid space • Evidence of indentation of medulla • Patient is symptomatic
RELATIVE CONTRAINDICATION	• Patient is asymptomatic AND • Chiari malformation type I is an incidental finding

- Contact sport participation should be limited only to patients with fusion of one or two levels at or below C3 with full ROM. There are other absolute contraindications to contact sports participation in for athletes with KFS (Table 27-3).
- The odontoid, in normal individuals, functions to hold the atlas from posterior translation and subsequent spinal cord stenosis or injuries. Athletes with Down syndrome or KFS may have congenital agenesis or hypoplasia of the odontoid. As previously discussed (see question 7), this can result in AAI and exclusion from high-risk sports.
- A Chiari malformation is a congenital condition characterized by herniation of the cerebellum through the foramen magnum. Depending on the degree of the herniation, patients are divided into subcategories (types I to IV), with type I being the mildest form. Only type I will be discussed in this chapter. Types II to IV are typically symptomatic, and sports participation is contraindicated in these patients. Patients with type I typically present to the clinic for increasingly frequent, long-lasting, throbbing headaches (occipital) or neck pain (nuchal area) that starts shortly after coughing, sneezing, or minor trauma. Current contraindications to the participation in contact sports by athletes with type I depend on the presence of symptoms and/or the presence of a specific radiographic findings (Table 27-4).

9. What Are Some Concerns That Should Be Addressed for Athletes Undergoing Rehabilitation for a Cervical Spine Injury?

- Relief of pain will be the focus during the initial phase of rehabilitation. Pain is likely the primary reason for decreased ROM, strength, or performance in the athlete. Therapists will likely employ a combination of manual therapy such as soft-tissue massaging, gentle stretching, and use of modalities. Modalities include, but are not limited to, the use of heat, ice, and electrical stimulation. The therapist will also use ultrasonography as either a deep heat conduction method or for iontophoresis.
- Once the pain has subsided, the next phase is to regain ROM. After the athlete achieves this, strength and stability of the cervical spine and upper extremities will be the focus to restore the patient's neck strength, upper back strength, and shoulder girdle stability, as well as to restore any related upper-extremity musculature deconditioning.

10. When Should I Refer an Athlete With a Cervical Spine Injury?

If the clinical history, examination, or imaging is consistent with a spinal cord injury, then referral to a specialist should be considered. If the athlete has persistent symptoms (greater than 4 to 6 weeks) from a cervical radiculopathy or peripheral nerve injury, such as a brachioplexopathy, the athlete should be referred to a specialist for electrodiagnostic studies. Other reasons for referral are incidental findings of congenital malformation and an athlete with Trisomy 21.

References

1. Mueller FO, Cantu R. National Center for Catastrophic Sport Injury research [twenty-fifth annual report]. Chapel Hill, NC: University of North Carolina; 2007.
2. Clarke KS. Epidemiology of athletic neck injury. *Clin Sports Med.* 1998;17(1):83-97.
3. Swartz EE, Decoster LC, Norkus SA, et al. Summary of the National Athletic Trainers' Association position statement on the acute management of the cervical spine-injured athlete. *Phys Sportsmed.* 2009;37(4):20–30.
4. Kleiner DM, Almquist JL, Bailes J, et al. Prehospital Care of the Spine-Injured Athlete. National Athletic Trainers' Association Web site. http://www.nata.org/sites/default/files/PreHospitalCare4SpineInjuredAthlete.pdf. Accessed April 6, 2012.
5. Waninger KN. Management of the helmeted athlete with suspected cervical spine injury. *Am J Sports Med.* 2004;32(5):1331–1350.
6. Hoffman JR, Mower WR, Wolfson AB, Todd KH, Zucker MI; National Emergency X-Radiography Utilization Study Group. Validity of a set of clinical criteria to rule out injury to the cervical spine in patients with blunt trauma. *N Engl J Med.* 2000;343(2):94–99.
7. American Academy of Pediatrics Committee on Sports Medicine and Fitness. Atlantoaxial instability in Down syndrome: subject review. *Pediatrics.* 1995;96:151.
8. Bull MJ, Committee on Genetics. Health supervision for children with Down syndrome. *Pediatrics.* 2011;128(2):393-406.
9. Samartzis DD, Herman J, Lubicky JP, Shen FH. Classification of congenitally fused cervical patterns in Klippel-Feil patients: epidemiology and role in the development of cervical spine-related symptoms. *Spine.* 2006;31(21):E798–E804.

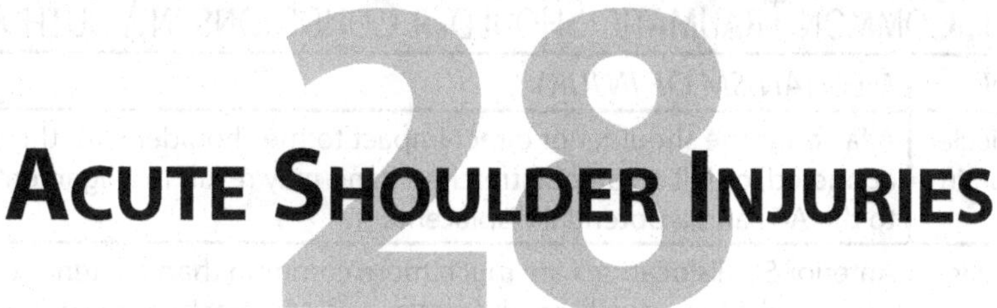

28 Acute Shoulder Injuries

John A. Schlechter, DO

1. A Child Falls and Suffers Immediate Shoulder Pain. What Are Some Potential Diagnoses?

Table 28-1 provides information on some painful injuries that may occur to the shoulder after a fall.

2. What Are the Physical Examination Components When Assessing an Acutely Injured Shoulder?

- A patient evaluation will be dictated by the degree of injury and the time that has transpired from the injury to the presentation. Many patients that are acutely injured have difficulty complying with an examination secondary to pain, apprehension, and guarding.
- An understanding of the relevant anatomy, innervation, and function of the nerve roots that arise from the cervical spine is of paramount importance for a complete neurovascular examination of the extremity (see Table 22-2).
- With anterior-inferior glenohumeral dislocations, the axillary nerve (which supplies cutaneous sensory innervation to the lateral superior aspect of upper arm) is at risk for injury.
- Palpation of the osseous structures for pain, crepitus, and deformity may allow the examiner to locate the specific location of injury (Figure 28-1).
- An assessment of glenohumeral motion and evaluation for ligamentous laxity may be extremely limited in the acute period secondary to pain, apprehension, and guarding, and this portion of the examination may have to be delayed.

3. What Are the Types of Sternoclavicular Injury, and Which Is a Potential Emergency?

- When evaluating a suspected sternoclavicular (SC) joint dislocation, consider the possibility of a medial clavicle physeal fracture in the adolescent patient. The clavicle is the last bone in the body to ossify with fusion of the epiphysis between 23 and 25 years of age[1]; therefore, tension across the SC joint may result in a growth plate fracture (Figure 28-2).
- Anterior SC dislocations commonly occur in a shoulder external rotation with a medially applied compressive force, and tend to lead to a medial clavicle prominence that typically heals with a mild permanent deformity without significant functional limitations. A reduction may be attempted; however, due to an inherent lack of bony stability, subsequent displacement typically occurs. A brief period in a sling or shoulder immobilizer is usually sufficient to allow adequate healing and is followed by a program to restore strength and range of motion (ROM). Surgical intervention is rarely indicated.
- Posterior SC dislocations can present as a life-threatening event due to the impingement of mediastinal structures (airway, great vessels, esophagus, or lungs). Up to 25% of patients

Koutures C, Wong V.
Pediatric Sports Medicine: Essentials for Office Evaluation (pp 183-191)

Table 28-1. Common Traumatic Shoulder Conditions in Youth Athletes

CONDITION	*MECHANISM OF INJURY*
Acromioclavicular joint (ACJ) sprain	A fall onto the shoulder or direct impact to the shoulder with the arm adducted, or fall on an outstretched hand may result in a ligamentous injury to the ACJ and a potential displacement.
Sternoclavicular (SC) joint injury	Anterior SC dislocations are much more common than posterior dislocations (10:1 ratio). They usually result from an indirect mechanism such as an anterior shoulder blow that rotates the shoulder. Direct posterior force to the medial clavicle may result in a posterior dislocation.
Clavicle fracture	A direct fall onto the outer/lateral shoulder, also by a direct blow to the clavicle or by a fall onto an outstretched hand.
Glenohumeral dislocation	Traumatic dislocations typically seen in older adolescents usually after the closure of the proximal humeral physis. They occur either in typical anterior-inferior direction secondary to direct trauma to an abducted externally rotated arm. Posterior dislocations are less common and can occur due to trauma from an anterior-to-posterior force or from a prolonged seizure.
Proximal humerus fracture	Direct blow or indirect trauma (fall onto an outstretched hand). May be associated with a physeal fracture/separation, and a metaphyseal fracture may also occur secondary to a benign bone cyst or lesion.

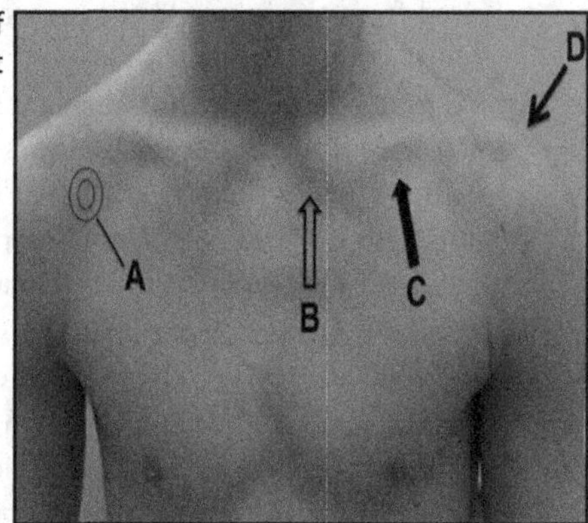

Figure 28-1. Topical shoulder anatomy. Key points of palpation: (A) coracoid process, (B) SC joint, (C) midshaft clavicle, and (D) ACJ.

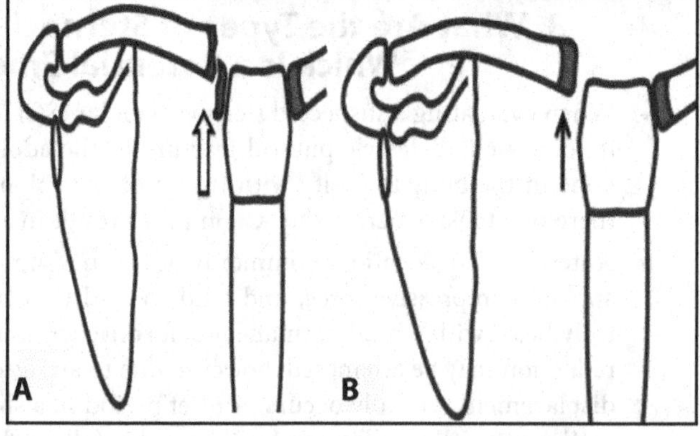

Figure 28-2. (A) Medial clavicle physeal injury with displacement (open arrow). (B) SC dislocation (solid arrow). (Adapted with permission from Wenger D, Pring M. *Rang's Children's Fractures*. 3rd ed. Philadelphia, PA: Lippincott Williams & Wilkins; 2005.)

present with concomitant injury of underlying vital structures; thus, a proper assessment for dysphonia, dyspnea, subcutaneous emphysema, or dysphagia is critical.[2] These findings require urgent stabilization and referral. Initial evaluation includes anteroposterior (AP), oblique, and 40-degree cephalic tilt radiographs, but computed tomography (CT) scan is

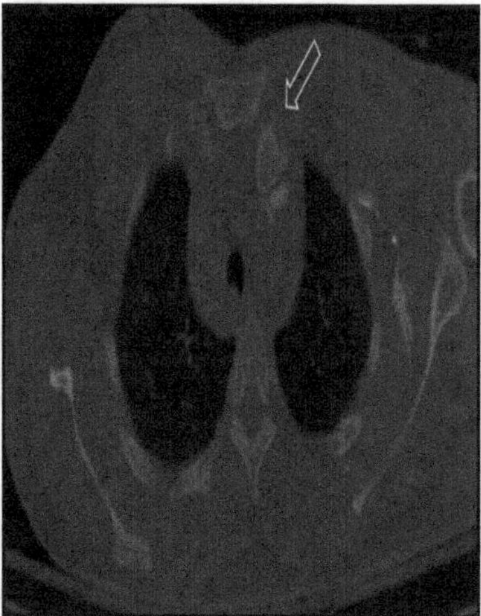

Figure 28-3. Computed tomography scan of an injured 16-year-old male motorcross rider showing a left posterior SC joint dislocation (open white arrow).

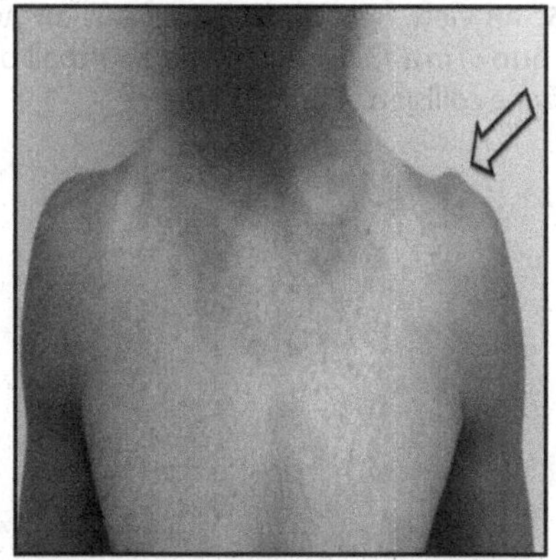

Figure 28-4. A left ACJ separation and apparent prominence (open black arrow) in a 15-year-old male football player.

the best modality for evaluation (Figure 28-3), and contrast allows the evaluation of possible associated vascular injury. Most attempts at external reduction are unsuccessful; thus, open reduction and soft-tissue reconstruction is the preferred treatment. A thoracic surgeon should be notified before beginning a reduction as a precaution for potential airway or vascular injury.

4. What Are the Most Common Acute Acromioclavicular Sprains, How Are They Identified, and Which Sprains Can Be Managed by a Primary Care Provider Versus a Specialist?

Acromioclavicular sprains typically occur after a fall onto the shoulder or a direct impact to the shoulder, causing capsular or ligamentous injury to the acromioclavicular joint (ACJ) or distal clavicle and potential displacement.

- True ACJ dislocations in the skeletally immature patient are rare due to the relatively weaker growth plate compared with the surrounding robust ligaments. Fracture or physeal separation has been referred to "pseudodislocation" of the ACJ.
- Physical examination is significant for tenderness over the affected area and at times a bony "step-off" or prominence at the distal clavicle/ACJ (Figure 28-4). Having the patient reach across his or her body toward the opposite shoulder loads the ACJ and may cause pain.
- Radiographs of the shoulder (AP, axillary, and cephalic tilt views) typically demonstrate increased distance between the coracoid process and the clavicle (Figure 28-5); comparison radiographs are quite useful. Magnetic resonance imaging can distinguish between a sprain, subluxation, dislocation, and physeal separation/distal clavicle fracture, but it is rarely necessary as the treatments for each of these conditions are similar.
- Grades I to III (Figure 28-6 [A through C]) injuries can be treated by a primary care physician, who should recommend that the patient use a sling for 2 to 3 weeks with early initiation of ROM exercises and avoid heavy activity for 6 weeks; healing is generally apparent at 4 to 6 weeks after sustaining the injury. Ample controversy exists regarding the treatment of grades IV to VI (Figure 28-6 [D through F]) injuries; orthopedic referral is appropriate in these cases.
- Most patients experience no functional long-term deficits and are able to fully return to sports.

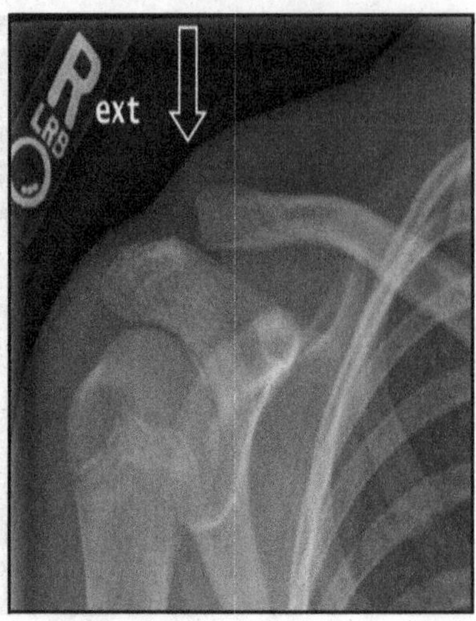

Figure 28-5. AP view right shoulder reveals an ACJ separation (open white arrow) in a 13-year-old female softball player that was sustained after a collision at home plate.

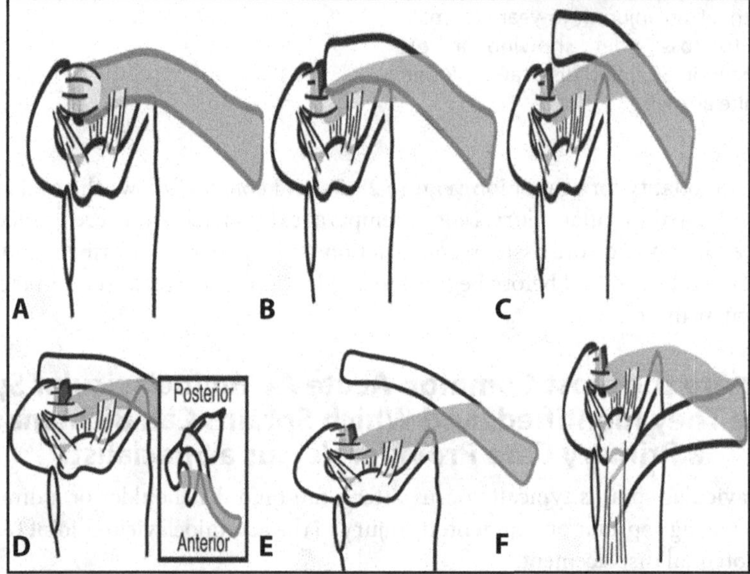

Figure 28-6. Pictoral description and grading of acromioclavicular joint sprains. (A) Grade I: sprain or minimal tear of the acromioclavicular ligament without widening of joint. (B) Grade II: small tear of the acromioclavicular ligament with stretching of the coracoclavicular ligaments and mild damage to the superolateral periosteal sleeve. The x-ray shows minimal acromioclavicular widening. (C) Grade III: complete disruption of the acromioclavicular and coracoclavicular ligaments and large disruption of the periosteal sleeve, resulting in superior displacement of the distal clavicle by 25% to 100%. (D) Grade IV: similar disruption as in grade III except that the distal clavicle is displaced posteriorly into the trapezius muscle. AP films may not identify posterior displacement, emphasizing the need of an axillary x-ray. (E) Grade V: similar tissue disruption as in grade III except that the superior periosteal sleeve is completely disrupted with 100% to 300% superior clavicle. (F) Grade VI: the distal clavicle is displaced inferiorly under the coracoid process. (Adapted with permission from Wenger D, Pring M. *Rang's Children's Fractures.* 3rd ed. Philadelphia, PA: Lippincott Williams & Wilkins; 2005.)

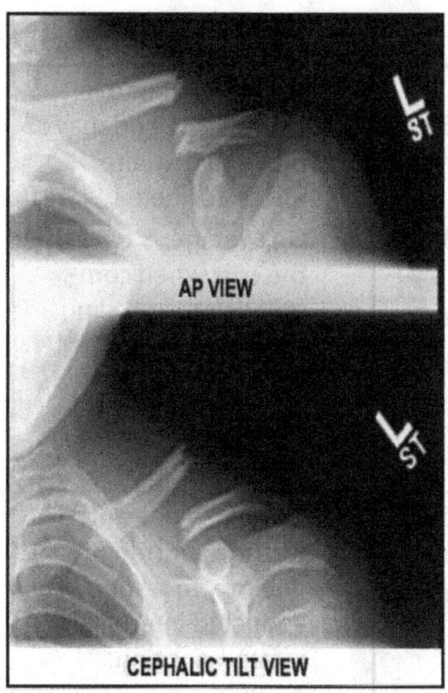

Figure 28-7. AP and cephalic tilt radiographs of a 12-year-old boy with a displaced midshaft clavicle fracture.

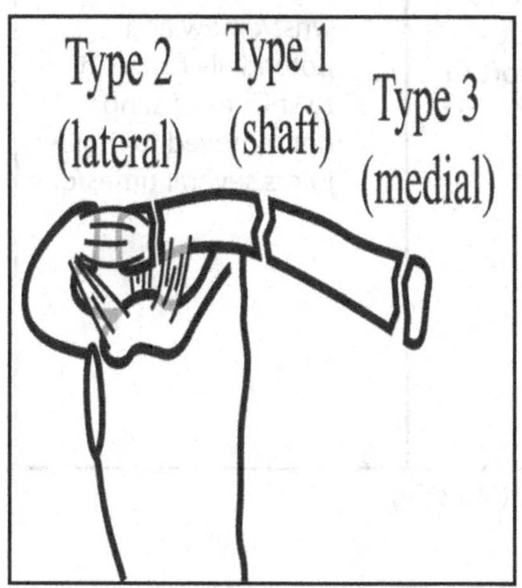

Figure 28-8. Clavicle fracture types. Type 1: fractures medial to the coracoclavicular ligaments and lateral to the sternocleidomastoid muscles. (76% to 85% of all pediatric clavicle fractures). Type 2: fractures lateral to the coracoclavicular ligament (10% to 21%). Type 3: fractures medial to the sternocleidomastoid muscle (3% to 5%). (Adapted with permission from Wenger D, Pring M. *Rang's Children's Fractures.* 3rd ed. Philadelphia, PA: Lippincott Williams & Wilkins; 2005.)

5. What Are the Best X-ray Views to Get for a Clavicle Fracture, and What Are Some Key Differences in Managing Proximal, Midshaft, and Distal Clavicle Fractures?

- X-rays: AP view centered on the clavicle and a cephalad-directed view which is helpful in evaluating degree of fracture displacement. These views can be taken with the x-ray beam angled 20 to 40 degrees cephalad to the clavicle, with the patient in a supine position (Figure 28-7).
- The clavicle is one of the most frequently fractured bones of the body accounting for greater than 90% of obstetrical fractures and 8% to 15% of all pediatric fractures.[2] Clavicular fractures are classified in to 3 types (Figure 28-8).
- Due to immense remodeling capacity of the immature skeleton, and if the periosteum remains intact and gross displacement does not exist, most patients can be treated with immobilization and early ROM exercises regardless of the fracture location. Immobilization is accomplished using a sling or figure 8 brace.
- General operative indications are severely displaced and irreducible fractures that threaten skin integrity or impinge upon the brachial plexus or upon structures within thoracic cavity, disrupted underlying vasculature, or having pierced overlying skin.

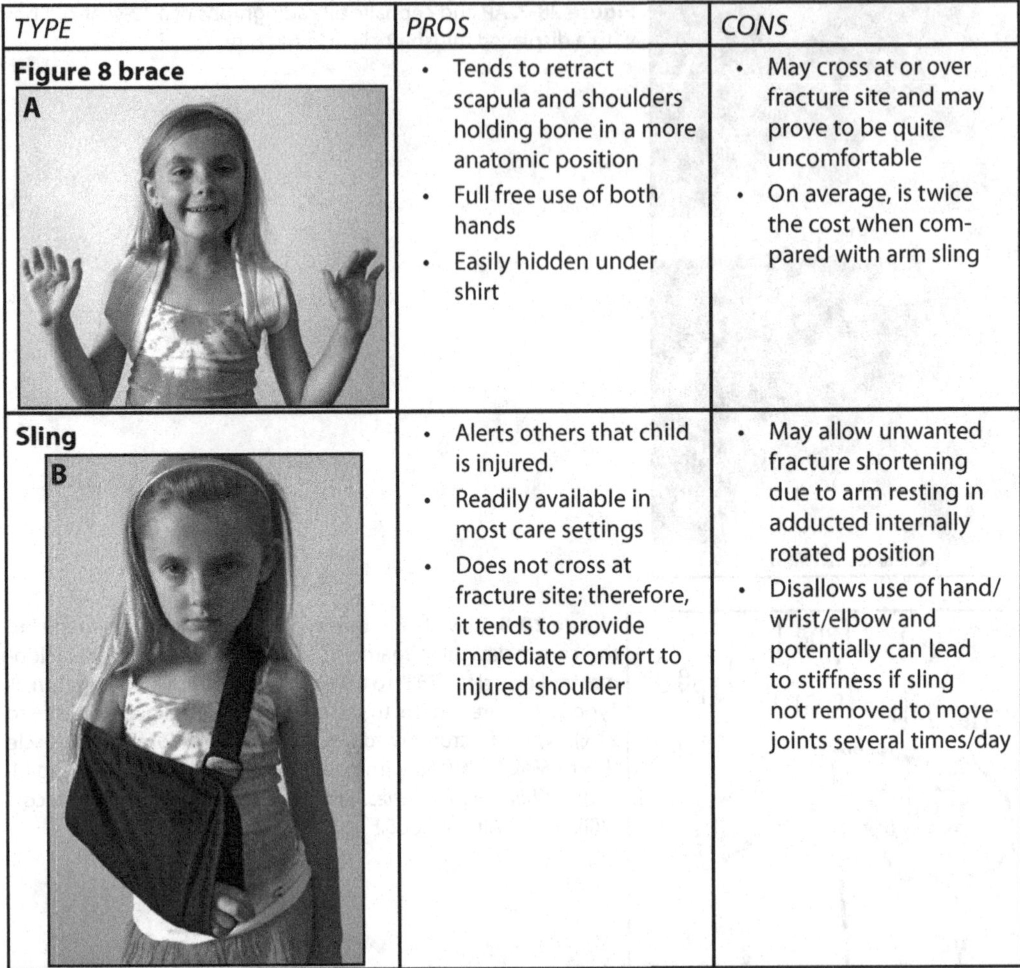

TYPE	PROS	CONS
Figure 8 brace A	• Tends to retract scapula and shoulders holding bone in a more anatomic position • Full free use of both hands • Easily hidden under shirt	• May cross at or over fracture site and may prove to be quite uncomfortable • On average, is twice the cost when compared with arm sling
Sling B	• Alerts others that child is injured. • Readily available in most care settings • Does not cross at fracture site; therefore, it tends to provide immediate comfort to injured shoulder	• May allow unwanted fracture shortening due to arm resting in adducted internally rotated position • Disallows use of hand/wrist/elbow and potentially can lead to stiffness if sling not removed to move joints several times/day

Figure 28-9. Eight-year-old girl wearing (A) a figure 8 brace and (B) a sling.

6. Which Is Better for Acute Clavicle Fractures: A Figure 8 Brace or a Sling?

See Figure 28-9 for information on the pros and cons of figure 8 braces and slings.

7. What Is a Surgical Role for Midshaft Clavicle Fractures in Children and Adolescents?

Absolute indications for open treatment and internal fixation of patients with midshaft clavicle fractures are open fractures or associated neurovascular or intrathoracic compromise. Relative indications include fracture displacement with "skin tenting" that threatens skin integrity and shortening > 1 to 2 cm that may lead to long-term dysfunction, especially if the dominant extremity is affected.

- Operative fixation may be accomplished by plate fixation over the superior or anterior aspect of the clavicle or by placing an intramedullary device. Complications may include implant migration (smooth pin fixation should not be used), infection, nonunion, and symptomatic hardware necessitating removal.
- A recent survey of the Pediatric Orthopaedic Society of North America members resulted in a near unanimous consensus for nonoperative treatment in nondisplaced and angulated midshaft clavicle fractures. For isolated segmental fractures, nearly half of the members

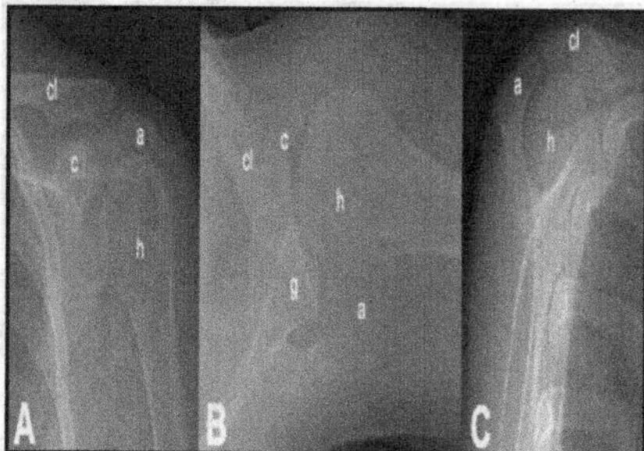

Figure 28-10. Normal left shoulder radiographic series. (A) AP view; (B) axillary view; (C) scapular "Y" view. Relevant anatomy: (a) acromion process; (c) coracoid process; (cl) clavicle; (g) glenoid; and (h) humeral head.

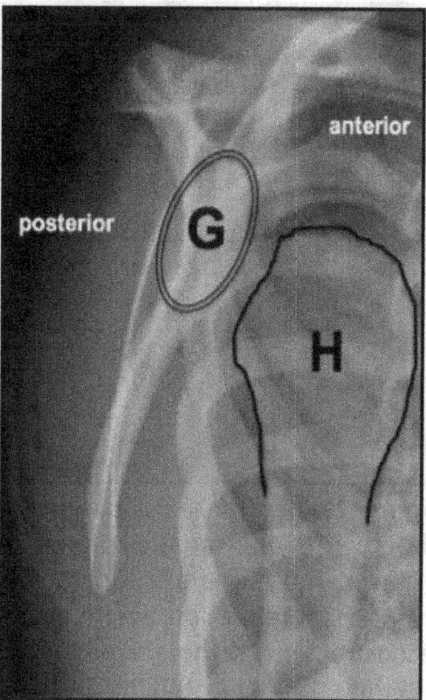

Figure 28-11. Lateral radiograph/scapular "Y" view of 16-year-old male athlete demonstrates anterior displacement of the humeral head (H) relative to the glenoid (G).

surveyed would opt for surgical treatment and were more inclined to operate on this type of fracture in older individuals.[3]

8. How Can One Determine the Difference Between an Acute Shoulder Subluxation and a Dislocation, and What X-ray Views Might Be Helpful in Making the Distinction?

- A dislocation occurs when neither of the 2 bones that create a given joint have normal articular contact, while a subluxation is an incomplete dislocation of a joint that retains some contact between the two bones.
- Subluxation is classically described as a feeling of pain or slipping, or a dead feeling in the arm. The patient may still maintain some ROM of the joint.
- A dislocation of the humeral head is characterized by gross displacement of the head and a severely limited ROM due to the bony constraint of the dislocated humeral head against the rim of the glenoid.
- X-rays: AP, axillary, and scapular "Y" views (Figure 28-10).
- Axillary views require passive abduction of the shoulder to 90 degrees, which may result in significant distress and pain. If the patient cannot comply, scapular lateral ("Y" view) or a transthoracic lateral view may be performed (Figure 28-11).

9. What Soft-Tissue and Bone Injuries May Occur After an Anterior Shoulder Dislocation?

- Hill-Sachs lesion: a posterolateral humeral head impression fracture that occurs from contact with the anterior glenoid rim. It may occur in anywhere from 40% to 90% of anterior dislocations and it approaches 100% in recurrent anterior instability.[4]
- Bankart lesion: the most common soft-tissue injury. Described as a tear of the glenoid labrum that can occur in isolation or may involve bony glenoid rim ("bony" Bankart; Figure 28-12).

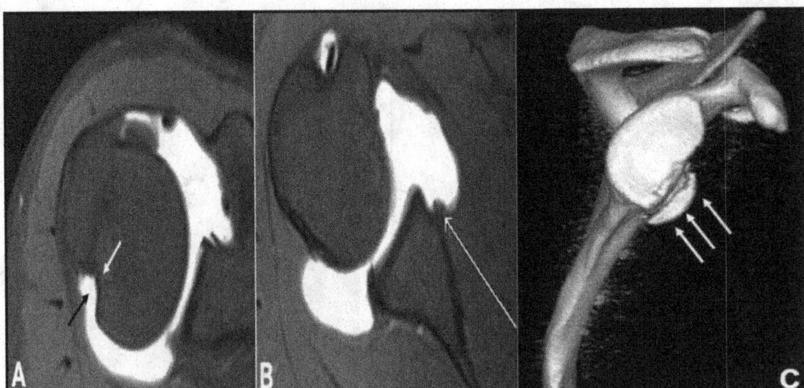

Figure 28-12. Transaxial magnetic resonance images of a 16-year-old football player with symptomatic anterior shoulder instability shows (A) a large Hill-Sachs lesion of the humeral head (black and white arrows) and (B) a Bankart lesion with medial retraction (white arrow). (C) A computed tomography scan with 3D reconstruction of the scapula of a 17-year-old male wrestler with symptomatic anterior shoulder instability and an osseous defect of the anterior inferior glenoid, consistent with "bony" Bankart lesion.

- Stretching or tearing of the glenohumeral ligaments and capsule.
- Humeral avulsion of the glenohumeral ligaments lesion.
- Superior labral anterior to posterior tear.
- Rotator cuff pathology.
- Greater or lesser tuberosity fracture.
- Nerve injury: the axillary nerve is the most commonly injured and, fortunately, most injuries are transient and resolve spontaneously.

10. After a First-Time Anterior Shoulder Dislocation, What Are the Risks/Benefits of Surgical Reconstruction Versus Nonoperative Rehabilitation in Allowing Return to High-Risk Sports and Lessening the Risk of Recurrent Dislocations?

- Nonoperative treatment of anterior dislocation typically entails closed reduction followed by immediate immobilization utilizing a sling or shoulder immobilizer in internal rotation. Immobilization in external rotation has been proposed in a 2007 study[5]; however, it may be awkward, not well tolerated, and may affect compliance.
- After 3 to 4 weeks of immobilization, physical therapy is indicated, with a potential return to high-risk activity 3 to 4 months postinjury with the use of a shoulder-stabilizing brace.
- The recurrence of instability following an anterior glenohumeral dislocation in a young active patient in his or her second decade of life is nearly a certainty.[6]
- Surgical intervention may reduce the risk of recurrent instability when compared with nonoperative treatment. Arthroscopic approaches appear to have similar results in terms of reducing recurrent instability when compared with open approaches.[7,8] Following a traumatic first-time dislocation, the athlete may be best served by orthopedic referral to discuss possible surgical management.

Table 28-2. Preferred Immobilization for Shoulder Injuries in the Youth Athlete

INJURY	*TYPE OF IMMOBILIZATION*	*DURATION*
Anterior glenohumeral dislocation	Shoulder immobilizer	~ 3 weeks
Posterior glenohumeral dislocation	Shoulder immobilizer	~ 3 weeks
Proximal humerus fracture	Arm sling/shoulder immobilizer	4+ weeks or until pain-free active ROM of the shoulder is possible
Humeral shaft fracture	Arm sling/shoulder immobilizer/humeral fracture brace/long arm cast	~ 6 weeks or until adequate subperiosteal new bone formation consistent with healing callus on follow-up radiographs
Acromioclavicular sprain/separation	Arm sling	1 to 3 weeks
Scapular fracture	Arm sling	2 to 4 weeks
Clavicle fracture	Sling or figure 8 brace	~ 4 weeks
SC dislocation	Arm sling	6 weeks

11. Should an Acute Shoulder Injury Be Immobilized? If So, in What Position, for How Long, and What Other Rehabilitation Tips Should Be Considered?

Table 28-2 provides information on the different types of injuries, such as an anterior glenohumeral dislocation, that should be immobilized and the types of immobilization that are most appropriate for that injury.

References

1. Ogden JA, Conlogue GJ, Bronson ML. Radiology of postnatal skeletal development. The clavicle. *Skeletal Radiol.* 1979;4(4):196–203.
2. Beaty J, Kasser J. *Rockwood and Wilkins' Fractures in Children.* 6th ed. Philadelphia, PA: Lippincott Williams & Wilkins; 2005.
3. Carry PM, Koonce R, Pan Z, Polousky JD. A survey of physician opinion adolescent midshaft clavicle fracture treatment preferences among POSNA members. *J Pediatr Orthop.* 2011;31(1):44–49.
4. Provencher MT, Frank RM, LeClere LE, et al. The Hill-Sachs lesion: diagnosis, classification and management. *J Am Acad Orthop Surg.* 2012;20:242–252.
5. Itoi E, Hatakeyama Y, Takeshi S, et al. Immobilization in external rotation after shoulder dislocation reduces the risk of recurrence: a randomized controlled trial. *J Bone Joint Surg Am.* 2007;89:2124–2131.
6. Marans HJ, Angel KR, Schemitsch EH, Wedge JH. The fate of traumatic anterior dislocation of the shoulder in children. *J Bone Joint Surg Am.* 1992;74:1242–1245.
7. Bottoni CR, Wilckens JH, DeBerardino TM, et al. A prospective, randomized evaluation of arthroscopic stabilization versus nonoperative treatment in patients with acute, traumatic, first-time shoulder dislocations. *Am J Sports Med.* 2002;30(4): 576–580.
8. Brophy RH, Marx RG. The treatment of traumatic anterior instability of the shoulder: nonoperative and surgical treatment. *Arthroscopy.* 2009;25(3):298–304.

Acknowledgment

I would like to express my gratitude to Ryan Shelden, BS, currently a third-year medical student, for his assistance with the preparation of this chapter.

29 Chronic and Overuse Shoulder Injuries

John A. Schlechter, DO

1. Can Adolescent Athletes Have Shoulder Impingement Syndrome? How Is the Presentation in an Adolescent Different From the Presentation in an Adult?

- Adolescent athletes can suffer from shoulder impingement, which is a decrease in the subacromial space available for the rotator cuff muscles due to bone spur (primary impingement) or scapula malposition (secondary impingement).
- Acromial apophysitis or an os acromiale (failure of the acromial ossification center to fuse to the acromium process) may contribute to impingement-like symptoms. An os acromiale is also a risk factor for rotator cuff tears.
- Overtraining, hypertrophy, and postural imbalance coupled with weak periscapular muscles can lead to an unopposed pull of the tight pectoralis minor attachment to the coracoid process, which can lead to secondary impingement as the acromium tilts forward, especially when the humeral head is in forward elevation of the arm[1] (Figure 29-1).

The classic presentation is a patient who sits or stands with a forward positioned head and neck, focal cervical lordosis (usually at C5 to C6), thoracic kyphosis, and protracted scapulae.[2] Lumbar lordosis with poor abdominal muscle control is frequently associated with shoulder impingement syndrome. An athlete with shoulder impingement syndrome typically reports pain with overhead activity (Figures 29-2).

- On examination, pain is elicited with forward elevation of the arm, with concomitant internal rotation of the humerus. The pectoralis minor should be assessed for shortening or tightness (Figure 29-3).
- Plain radiographs can assess osseous structures, especially the morphology of the acromion process. In primary impingement, there may be a hooked shaped or a curved acromion and/or a bone spur on the undersurface of the acromion (Figure 29-4). An outlet view of the shoulder is most useful in assessing acromial morphology. Magnetic resonance imaging (MRI) can assess the rotator cuff and is indicated if rotator cuff dysfunction is detected on physical examination.
- Patients with secondary shoulder impingement are candidates for formal physical therapy (PT) that focuses on scapular stabilization and soft-tissue modalities. Surgery is rarely indicated.

2. What Is Youth Thrower's Shoulder?

- *Youth thrower's shoulder* is an inflammatory condition of the proximal humeral growth plate or physis that occurs in skeletally immature children and adolescents who engage in various overhead sports that require a repetitive shoulder motion such as baseball, tennis,

Koutures C, Wong V.
Pediatric Sports Medicine: Essentials for Office Evaluation (pp 192-199)

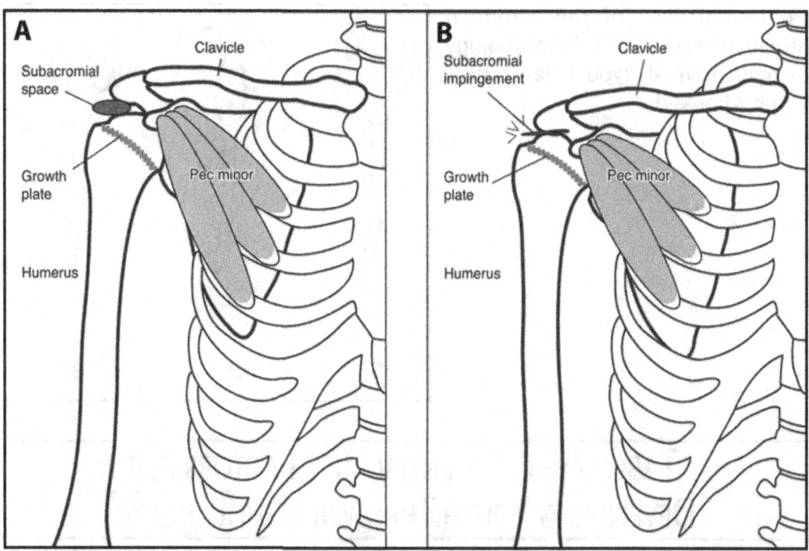

Figure 29-1. (A) Normal pectoralis minor length with preservation of the subacromial space. (B) Secondary impingement due to scapular malposition from a tight pectoralis minor.

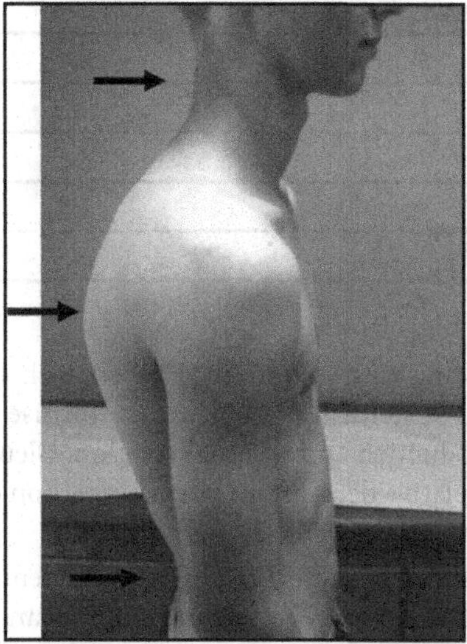

Figure 29-2. Postural imbalance. Arrows (from top down) depict forward head and neck, focal cervical lordosis, thoracic kyphosis, and protracted scapulae and increased lumbar lordosis.

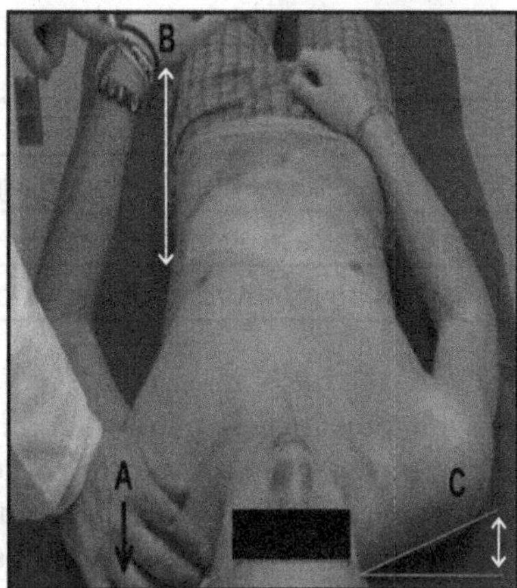

Figure 29-3. Pectoralis minor assessment. Posterior force is applied to the left shoulder (A, black arrow) and the forearm, wrist, and hand involuntarily elevate and externally rotate, (B) indicating significant pectoralis minor tightness. (C) Depicts the resting anterior tilt of the right shoulder.

and water polo. The risk factors for developing youth thrower's shoulder include pitching more than 100 innings per year (Table 29-1).[3,4]

- A growth plate is composed of cartilage cells arranged in nests and columns, with transformational growth progressing from cartilage to bone, which adds length to the extremity. The growth plate cartilage is weaker than bone, making it more vulnerable to injury, especially during periods of maximal growth. In severe cases, the stress may lead to a small break or fracture of the growth plate.

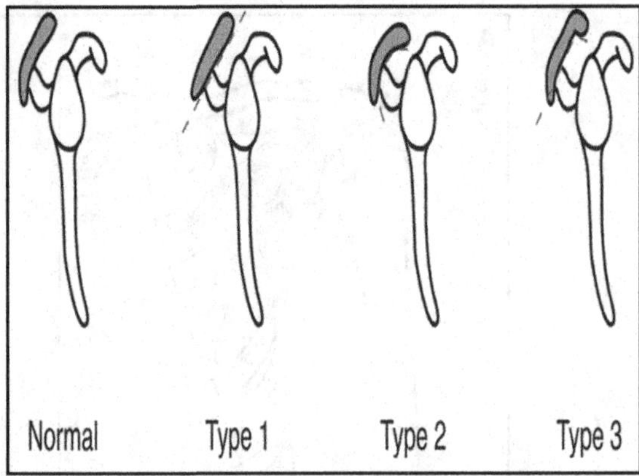

Figure 29-4. Lateral view of the acromion, depicting the variations in acromial morphology. From left to right: normal, type I flat, type 2 curved, and type 3 hooked.

Table 29-1. Potential Risk Factors for Developing Youth Thrower's Shoulder[3,4]
• Year-round participation in a single overhead throwing sport
• Pitchers who concomitantly play catcher in the same season • Moving a participant from pitcher to catcher or vice versa in the same contest/game
• Weekend tournaments, with little or no rest between games
• Pitching > 100 innings per year
• Poor throwing mechanics
• Pitch type (curveball throwing at a young age)
• Participating in showcase events
• Use of a radar gun to measure throwing velocity

- Typical symptoms include pain when throwing with less strength or control. There may be swelling or tenderness, typically located posterolateral, but can be diffuse along the proximal humerus. Pain is exacerbated in abduction and external rotation. Glenohumeral external rotation may be increased, with a relative decrease in internal rotation compared with the contralateral shoulder.
- Plain radiographs are usually negative; however, in advanced cases, widening of the growth plate may be observed (Figure 29-5). MRI is rarely necessary, but it can detect the degree of physeal disturbance and reveal signal changes in the periphyseal region.

Treatment

- Youth thrower's shoulder typically resolves if it is properly treated, but if it is ignored, it can limit a young athlete's career and cause chronic shoulder pain as an adult.
- The best treatment is prevention. In youth throwers, pitch counts should be monitored.[5] Adequate rest between appearances is of paramount importance. To reference age-appropriate pitch count and rest recommendations, please visit www.littleleague.org/Assets/forms_pubs/media/PitchingRegulationChanges_BB_11-13-09.pdf
- Youth pitchers should avoid throwing breaking pitches[6] (curves, sliders) until they reach physical maturity, and they should avoid multiple appearances in a single game. Pitchers need a period of "active rest" after the season ends and before the next preseason begins. For a minimum of 3 months per year, pitchers should NOT play any baseball or participate in throwing drills or other stressful overhead activities. Instruction in proper mechanics

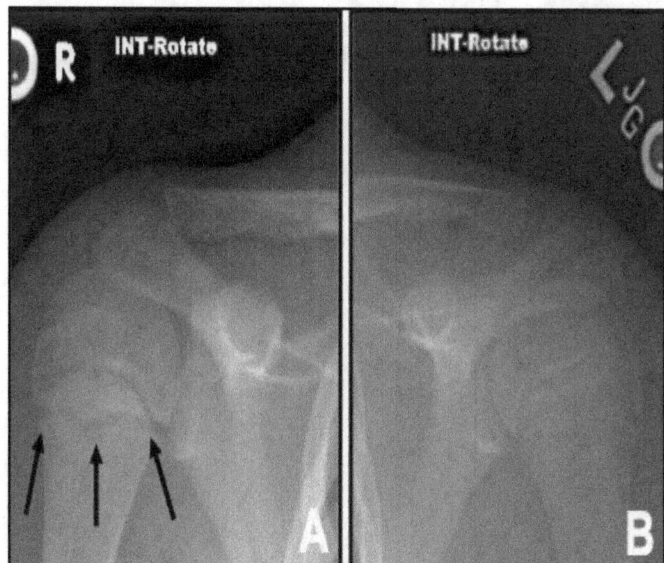

Figure 29-5. 12 year old male pitcher with right shoulder pain. (A) AP x-ray of the symptomatic shoulder in internal rotation shows subtle proximal humeral physeal widening (solid arrows). (B) Comparison radiograph of the contralateral shoulder is with normal physeal morphology.

should be initiated as early as possible. Year-round physical/core conditioning should be emphasized as the body develops.

- For children with active symptoms, stop the aggravating activity so that the growth plate can heal. To prevent re-injury, formal PT can improve shoulder muscle strength, assess throwing mechanics, and functionally progress the athlete back to competition. Youth throwers should not throw with pain.

3. Do Children Get Rotator Cuff Injuries?

- Rotator cuff injuries are less frequent in children than in adults, and are rarely complete tears.
- The SITS (Supraspinatus, Infraspinatus, Teres minor, and Subscapularis) muscles coalesce to form the rotator cuff. The first three insert on the greater tuberosity of the humerus, while the subscapularis inserts on the lesser tuberosity. The humeral tuberosities each have growth plates that provide appositional growth.
- Rotator cuff injuries range from incomplete tendon tears/fraying (typically from overuse) to traumatic complete tears, and apophyseal avulsion fractures of the humeral tuberosities, particularly subscapularis avulsion of the lesser tuberosity.[7]
- A high index of suspicion is required to promptly diagnose rotator cuff pathology in youth athletes. Athletes typically report activity-related pain and dysfunction, and may have weakness or limitations with elevation, abduction, and internal and/or external rotation. X-rays can assess for osseous abnormalities including apophyseal avulsion fractures. Radiographs can be falsely negative; MRI remains the gold standard for imaging the rotator cuff and proximal humeral tuberosities.
- Suspected or proven rotator cuff pathology should be referred for a formal orthopedic evaluation. Primary treatment for partial thickness tears includes activity modification, ice, anti-inflammatory medications as necessary, and referral to PT. Operative treatment is reserved for cases where there is failure to progress with adequate PT, complete and/or retracted tears, and displaced avulsion fractures.

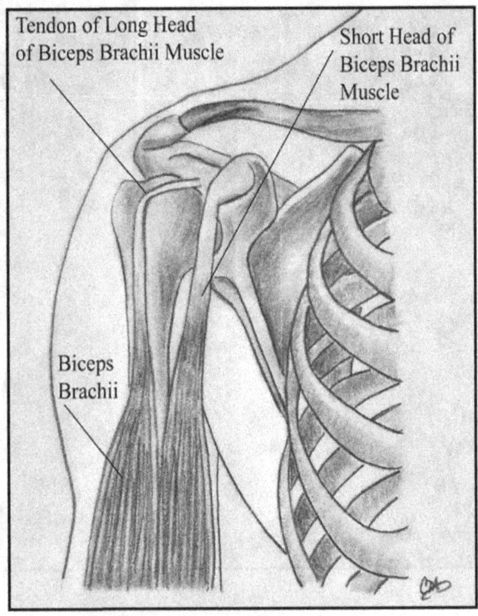

Figure 29-6. The proximal biceps has two origins: the long head on the superior aspect of glenoid and the short head on the coracoid process. (Graphite Pencil-Copyright © 2012 Cora Maglaya, PT, ATC, CSCS.)

4. A 12-Year-Old Pitcher Presents With Pain at the Anterior Region of His or Her Shoulder After Pitching in a Tournament Over the Weekend. The Pain Worsens With Throwing, but Improves With Rest. What Could This Be?

- Amongst the many causes of anterior shoulder pain, this scenario is a typical presentation of an inflamed biceps tendon (Figure 29-6).
- Biceps tendonitis almost exclusively occurs from overuse, causing inflammation of the sheath or lining of the tendon and leading to pain and dysfunction. Other causes include a sudden increase in the amount or intensity of training and direct trauma. Athletes with biceps tendonitis will have activity-related anterior pain and loss of throwing velocity.
- Examination findings are pain over the anterior shoulder and with biceps testing.
- X-rays can rule out any osseous processes; MRIs are reserved for atypical cases.
- The best treatment for biceps tendonitis is prevention. Appropriate warm-up and stretching before activity with adequate rest and recovery between events are important. In symptomatic athletes, stop aggravating activity. To prevent reinjury, PT can improve the athlete's shoulder strength, assess their throwing mechanics, and functionally progress him or her back to competition. Referral to an orthopedic or sports medicine specialist is appropriate in cases with extreme dysfunction and/or severe symptoms.

5. What Are Proper Throwing and Swimming Techniques for Young Athletes?

- For youth throwers, proper throwing technique involves maintaining soft-tissue homeostasis in the periscapular and shoulder girdle musculature while adhering to a core-strengthening program.
- The athlete should position his or her throwing arm in the plane of the scapula (Figure 29-7).
- Youth swimmers can benefit from maximizing body roll during their swim stroke and from using larger core muscles, early catch and exit, and straight-through arm pulls, all of which create a sleeker bodyline or "vessel" to decrease drag and resistance.
- Efficient swimming can be assessed by the number of strokes necessary (stroke rate) to complete a single lap or pool length. Decreasing one's stroke rate while increasing stroke

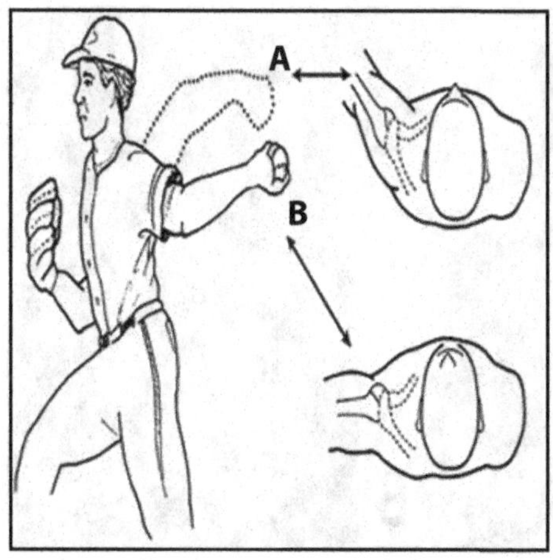

Figure 29-7. (A, dotted line). Proper mechanics with arm position in abduction in the plane of the scapula with the elbow high enough to keep the upper arm at or above the horizontal plane. (B) Improper mechanics represented by a "dropped elbow" (solid line), with hyperangulation posterior to the scapula plane. (Adapted with permission from Burkhart S, Morgan C, Kibler WB. The disabled throwing shoulder: spectrum of pathology part III: the SICK scapula, scapular dyskinesis, the kinetic chain, and rehabilitation. *Arthroscopy.* 2003;19(6):641-661.)

length through extension and body roll will maximize efficiency. Limiting thumb-first hand entry that crosses midline may decrease the risk of impingement. Unilateral breathing and asymmetric body roll may increase the risk of developing symptoms.

6. A 12-Year-Old Swimmer Presents With Painless Popping in His or Her Shoulders and Intermittent Sensations That His or Her "Shoulder Is Slipping Out of Place." He or She Denies Any Trauma. Is It Possible That the Athlete Has Repetitive Mild Joint Instability?

- Multidirectional instability (MDI) may have unilateral symptoms, but athletes often have bilateral laxity. The physical examination should evaluate for generalized hyperlaxity and can be graded using the Beighton scale.[8]
- MDI may have unilateral symptoms, but athletes often have bilateral laxity. The physical examination should evaluate for generalized hyperlaxity and can be graded using the Beighton scale[8] (see Figure 14-3).
- Other findings are sulcus sign and load and shift testing (Figures 29-8 and 29-9).
- Imaging includes a standard shoulder series; MRI should be reserved for atypical cases. Atraumatic MDI is treated primarily with PT; a prolonged course is sometimes necessary. Surgery should be reserved for those who have had multiple failures at nonoperative treatment and activity modification.

7. Many Athletes Have Recurrent Shoulder Subluxations or Actual Dislocations. What Are the Management/Rehabilitation Recommendations for Both of These Issues, and When Should These Athletes Be Referred? Does Bracing Help?

- A shoulder subluxation occurs when the humeral head ("ball") partially comes out of the glenoid ("socket") with minimal trauma and then spontaneously relocates.
- A shoulder dislocation occurs when the humeral head moves completely beyond the anatomic extent of the glenoid, characteristically occurring in an anterior-inferior direction. Dislocations occur from a rather forceful fall or a direct blow to an abducted and externally rotated arm, are more painful, and often require medical care for reduction.
- The physical examination of a patient with only subluxation of the joint may be rather normal. The examination should assess the athlete's overall range of motion (ROM), manual muscle testing of the rotator cuff and periscapular muscles, and assessment for generalized hyperlaxity and glenohumeral stability using the sulcus sign and the load and shift and apprehension tests (Figure 29-10).

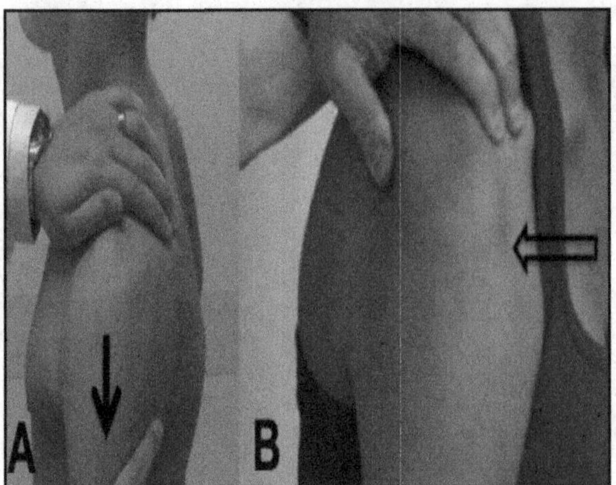

Figure 29-8. (A) Sulcus sign. Apply downward traction (solid black arrow) through humeral shaft with arm at the patient's side. A positive test will result in a sulcus being formed between the acromion and the humeral head. Displacement > 2 cm is abnormal, and 3 cm or greater is considered severe. The sulcus sign is felt to be pathognomonic of multidirectional instability. (B) Apparent sulcus (open arrow) in an adolescent athlete with MDI.

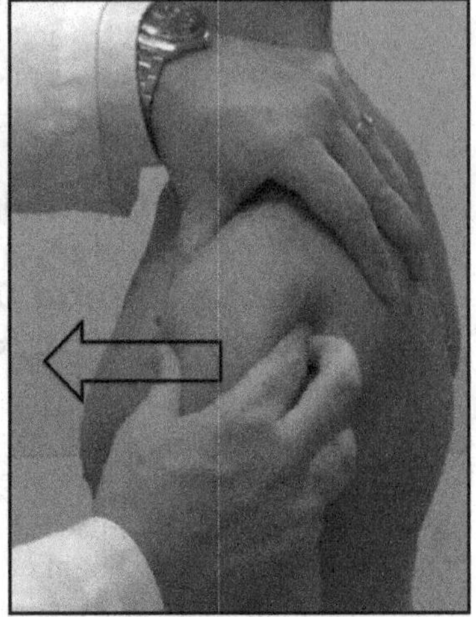

Figure 29-9. Load and shift test. With the patient in a seated position, the examiner stabilizes his or her shoulder and applies an anterior (open arrow) and/or posterior force with the humeral head loaded on to the glenoid to determine the amount of "shift" of the humeral head relative to the socket. The examination should be performed on both shoulders and can be graded as mild (0- to 1-cm translation), moderate (1 to 2 cm or translates to glenoid rim), or severe (> 2-cm translation or over glenoid rim).

- In recurrent laxity, MRIs with intra-articular contrast and noncontrast computed tomography scans assess soft tissues and osseous integrity, respectively.
- Management of recurrent shoulder instability is primarily nonoperative and relies on PT to strengthen the shoulder girdle and dynamic stabilizers and improve scapular control.
- Orthopedic referral and potentially surgical repair and stabilization are indicated in recurrent instability that has failed nonoperative treatment and conceivably for contact athletes who have suffered traumatic dislocation(s).
- Prefabricated braces are available that restrict ROM; however, there is no brace that will completely prevent traumatic dislocation. Many find such braces to be too restrictive and not compatible with their position or sport.

8. Why Is the Stability of the Scapula Important in Overhead Athletes? How Does the Scapula Become "Unstable," and What Is "SICK Scapula Syndrome?"

- SICK (actually an acronym) scapula syndrome[9] is typically seen in overhead throwing athletes and is related to an overuse muscle fatigue syndrome. It can be secondary to intrinsic shoulder pathology.
  - S—Scapular malposition.
  - I—Inferior medial scapular border prominence.

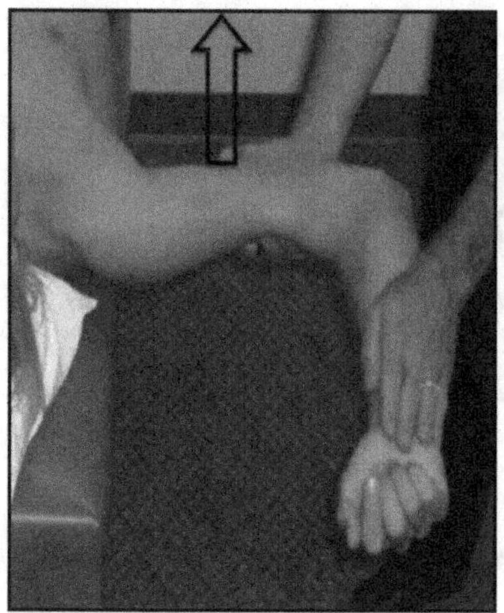

Figure 29-10. Apprehension test performed with the patient's supine and the scapula stabilized by the examination table. The arm is abducted and externally rotated, and an anteriorly directed force (open arrow) is applied. A positive examination will elicit "apprehension" from the patient and a sensation of impending subluxation of the joint.

  - C—Coracoid pain and malposition.
  - K—Dyskinesis of scapular movement.
- The classic physical examination finding is scapula malposition in the dominant arm, which usually appears as if one shoulder is lower than the other.
- Other causes for shoulder height asymmetry should be excluded, especially in younger adolescents (scoliosis, pelvic obliquity, and limb length discrepancy).
- Imaging should include standard shoulder series; one should reserve MRI for atypical cases.
- Treatment is almost always nonoperative. Referral to a physical therapist who is familiar with SICK scapula syndrome is necessary to help the patient retrain movement patterns of his or her shoulder girdle, obtain soft-tissue balance, and re-educate his or her periscapular muscles. Referral to an orthopedic surgeon/sports medicine specialist should be considered in refractory cases to rule out contributing shoulder pathology.

References

1. Borstad JD, Ludewig PM. The effect of long versus short pectoralis minor resting length on scapular kinematics in healthy individuals. *J Orthop Sports Phys Ther.* 2005;35(4):227–238.
2. Greenfield B, Catlin PA, Coats PW, et al. Posture in patients with shoulder overuse injuries and healthy individuals. *J Orthop Sports Phys Ther.* 1995;21:287–295.
3. Fleisig GS, Andrews JR, Cutter GR, et al. Risk of serious injury for young baseball pitchers: a 10-year prospective study. *Am J Sports Med.* 2011;39(2):253–257.
4. Kerut EK, Kerut DG, Fleisig GS, et al. Prevention of arm injury in youth baseball pitchers. *J La State Med Soc.* 2008;160(2):95–98
5. Andrews JR, Fleisig GS. How many pitches should I allow my child to throw? *USA Baseball News.* 1996.
6. Lyman S, Fleisig GS, Andrews JR, Osinski ED. Effect of pitch type, pitch count, and pitching mechanics on risk of elbow and shoulder pain in youth baseball pitchers. *Am J Sports Med.* 2002;30(4):463–468.
7. Vezeridis PS, Bae DS, Kocher MS, et al. Surgical treatment for avulsion injuries of the humeral lesser tuberosity apophysis in adolescents. *J Bone Joint Surg Am.* 2011;93:1882–1888.
8. Beighton P, Horan F. Orthopaedic aspects of the Ehlers-Danlos syndrome. *J Bone Joint Surg Br.* 1969;51:444–453.
9. Burkhart S, Morgan C, Kibler WB. The disabled throwing shoulder: spectrum of pathology part III: the SICK scapula, scapular dyskinesis, the kinetic chain, and rehabilitation. *Arthroscopy.* 2003;19(6):641–661.

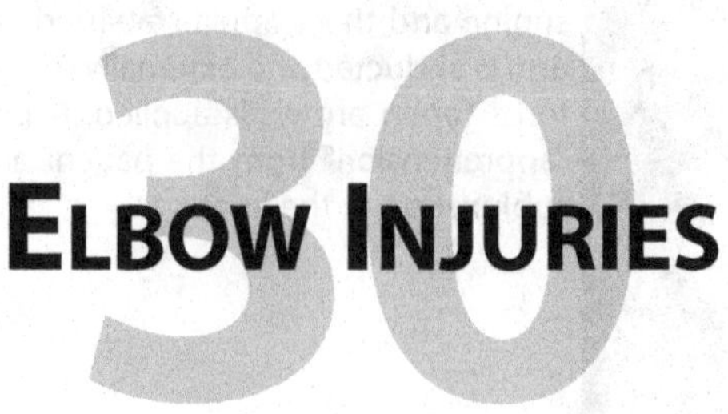

30 Elbow Injuries

Greg Landry, MD

1. What Is the Significance of an Intra-articular Effusion of the Elbow, How Can One Tell if It Is Present, and What Initial X-ray Evaluations and Referrals Should Be Considered?

An intra-articular effusion will be best appreciated by examining the dimple adjacent to the lateral epicondyle and comparing it with the uninjured side. The dimple is more prominent with the elbow extended. If the dimple is gone, that means that there is fluid in the elbow joint. In the setting of an acute injury, its presence means a hemarthrosis and should lead to x-ray examinations. It is usually adequate to order two views: anteroposterior and lateral. Sometimes, a radiocapitellar view will be necessary to see a radial head fracture. On the lateral view, the anterior fat pad may be seen as being pushed away from the bone just anterior to the coronoid fossa. This is known as the "sail" sign. If a fat pad is seen posterior to the olecranon, this too is an indication of a hemarthrosis. The presence of a hemarthrosis is usually a sign of a fracture. Orthopedic consultation should be considered if there is a hemarthrosis, normal x-ray findings, and the patient has significant loss of motion.

If the effusion is of a more insidious onset, a rheumatologic cause should be considered. X-ray examinations should be performed to look for osteochondritis dissecans and similar disorders that might account for the effusion. Magnetic resonance imaging (MRI) should be considered if the rheumatologic evaluation is totally negative to look for any articular cartilage abnormality or loose body.

2. What Is a Supracondylar Fracture, Which Age Groups Are at the Highest Risk, How Can It Be Identified on X-ray, and What Are the Initial Immobilization and Referral Guidelines?

Supracondylar fractures occur just proximal to the condyles where the humerus flattens and flares. They are most common from age 5 to 8 years. They are usually seen easily on x-rays, and the degree of displacement is determined on the lateral view. Supracondylar fractures should be immobilized in a long posterior splint with the elbow flexed to 90 degrees and the forearm rotation neutral. If there is any neurovascular compromise, the elbow should be extended until the neurovascular function returns to normal. Immediate orthopedic consultation is indicated for any neurovascular compromise, while urgent referral to an orthopedic surgeon is recommended for all other supracondylar fractures due to the high risk of early or late neurovascular compromise.

Koutures C, Wong V.
Pediatric Sports Medicine: Essentials for Office Evaluation (pp 200-205)

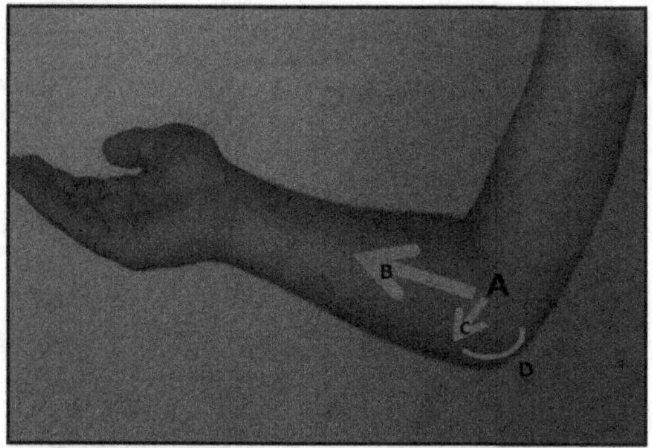

Figure 30-1. Key structures of the medial elbow. (A) Medial epicondyle; (B) flexor-pronator muscles; (C) ulnar collateral ligament; and (D) ulnar nerve.

3. What Is the Usual Mechanism of an Elbow Dislocation/Subluxation, and What Are Both Short-Term and Long-Term Concerns With Such an Injury?

Elbow dislocations/subluxations are relatively common in young athletes and are usually due to a fall on an outstretched arm. The injury normally results in the complete disruption of the ligaments around the elbow. X-rays should always be performed to make sure that there is no associated fracture. A good neurovascular examination should be performed both prereduction and postreduction. The biggest long-term problem with an elbow dislocation is the loss of motion. It is important to work diligently on range of motion (ROM) early and not immobilize longer than 2 to 3 weeks.

4. An Athlete Presents With Swelling of the Olecranon Bursa. What Are the Pros and Cons of Drainage, and What Are the Criteria for Return to Play?

Olecranon bursitis can occur due to acute trauma and bleeding into the bursa or from repetitive trauma. It can usually be managed with compression, ice, and the judicious use of a nonsteroidal anti-inflammatory drug. It rarely requires drainage. Draining of the bursa risks infection, and fluid usually reaccumulates. The bursa should be tapped if there is any suspicion for infection (increased warmth of the area or rapid increase in pain and swelling). Olecranon bursitis should rarely affect the ability of an athlete to return to play. In collision sports, the area can be protected with a doughnut pad. Rarely, the bursitis becomes chronic and a bursectomy will be indicated.

5. A Throwing Athlete Comes to Your Clinic With Medial Elbow Pain. What Structures Are Potentially at Risk, and What Examination/X-ray Findings Can Help One Make a Proper Diagnosis?

In the growing athlete, medial elbow pain can represent either acute or chronic overuse injury to the medial apophysis, ulnar collateral ligament (UCL), flexor-pronator tendon, ulnar nerve, or any combination (Figure 30-1). The diagnosis can usually be made by a careful physical examination and x-rays.

- An avulsion or irritation of the medial apophyseal growth plate can be at risk for nonunion and persistent pain (Figure 30-2). An apophyseal injury should be suspected when there is bony tenderness and pain with resisted pronation and wrist flexion. X-rays may show some widening of the growth plate, and comparison views to the uninjured elbow are often helpful. If injury to a growth plate is suspected, total rest from throwing activities is indicated for about 6 weeks, or until the elbow is no longer tender.

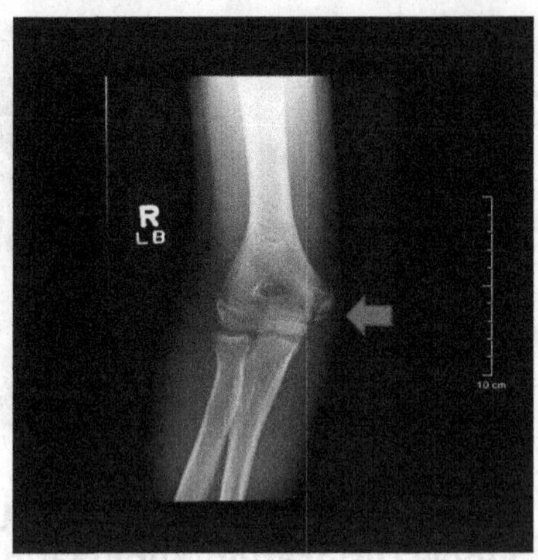

Figure 30-2. Avulsion of medial apophysis.

- UCL tears may result in chronic pain and instability. The UCL is assessed by applying valgus stress to the elbow in 30 degrees of flexion and comparing it with the uninjured side. If a ruptured UCL injury is suspected, an ultrasonography or MRI arthrogram can assess the integrity of the ligament (see question 7).
- A more benign injury would be a flexor-pronator strain, which is less likely to cause persistent pain if treated properly with relative rest and rehabilitation. This injury will cause tenderness over the tendon just distal to the medial apophysis, and the patient will experience pain (and sometimes weakness) with resisted pronation and wrist flexion.
- Any of these injuries can also irritate the ulnar nerve, as occasionally a medial injury will result in a dislocating ulnar nerve. This is usually diagnosed by manually pulling the ulnar nerve out of the cubital tunnel. When there is inflammation of the ulnar nerve, the patient may report intermittent numbness and tingling in the medial forearm, radiating into the fourth and fifth fingers. This is thought to be from compression of the nerve in the cubital tunnel (cubital tunnel syndrome). Tapping the ulnar nerve (positive Tinel sign) can reproduce the symptoms. Manual muscle testing should be performed for the flexor carpi ulnaris, adductor pollicus, and intrinsic muscles of the hand, as they are supplied by the ulnar nerve. It is unusual to have weakness. Sleeping with the elbow extended and wrapped in a towel will often help the symptoms of ulnar neuritis. This problem is often treated surgically by permanently transposing the nerve anterior to the cubital tunnel.

6. What Are the Risk Factors for Developing "Thrower's Elbow," and What Anticipatory Guidance Can Help Prevent This Injury?

Throwers can develop medial elbow pain due to valgus overload. The act of throwing tends to open the medial side of the elbow while compressing the lateral side. Medial pain may occur from an injury to any of the medial structures previously mentioned. Risk factors for developing elbow injuries in throwers include pitching for more than 8 months of the year and pitching more than 80 pitches per game. Poor throwing mechanics, arm fatigue, and weight lifting have also been discussed as risk factors.[1] Issues with the ipsilateral shoulder (limited glenohumeral internal rotation, poor scapular position, and rotator cuff weakness), lumbosacral region (limited lumber flexion and rotation, and weak gluteal and abdominal muscles) and contralateral hip (limited internal rotation),[1] can contribute to medial elbow pain. Breaking balls (curve balls and sliders) may increase one's chance of developing elbow pain, but there is little scientific evidence to support that recommendation. The USA Baseball Medical/Safety Advisory Committee and Little League Baseball have created guidelines for young pitchers, and recommendations for the appropriate

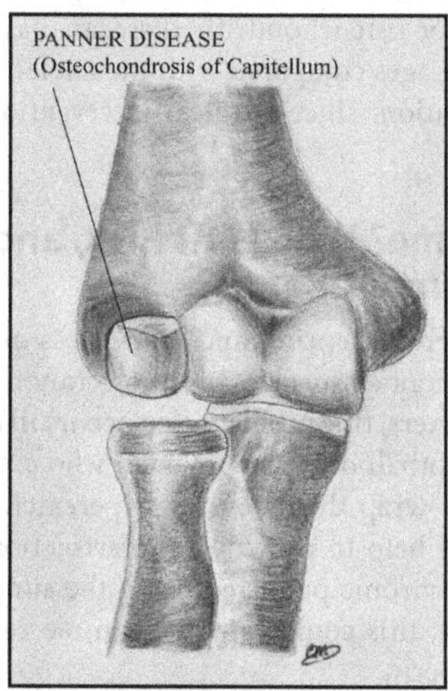

Figure 30-3. Panner osteochondrosis of the capitellum. (Graphite Pencil-Copyright © 2012 Cora Maglaya, PT, ATC, CSCS.)

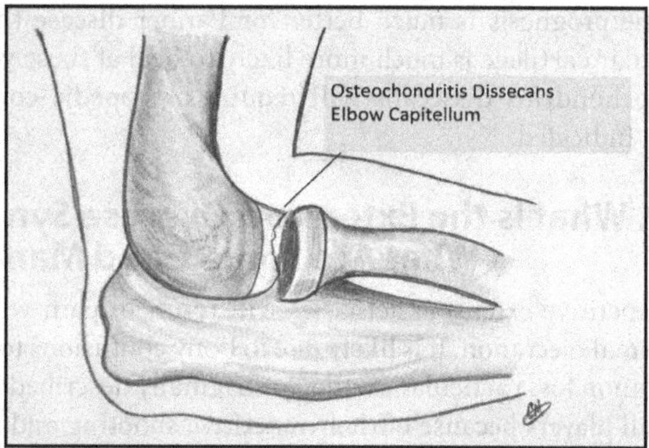

Figure 30-4. Osteochondritis dissecans of the capitellum. (Graphite Pencil-Copyright © 2012 Cora Maglaya, PT, ATC, CSCS.)

number of pitches and ages can be referenced at www.littleleague.org/Assets/forms_pubs/media/PitchingRegulationChanges_BB_11-13-09.pdf

7. What Is "Tommy John Surgery" for a Torn Ulnar Collateral Ligament? Can It Be Performed in Children, and What Is the Long-Term Prognosis?

Tommy John surgery is the reconstruction of the UCL, usually done using the palmaris longus tendon. The original surgery was described by Jobe, who operated on major league pitcher Tommy John, who was able to return to professional pitching after his surgery.[3] Surgeons continue to modify the technique to improve their results. Most UCL injuries in young throwers should be treated nonsurgically with rest and rehabilitation for at least 6 weeks. If conservative management fails, surgery can be an option if the young athlete will participate in the extensive postoperative rehabilitation program.[2] The results for adult throwers are better than their adolescent counterparts. One report of 743 patients aged 14 to 59 stated that 83% were able to return to previous or higher level of competition in less than 1 year.[4] In a series of 27 adolescent throwers, 73% were able to return to baseball at the same or higher level.[5]

8. How Can One Differentiate the Diagnosis and Treatment for Panner Disease From That for Osteochondritis Dissecans of the Capitellum in a Thrower With Lateral Elbow Pain?

Lateral elbow pain in a thrower is due to compression of the capitellum against the radial head due to valgus elbow overload.

- Panner disease is an osteochondrosis (general disruption of the ossific nucleus) of the capitellum that occurs between the ages of 5 and 10. It is not associated with trauma (Figure 30-3).
- Osteochondritis dissecans is focal fragmentation of the articular cartilage of the capitellum in a thrower who is aged 13 years or older (Figure 30-4).

The prognosis is much better for Panner disease than for osteochondritis dissecans, as the articular cartilage is much more likely to heal at these young ages compared with the adolescent. Osteochondritis dissecans will require orthopedic consultation, since surgical intervention is often indicated.

9. What Is the Extension Overuse Syndrome? Who Is At Risk, and What Are Some Good Management Pearls?

Repetitive extension activities will result in pain with hyperextension and tenderness of the proximal olecranon. It is likely due to bony contusions to the contact surfaces of the olecranon and olecranon fossa articular cartilage. Originally described in boxers, this problem also occurs in basketball players because of their repetitive shooting and in football offensive linemen who extend their arms when they block. Any device such as a sleeve or wrap that prevents hyperextension will help. Strengthening exercises for the elbow flexors will help to provide countertraction to hyperextension. Occasionally, an osteophyte develops with chronic pain, requiring the surgical removal of the osteophyte. In a skeletally immature athlete, this could represent an olecranon apophysitis, which can go on to nonunion if not treated properly.

10. What Is "Tennis Elbow" (Lateral Epicondylitis), Does It Present in Children, and How Can It Be Diagnosed and Managed?

Tennis elbow is lateral elbow pain and tenderness of the lateral epicondyle associated with overuse in an adult athlete. It is common in racquet sports such as tennis that involve firm grip, but is probably more common in adults in the workplace. It is the overuse of extensor carpi radialis brevis muscle and tendon with microscopic breakdown of the tendon, resulting in hypervascularization and active fibroblasts. It should be called a tendinosis rather than tendinitis since there is very little inflammation involved. It is rare in children. Lateral elbow pain in a child is usually due to capitellar damage; therefore, a child with lateral elbow pain should always have x-ray examinations performed.

Management of lateral epicondylitis includes relative rest (reducing the stress to the extensor muscles, ice, and analgesic for comfort). A tennis elbow strap will be helpful for patients who still have to use their extensors frequently. If there is morning pain, a cock up wrist splint should be worn at night. Some patients unknowingly stress the extensors while sleeping. In racquet sports, an evaluation of the size of the grip on the racquet should be done. A physical therapy consult will be helpful so that the athlete can learn appropriate extensor muscle stretching and strengthening exercises.[6]

11. What Are Suspicious Findings for Radial Head or Neck Fractures, and How Are They Managed?

Radial head or neck fractures often present with focal pain on the radial side of the proximal forearm and limitations in elbow extension and forearm pronation and supination after a fall on an outstretched arm. There may be an intra-articular effusion noted on examination. Children with an open radial head physis tend to suffer from Salter-Harris type II fractures of the radial neck, whereas adults are more apt to have a radial head fracture. Plain anteroposterior and lateral elbow radiographs are usually sufficient to identify radial head or neck fractures, but sometimes a radiocapitellar view will be necessary. Fractures without significant displacement or comminution are initially treated with a posterior elbow splint or an arm sling for 1 to 2 weeks, followed by a gradual increase in ROM. More complicated fractures with significant displacement or comminution require orthopedic surgical consultation. Loss of elbow extension is a common finding and may require physical therapy consultation to best regain full elbow ROM.

12. What Types of Injuries Should Be Referred for Specialty Care, and on What Basis (Routine, Urgent, or Emergent)?

Acute elbow fractures have a high risk for permanent deformity and loss of motion, so the practitioner should have a low threshold for orthopedic consultation. An emergent orthopedic consultation is necessary for any fracture that is causing neurovascular compromise. Any displacement of an elbow fracture usually warrants urgent orthopedic consultation. Osteochondritis dissecans and a dislocating ulnar nerve require a nonurgent orthopedic consultation.

References

1. Fleisig GS, Weber A, Hassell N, Andrews JR. Prevention of elbow injuries in youth baseball pitchers. *Curr Sports Med Rep.* 2009;8(5):250–254.
2. Hariri S, Safran MR. Ulnar collateral ligament injury in the overhead athlete. *Clin Sports Med.* 2010;29(4):619–644.
3. Jobe FW, Stark H, Lombardo SJ. Reconstruction of the ulnar collateral ligament in athletes. *J Bone Joint Surg Am.* 1986;68(8):1158-1163.
4. Cain EL, Andrews JR, Dugas JR, et al. Outcome of ulnar collateral ligament reconstruction of the elbow in 1281 athletes. Am J Sports Med. 2010;38(12):2426–2434.
5. Petty DH, Andrews JR, Fleisig GS, Cain EL. Ulnar collateral ligament reconstruction in high school baseball players: clinical results and injury risk factors. *Am J Sports Med.* 2004;32(5):1158-1164.
6. VanHofwegen C, Baker CL, Baker CL Jr. Epicondylitis in the athlete's elbow. *Clin Sports Med.* 2010;29:577–597.

31

Wrist and Forearm Pain

Joel S. Brenner, MD, MPH, FAAP and David V. Smith, MD, FAAP

1. What Are the Key Anatomical Landmarks in the Wrist and Forearm in Terms of Sports Injuries?

- The key landmarks include the following (Figure 31-1):
  - A = Distal radial physis
  - B = Distal ulnar physis
  - C = Anatomic snuffbox (Figure 31-2)
  - D = Triangular fibrocartilage complex (TFCC)
  - E = Metacarpal bone
  - F = First metacarpal and ulnar collateral ligament
  - G = Radius
  - H = Ulna

2. What Is a Wrist Sprain?

- A wrist sprain is a tear (partial or complete) of any of the ligaments connecting the radius and ulna with the metacarpals. It usually occurs after a hyperflexion or hyperextension mechanism and will present with no swelling or minimal to moderate swelling. It is a diagnosis of exclusion; one should remember to consider possible fractures.
- Physical examination findings in a patient with a wrist sprain include the following:
  - Pain to palpation over the wrist joint
  - Decreased active range of motion (ROM) of the wrist
  - Pain with passive ROM of the wrist
  - Decreased strength against resistance testing

3. Skeletally Immature Gymnasts Often Present With Distal Radial Pain. What Is a "Gymnast's Wrist?" How Should This Be Worked Up and Initially Managed, and When Is a Referral Necessary?

- A "gymnast's wrist" is a stress injury to the distal radial physis. It is an overuse injury resulting from repetitive weight bearing on the wrist joint. This should be suspected in any gymnast or cheerleader who presents with wrist pain. A patient with gymnast's wrist will have pain to palpation at the distal radial physis, decreased wrist extension, pain with hyperextension of the wrist, and pain with weight bearing of the wrist, also also called distal radial epiphysiolysis or a Salter 1 fracture of the distal radius. (The health care provider

Koutures C, Wong V.
Pediatric Sports Medicine: Essentials for Office Evaluation (pp 206-210)

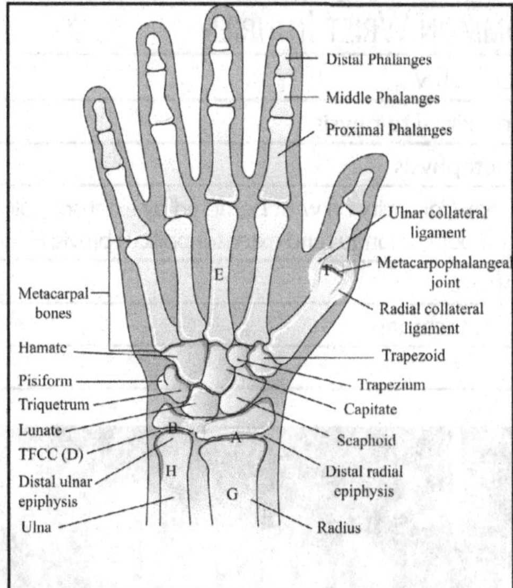

Figure 31-1. Anatomic landmarks of the wrist.

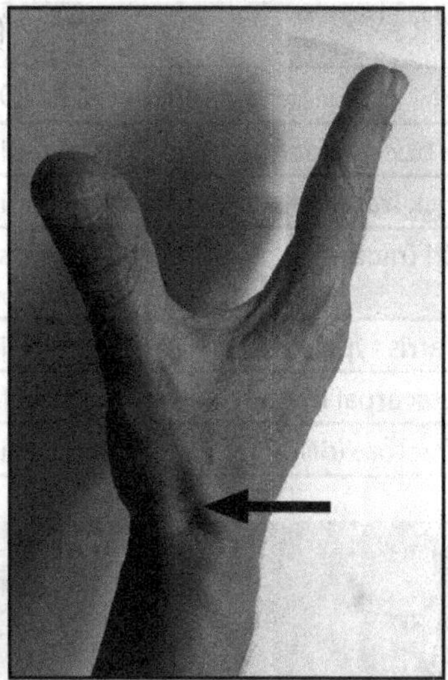

Figure 31-2. Anatomic snuffbox.

should ask the patient to push him- or herself up while sitting on the examination table to test his or her pain level.)

- Radiographs of both wrists (posteroanterior [PA] and lateral views) should be obtained; they will show the following in a patient with gymnast's wrist (refer to Chapter 20, Figure 20-3):
  - A widening and irregularity of the radial growth plate
  - Sclerosis of the metaphysis
  - Cystic changes of the metaphysis
- Initial management includes the following:
  - Stopping upper-extremity weight bearing activity
  - Using an over-the-counter wrist brace for pain control and to prevent the use of the wrist in weight bearing
  - Consider physical therapy to increase wrist strength and flexibility
- A referral to a sports medicine specialist should occur in the following situations:
  - If the pain does not resolve with rest
  - If the athlete is unable to progress back to activities pain free
  - If the diagnosis is uncertain
  - If the health care provider is not comfortable managing the problem

4. Pain in the Distal Radial Aspect of the Wrist Is Common After a Fall on the Outstretched Hand. What Are the Most Common Injuries, and How Can They Be Differentiated on Palpation of Surface Anatomy?

Table 31-1 provides information on common injuries to the wrist.

5. What Is a Torus Fracture? Can They Be Managed by the Primary Care Provider Versus Referral to an Orthopedist or Sports Medicine Specialist?

- A torus or buckle fracture is a plastic deformation of the weak metaphyseal cortex caused by an axial load (eg, fall on an outstretched hand; Figure 31-3).

Table 31-1. Common Wrist Injuries	
INJURY	*LOCATION OF PAIN*
Torus or buckle fracture	Distal radius proximal to physis
Greenstick fracture	Distal radial metaphysis
Scaphoid fracture	Anatomic snuffbox (concavity on wrist bordered by extensor pollicus longus and abductor pollicus longus and extensor pollicus brevis; Figure 31-2)
Salter-Harris type I fracture	Distal radial physis
First metacarpal fracture	Proximal first metacarpal
Colles' fracture (distal radius)	Distal radius

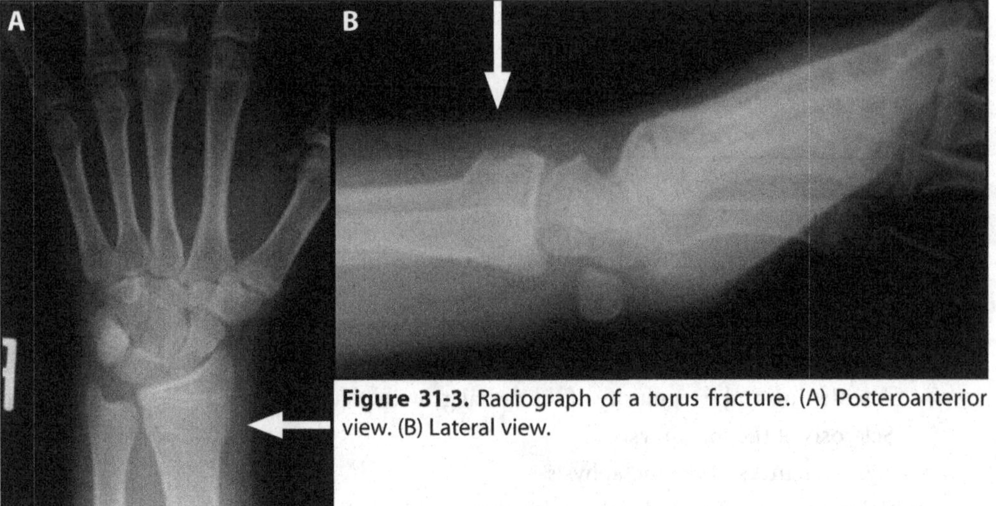

Figure 31-3. Radiograph of a torus fracture. (A) Posteroanterior view. (B) Lateral view.

- This type of fracture can only occur in the pediatric (skeletal immature) athlete.
- Torus fractures can be managed by the primary care provider using an over-the-counter wrist brace, volar splint, or short arm cast for 4 weeks.

6. What Criteria Are Used to Differentiate Lower-Risk Versus Higher-Risk Distal Radius Fractures, and How Should They Be Initially Splinted?

- Multiple classification systems have been reported for distal radius fractures. However, none of the systems "include 3-dimensional assessment of the fracture, is user-friendly, and have a high inter- and intra-observer agreement."[1] Low-risk fractures that most pediatricians should feel comfortable managing without a referral to a specialist are nonangulated, single-bone forearm fractures, including a Salter-Harris type I fracture. Patients with any angulation, dual-bone fractures, or higher-grade Salter-Harris fractures should be referred on an urgent basis. While awaiting referral to a specialist, the patient's arm should be placed in a "volar or sugartong splint with the wrist in slight flexion and ulnar deviation, forearm in neutral position and the elbow at 90 degrees."[2]

7. Why Is It Essential to Palpate in the "Anatomic Snuffbox" in any Case of Wrist/Hand Pain? What Are Scaphoid Fractures, and Why Can They Be So Difficult to Identify and Treat? Do Children With Scaphoid Fractures Have a Better Outcome Than Adults With This Type of Fracture?

- Scaphoid fractures can be difficult to diagnose initially; therefore, palpating the anatomic snuffbox is essential in anyone with wrist/hand pain (see Figure 31-2).
- A fracture of the scaphoid bone can occur after a fall on an outstretched hand; the patient can have pain and swelling near the distal radius, but it may be more diffuse, making the diagnosis difficult. This type of fracture can occur at the proximal third, midbody, or distal third portion of the scaphoid. Radiographs can often be normal on initial presentation, requiring a high index of suspicion. Children and adolescents have similar outcomes as adults, with 90% of cases healing with casting alone.[3]

8. If an Athlete Has Snuffbox Tenderness After Sustaining an Acute Injury, What Are the Recommended Initial Radiologic Views? How Should the Wrist Be Splinted? What Is the Proper Follow-Up?

- Any athlete with anatomic snuffbox tenderness should have PA, lateral, and oblique radiographs of the wrist, along with a special scaphoid view that helps to isolate the scaphoid bone.
- If the radiographs are negative but a scaphoid fracture is still suspected, the athlete's wrist and thumb should be immobilized in a short-arm thumb spica splint (or over-the- counter brace) or a short-arm cast.
- Repeat radiographs should occur in 2 to 3 weeks to determine if a fracture is present. If these radiographs are still normal but the suspicion is still high for a fracture, magnetic resonance imaging or a computed tomography scan could be considered.
- Nondisplaced or distal scaphoid fractures can be managed by primary care providers using short-arm thumb spica cast for 6 to 10 weeks. All other cases of scaphoid fractures or suspected fractures with normal radiographs should be referred to a sports medicine specialist or an orthopedic surgeon.

9. What Is the Triangular Fibrocartilage Complex, and How Is It Usually Injured?

- The triangular fibrocartilage complex (TFCC) is comprised of the triangular fibrocartilage articular disc, the dorsal radioulnar ligament, the volar radioulnar ligament, the ulnolunate ligament, the ulnotriquetral ligament, the extensor carpi ulnaris sheath, and the meniscus homologue. The meniscus homologue connects the triquetrum and the articular disc.
- The function of the TFCC is to help stabilize the distal radioulnar joint and bear a small portion of the force transmitted across the wrist.
- The typical mode of injury is from repetitive axial loading of the wrist, such as during gymnastics or racquet sports. It may also occur from a fall onto an outstretched hand.
- The patient will present with ulnar-sided wrist pain that is worse with weight bearing on the wrist or activities that stress the ulnar side of the wrist (eg, opening doors or jars). There is frequently a report of "popping" in the lateral wrist.
- The physical examination will reveal no swelling or minimal (if presenting acutely with a fall onto an outstretched hand). The athlete will have pain to palpation in the ulnar fovea (just distal and radial to the ulnar styloid) and pain with axial loading and circumducting

the wrist in an ulnar-deviated position. He or she will also have ulnar-sided wrist pain when pushing him- or herself off of the table while sitting.

- PA and lateral radiographs of the wrist should be performed to rule out fractures of the distal ulna or carpal bones. Positive ulnar variance (ulna is longer than the radius) may be seen, which is a risk factor for a TFCC injury. Magnetic resonance arthrogram may be performed, but this should only be ordered by a sports medicine specialist or an orthopedic surgeon.
- Wrist arthroscopy can be both diagnostic and therapeutic in cases that are resistant to conservative management.
- The primary care provider can initiate treatment with rest from the activities that cause the pain and a wrist brace for 4 to 6 weeks. If the pain persists at the follow-up visit, the patient should be referred to a sports medicine specialist.

10. What Are Some Concerns That Should Be Addressed for Athletes Undergoing Rehabilitation for Wrist and Forearm Injuries?

- Athletes who have sustained a wrist or forearm injury and have been treated with any form of immobilization will have a decrease in strength and range of motion. As part of the treatment plan, athletes should be prescribed a rehabilitation program that works on increasing their functional strength and returning their range of motion back to normal. This can be performed as part of a home exercise program or, for more extensive injuries, it is helpful to prescribe a formal physical therapy program. A lack of normal range of motion in young athletes can lead to significant long-term or permanent problems in the wrist/forearm. This can also cause secondary problems in other joints (eg, the elbow or the shoulder) due to the athlete compensating for his or her wrist/forearm deficits.

References

1. Kural C, Sungur I, Kaya I, Ugras A, Ertürk A, Cetinus E. Evaluation of the reliability of classification systems used for distal radius fractures. *Orthopedics*. 2010;33(11):801.
2. Eiff MP, Hatch RL, Calmbach WL. *Fracture Management for Primary Care*. 2nd ed. Philadelphia, PA: Saunders, 2003:331–352.
3. Gholson JJ, Bae DS, Zurakowski D, Waters PM. Scaphoid fractures in children and adolescents: contemporary injury patterns and factors influencing time to union. *JBJS*. 2011;93(13):1210-1219.

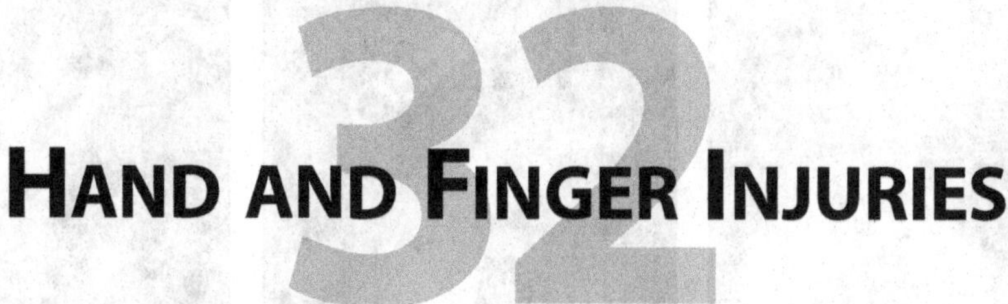

Hand and Finger Injuries

Philip J. Cohen, MD

1. What Are Malrotated or Angulated Finger Injuries, and What Screening Examination Techniques Can Identify These Issues?

Malrotation

Occurs when fragments of bone on either side of a fracture rotate away from each other in such a way as to impair or prevent proper healing.

- Malrotation is more common in oblique and spiral fractures of the proximal and middle phalanges, as these fractures tend to be unstable.[1]
- If present, it is most apparent when the patient attempts to make a fist and flex his or her fingers toward his or her palm.

Normally, the tips of the second through fourth fingers will remain parallel to each other and point toward the scaphoid bone. With malrotation, the flexed affected finger may overlap with the adjacent finger (also known as scissoring) rather than point toward the scaphoid bone (Figure 32-1).

- If malrotation is not properly reduced, a debilitating rotational malunion may ensue.

Angulation

Angulation describes the relationship of fracture fragments to one another in the long axis of the finger.

- In an angulated fracture, the central aspect of the fracture site "points" dorsally, volarly, or laterally.
- Fracture angulation may be detected on physical examination by seeing or palpating this point.
- Lateral angulation may be accompanied by malrotation.[2]

2. How Should Angulation of Metacarpal Fractures Be Measured on X-rays, and What Is Acceptable Angulation for Each of the Five Metacarpals?

Angulation of fractures should be measured on a true lateral x-ray. There is usually about 15 degrees of angulation at each metacarpal neck, so this must be taken into account when determining the degree of additional angulation caused by the fracture (Figure 32-2).[3] No hard and fast evidence-based rules exist with regard to how much angulation is truly acceptable for metacarpal neck fractures.

Koutures C, Wong V.
Pediatric Sports Medicine: Essentials for Office Evaluation (pp 211-217)

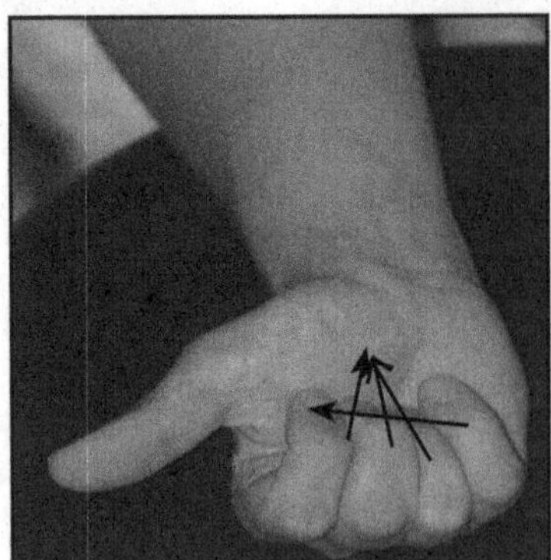

Figure 32-1. Malrotation of the fifth finger.

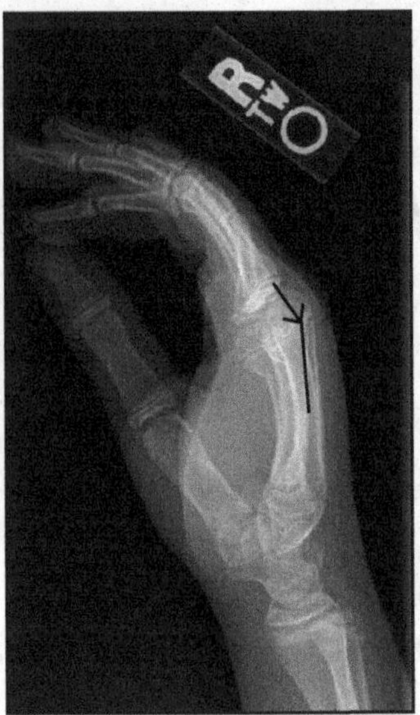

Figure 32-2. Boxer's fracture of the fifth metacarpal with angulation measurement.

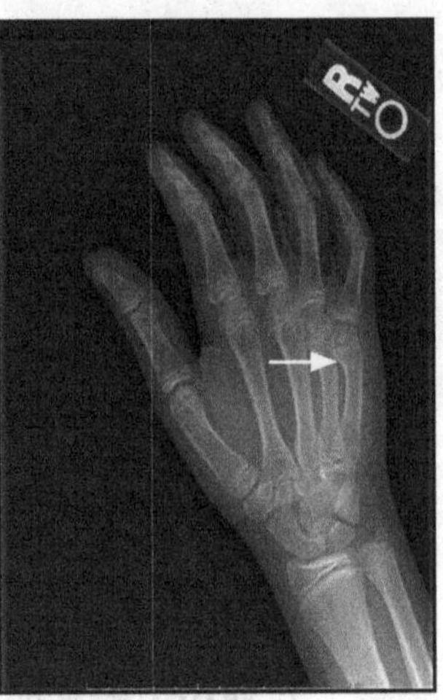

Figure 32-3. Boxer's fracture of the fifth metacarpal.

- Generally, experts feel that up to 30 to 45 degrees of angulation is tolerable at the fourth and fifth metacarpals, whereas only 10 to 15 degrees of angulation can typically be accepted at the second and third metacarpals.[4]
- The more proximal the injury, the less angulation is acceptable.
- Keep in mind that the measurement of angulation is subject to significant inter- and intraobserver variability.[5]

3. What Is a Boxer's Fracture, and Can General Pediatric Health Care Providers Manage This Injury?

A boxer's fracture usually refers to a fracture of the fourth or fifth metacarpal neck, although a variant has been described involving the fourth metacarpal shaft (Figures 32-2 and 32-3).

- A boxer's fracture typically occurs when the patient punches a wall or another hard object, usually making contact with the distal fourth and/or fifth metacarpal head.
- As these bones and supporting structures are relatively weak, the force transmitted through them tends to cause a fracture at the metacarpal neck.
- Due to the pull of surrounding musculature, these fractures usually have apex dorsal angulation. The volarly displaced metacarpal head is often palpable as a tender mass in the palm.

In most cases, as long as the angulation is less than 45 degrees and no associated pathology is noted, patients will regain good function with conservative treatment (ie, an ulnar gutter splint). If more severe angulation is present, many experts feel that reduction is indicated to prevent pseudoclawing (inability to fully extend the proximal and distal interphalangeal joints) and functional compromise.[3]

- However, one study reported excellent results with the use of a soft wrap and buddy taping in patients with angulation up to 70 degrees.[6]
- An experienced pediatrician who is well versed in splinting techniques may be able to manage many patients who present with this injury. For patients who are high-demand upper extremity athletes or musicians, a referral to a hand specialist may be warranted.

It is important to realize that, due to the mechanism of most of these injuries, further psychosocial evaluation is recommended. A boxer's fracture may be a blessing in disguise, as it alerts the astute physician to the possibility of an underlying anger management condition, alcohol or other substance abuse, or other psychologic or psychiatric disorder. If these issues are tactfully explored with the patient (not necessarily at the first visit), it may open up a dialogue that would never have otherwise taken place, allowing for better evaluation and management of the underlying condition. Thus, even if the patient is referred to orthopedics for fracture management, the pediatrician should not miss this opportunity to evaluate for these underlying conditions.

4. A Patient Has Pain on the Ulnar Aspect of the First Metacarpophalangeal Joint. How Should One Evaluate for an Ulnar Collateral Ligament Tear, and What Findings Require Urgent Surgical Referral?

- Ulnar collateral ligament (UCL) tear is classically known as gamekeeper's thumb in reference to the chronic, attritional UCL tear from wringing the necks of game animals such as rabbits.
- In this day and age, most UCL injuries are acute in nature, and occur as the result of a direct hyperabduction force to the thumb (ie, skier's thumb, resulting from hyperabduction of the thumb by a ski pole during a fall).[7]

Physical examination usually discloses edema and sometimes ecchymosis around the first metacarpophalangeal (MCP) joint and often at the thenar eminence. The UCL itself and surrounding tissues are typically tender, and range of motion (ROM) is limited.

- Stress testing of the collateral ligaments and volar plate are required to assess the stability and integrity of the joint.
- Stress testing in extension is generally considered positive for UCL tear if there is more than 30 degrees of valgus laxity or greater than 15 degrees of increased laxity compared with the uninjured thumb.
- Some clinicians worry that stability testing may convert an incomplete UCL tear to a complete one, causing a Stener lesion (defined next). It seems unlikely, however, that firm but gentle stability testing would cause this to happen.[8]

If there is significant laxity of the UCL on stress testing, one must maintain a high index of suspicion for a complete rupture of the ligament. With a complete UCL tear, the adjacent adductor aponeurosis may become interposed between the torn ends of the UCL (Stener lesion), thereby preventing the ligament from ever fully healing without surgical intervention.

- Stener lesions occur in 20% to 70% of UCL tears.[9]
- In some cases, there may be an avulsion fracture where the UCL inserts onto the bone. An intact yet avulsed and displaced UCL may retract, allowing the interposition of the adductor aponeurosis and essentially forming a Stener lesion.
- Thumb x-rays should be obtained in all cases of suspected UCL injury, and the films should be scrutinized for tiny avulsion fractures and for larger lesions. Any patient suspected of having a complete UCL tear or an avulsion injury should be referred expeditiously to a hand specialist.

5. After a Patient Relocated a Dislocated Finger Joint, Should I Order X-rays? If So, Which Views Are Appropriate and What Findings Are of the Most Concern?

It is generally advisable to obtain a standard finger series (anteroposterior, lateral, and oblique views) in this setting. This ensures that proper reduction has been achieved, and also allows detection of associated fractures (Figure 32-4). Some authors advocate obtaining stress views to better

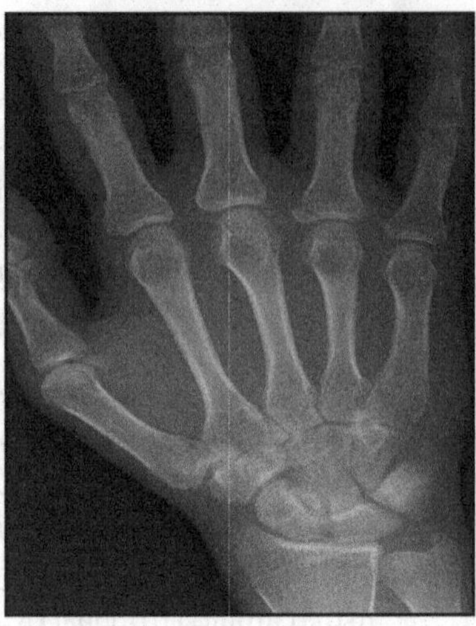

Figure 32-4. Intra-articular fracture, proximal phalanx of the fourth finger.

evaluate for instability. Indications for referral include the inability to obtain complete reduction, significant instability, and associated fracture, including physeal injury.

6. Are There Any Good Examination Techniques to Differentiate a Finger Fracture From a Joint Sprain Without Getting X-rays?

- Gross deformity (not caused by a dislocation) clearly implies a fracture.
- Bony point tenderness, bony step-off, and bony crepitus all strongly suggest a fracture. However, the absence of these findings is not enough to rule out a fracture.
- The pain level and loss of function are also not sufficiently sensitive to rule out a fracture.[10]
- Many apparent "sprains" turn out to involve a fracture, and sometimes (albeit infrequently) this alters management.
- Imaging is warranted in any case in which a significant sprain or possible fracture is suspected.

7. What Are Some Management Tips and Expectations for Healing After a Sprained Distal Interphalangeal or Proximal Interphalangeal Joint, and What Are the Return-to-Play Criteria?

Isolated distal interphalangeal (DIP) and proximal interphalangeal (PIP) sprains usually heal well with conservative treatment (buddy taping and/or splinting; Figure 32-5).

- Exceptions include a complete rupture of the radial collateral ligament of the index finger of the dominant hand, as instability at this location may interfere with the ability to write and pincer grasp.
- Similarly, volar plate ruptures may be associated with persistent instability and dysfunction, which are indications for surgical referral. They are suspected clinically by increased PIP or DIP passive hyperextension or suspected on lateral radiographs by fleck fractures on the volar (palmar) aspect of the DIP/PIP or loss of usual DIP/PIP alignment.
- Children typically tolerate splinting better than adults, but care must be taken to ensure that the joints are maintained in proper position (see Section 11 for more detail).
- It is important to ensure that uninvolved joints are not unnecessarily immobilized.
- Return to play can generally be allowed once ROM, strength, and stability have been restored, and stability has been confirmed.

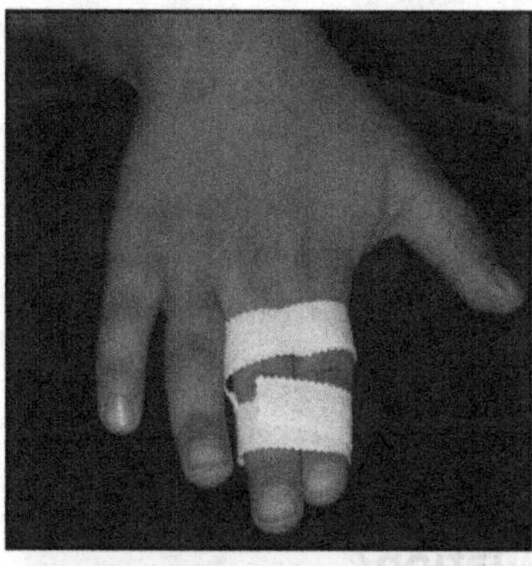

Figure 32-5. Buddy taping (the tape is applied proximal and distal to the involved joint).

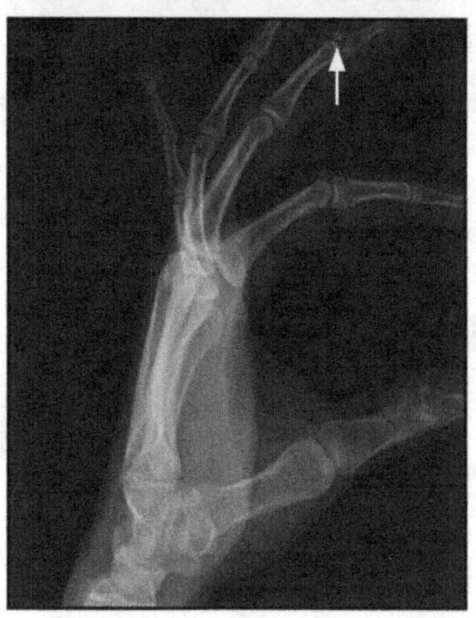

Figure 32-6. Bone mallet finger with subluxation, distal phalanx.

- The patient and parents should be informed that it is very common to have persistent stiffness and mild swelling or thickening at the involved joint, but ongoing significant pain or functional disability requires further investigation by a health care provider.

8. A Patient Presents With Direct Trauma to the Tip of a Finger and Inability to Fully Extend the Distal Interphalangeal Joint. What Is the Proper Evaluation and Management for This Injury?

- Injury to the extensor tendon insertion into the distal phalange can create the above presentation, known as mallet finger.
- X-rays should be obtained to evaluate for an associated fracture (Figure 32-6).
  - If there is a large fracture (involving ≥ 30% of the articular surface), significant fragment displacement, or volar displacement of the distal fragment, hand specialist referral is indicated.
    - If there is a small avulsion fracture without the above complications, or if no fracture is present, then treatment consists of splinting the DIP in full extension for approximately 6 to 8 weeks, until healing has occurred.[11]
    - Emphasize the need to maintain the fully extended position. Do not allow the DIP to move into flexion during cleaning or splint changes.
- Rest, ice, gentle compression, and elevation can be utilized in the acute setting.
- Patients who are not improving despite adequate conservative treatment should be referred for hand surgeon consultation.

9. A Patient Gets His or Her Finger Caught in an Opponent's Jersey. What Is the Initial Management for Jersey Finger, and How Should This Injury Be Referred?

Jersey finger is rupture of the flexor digitorum profundus tendon and/or its bony insertion.

- It requires urgent hand surgeon referral because it will not heal on its own.
- If excessive delay (more than 7 to 10 days) occurs prior to surgical treatment, primary repair may not be possible and a fusion procedure or other salvage procedure may be required.

10. Which Finger Injuries Require Urgent or Emergent Hand Specialty Evaluation?

Urgent hand surgeon referral is indicated for the following:

- Jersey finger.
- Large intra-articular fracture (see Figure 32-4).
- Displaced, severely angulated, or rotated fractures.
- Large avulsion fractures.
- Multiple fractures.
- Fractures associated with dislocations or significant instability, including volar plate.

Emergent referral is indicated for the following:

- Suspected septic joint.
- Neurovascular compromise.
- Open fracture or dislocation.
- Fracture or dislocation that cannot be reduced.
- Bite wounds to the hands are at high risk for infection.
    - Copious irrigation, prophylactic antibiotics, and updating tetanus status are recommended.

11. How Should the General Pediatric Health Care Provider Splint a Suspected Serious Hand Injury While the Patient Is Awaiting Specialty Evaluation?

Initial splinting of hand injuries depends on the type and severity of injury.

- In general, the wrist and hand should be placed in the position of function, with the wrist in slight extension and the fingers positioned as though they are holding a drinking glass.
- For a suspected second, third, or fourth metacarpal fracture, a volar splint ending at the distal palmar crease can be employed.
- For a fourth or fifth metacarpal fracture, an ulnar gutter splint with the MCP joint in 70 to 90 degrees of flexion and the interphalangeal (IP) joints extended is another good option.
- A radial gutter splint can be utilized for a first metacarpal fracture.
- A thumb spica splint or brace can be used for a thumb UCL injury.
- Nondisplaced phalangeal fractures and IP joint sprains can be buddy taped or treated with various splints (ie, aluminum/foam splint).
- For volar plate sprains, keep the involved joint in slight (30 degrees) flexion.
- For mallet finger or central slip injuries, keep the involved joint in complete extension.

12. What Are Some General Rehabilitation Tips After a Hand/Finger Injury?

- The IP and MCP joints get stiff easily with prolonged immobilization. Fortunately, children tend to rapidly regain ROM once immobilization is discontinued.
- Initially, patients are encouraged to perform gentle, pain-free, active range of motion exercises. Often, immersing the injured hand in warm (NOT HOT) water makes the joint feel less stiff and may aid in regaining motion.
- As range of motion improves and pain and swelling have subsided, gentle strengthening exercises can be performed. Hand strengthening can involve opening and closing the fist in the air or underwater, as well as gripping a stress ball or old racquetball or using commercial grip strengtheners.
- Wrist strengthening can be achieved by performing wrist curls against gravity at first, and then gradually adding resistance (eg, 1 to 2 lb dumbbell, can of soup).
- Passive range of motion/stretching exercises can be added for persistent stiffness. Severe stiffness and flexion contractures may require tension splinting. In these situations, working with a hand specialist and occupational therapist may be helpful.

References

1. Lakshmanan P. Malunion of hand fracture. Medscape Web site. http://emedicine.medscape.com/article/1243899-overview#a0104. Updated February 15, 2012. Accessed August 2, 2012.
2. Leggit JC, Meko CJ. Acute finger injuries: part II. Fractures, dislocations, and thumb injuries. *Am Fam Physician.* 2006;73:827-834.
3. Wheeless CR. Boxer's fracture (metacarpal neck). www.wheelessonline.com/ortho/boxers_fracture_metacarpal_neck_1. Accessed August 2, 2012.
4. Dye MT. Metacarpal fractures treatment and management. Medscape Web site. http://emedicine.medscape.com/article/1239721-treatment. Accessed August 2, 2012.
5. Leung YL, Beredjiklian PK, Monaghan BA, Bozentka DJ. Radiographic assessment of small finger metacarpal neck fractures. *J Hand Surg Am.* 2002;(27):443–448.
6. van Aaken J, Kämpfen S, Berli M, Fritschy D, Della Santa D, Fusetti C. Outcome of boxer's fractures treated by a soft wrap and buddy taping: a prospective study. *Hand.* 2007;2(4):212–217.
7. Hannibal M. Gamekeeper's thumb. *Medscape Reference.* http://emedicine.medscape.com/article/97679-overview. Accessed August 2, 2012.
8. Adler T, Eisenbarth I, Hirschmann MT, Müller-Gerbl M, Fricker R. Can clinical examination cause a Stener lesion in patients with skier's thumb? A cadaveric study. *Clin Anat.* 2012;25(6):762–766.
9. Louis DS, Huebner JJ Jr, Hankin FM. Rupture and displacement of the ulnar collateral ligament of the metacarpophalangeal joint of the thumb. Preoperative diagnosis. *J Bone Joint Surg Am.* 1986;68:1320–1326.
10. Rimmer CS, Burke D. Proximal interphalangeal joint hyperextension injuries in children. *Emerg Med J.* 2009;26:854–856.
11. Anderson D. Mallet finger—management and patient compliance. *Aust Fam Physician.* 2011;40:47–48.

33 Thoracic and Lumbar Spine Injuries and Sacroiliac Region Pain

David Olson, MD; Austin Krohn, MD; and Robby S. Sikka, MD

1. What Are the Findings for Back Pain That Are More Concerning and Warrant Further Work-Up?

- Further work-up of back pain should be considered when any of the following red flag signs or symptoms are present: signs of infection (fever, malaise), pain unrelated to activity or nighttime pain, neurologic signs or symptoms (weakness, paresthesias), unintentional weight loss, or pain that fails conservative management and persists for greater than 1 month.[1]

2. A Parent Has the Complaint That His or Her Child Has "Poor Posture." On Examination, It Is Found That the Child Has a Thoracic Kyphosis (eg, Appears to Have a "Hunchback") but Is Otherwise a Normal Teenager. What Is a Possible Diagnosis?

- The appearance of a "hunchback" should key the health care provider to think about 2 things immediately: postural kyphosis and Scheuermann's kyphosis (SK). Patient's with a postural kyphosis will typically have a flexible deformity of the thoracic spine and lack the rigid, abrupt posterior angulation (gibbus deformity) that is characteristic of SK. The prevalence of SK is 0.4% to 10% in adolescents age 13 to 17 years (typically affecting the skeletally immature).[2,3]
- Patients will present with increased rounding/deformity of the thoracic spine, with pain as the presenting report 20% to 60% of the time. The pain is usually located in T7 to T9 or in the lumbar area because of excessive lordosis. The "rounding" is a rigid hyperkyphosis in SK (not flexible as in postural kyphosis).[2]
- Work-up—Adam's forward bend test, assessment for hamstring tightness (common), a thorough neurologic examination, and an assessment of range of motion should be part of the routine work-up. An obvious kyphotic deformity may be noted. Radiographic examinations should include standing posteroanterior and lateral radiographs of spine.
- Radiographic findings of thoracic kyphosis are provided in Table 33-1.

3. What Are the Management Options for Scheuermann's Kyphosis? When Is Referral Necessary?

- SK can be managed both nonoperatively and with surgery. Nonoperative management has been shown to have a 40% to 60% correction of kyphosis.[2,4] The 2 main goals of nonoperative management are to control the deformity (and/or prevent progression) and to

Koutures C, Wong V.
Pediatric Sports Medicine: Essentials for Office Evaluation (pp 218-225)

Table 33-1. Radiographic Findings of Scheuermann's Kyphosis
• Increased thoracic kyphosis (> 45 to 50 degrees between T5 and T12) with compensatory lumbar and/or cervical hyperlordosis.
• Vertebral wedging of three or more consecutive levels of the spine.
• End plate irregularities, loss of disc space height, and Schmorl's nodes.
• Posteroanterior plain films usually show a mild scoliosis that rarely measures < 25 degrees.
• Lateral bolster radiograph (lie supine on the table with a bolster at or below the apex of the kyphotic deformity). This can show the degree to which the kyphosis is expected to correct with bracing and/or surgery.

Table 33-2. Nonoperative Management of Scheuermann's Kyphosis
• Hamstring stretching and anterior shoulder stretching
• Kyphosis that is < 55 degrees: physical therapy for hamstring stretching, anterior shoulder stretching and postural training
• Kyphosis that is 55 degrees to 70 degrees: orthosis that is worn full time (18 to 23 hr/day); 50% correction expected[1,2]
• Follow clinically and radiographically every 6 months until growth is complete
• If bracing is not working, serial casting may be performed, which may be extremely effective, but less well tolerated. This is done for 6 to 9 months and followed by orthosis until skeletal maturity (40% to 60% correction of kyphosis[1,3])

reconstitute the anterior vertebral height by applying hyperextension forces. See Table 33-2 for information on the nonoperative management of SK.

- Surgical—Referral to a pediatric spine surgeon is generally reserved for patients with progressive or rigid curve > 70 to 75 degrees, persistent back pain, and an unacceptable cosmetic appearance[2] (Figure 33-1).

4. Adolescent Athletes Commonly Present With Back Pain When They Go Into Forward Flexion. What Are Some Diagnostic Considerations in a Patient With Flexion-Based Back Pain?

- In addition to the common etiologies of low-back pain, flexion-based back pain in an athlete should key the provider to consider disc herniation, wedge-type compression fractures (most common thoracolumbar fractures in young athletes), and burst fractures.

5. Do Adolescent Athletes Get Back Pain From Disc Herniation or Protrusion? What Are the Best Imaging Tests and Management Plan for a Disc Herniation?

- Disc herniation in adolescents is much less frequent than in adults, and typically is preceded by trauma. There is a history of trauma in 30% to 60% of children with symptomatic lumbar disc herniation (LDH); however, trauma may just be the inciting event, as genetic factors are also thought to play a role (13% to 57% of adolescents with LDH have a first-degree relative with the same disorder).[5,6]
- Clinical presentations of pediatric LDH are generally similar to those observed in adults. One distinctive feature is that up to 90% of patients have a positive straight leg raise test, which can be explained by the finding that children and adolescents tend to have a greater

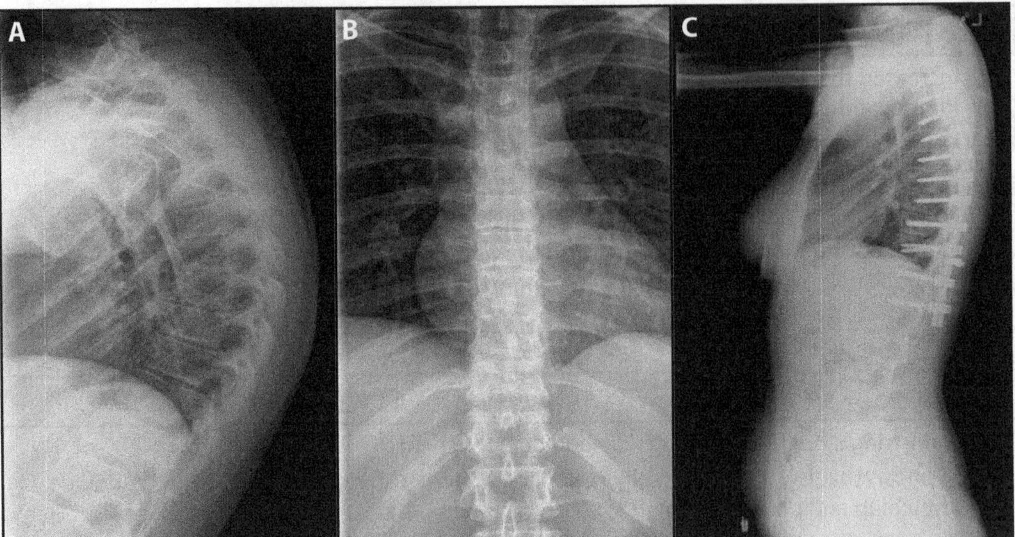

Figure 33-1. (A,B) AP and lateral radiographs are seen prior to spinal fusion. (C) Postoperative lateral radiograph following spinal fusion.

nerve root tension than adults. However, children and adolescents are less often seen with neurologic symptoms such as numbness and weakness.[5,6]

- The imaging study of choice is magnetic resonance imaging (MRI; Figure 33-2); however, plain radiographs must be obtained to exclude a pars defect or other spinal lesions.[5,6]
- Pediatric patients tend to respond less favorably to conservative treatment when compared with adults; however, outcomes of surgery remain satisfactory at 10-year follow-up. Conservative treatment is still generally recommended as the first-line treatment for LDH in children without neurologic deficits. This primarily consists of 1 to 2 weeks of relative rest, analgesic therapy, and avoiding strenuous physical activities.[5,6]
- Referral for chemonucleolysis (a procedure to treat a herniated disk that involves an enzyme being injected into the gelatinous center of the disk to dissolve it) or surgery should be made for any of the following:
  - Severe pain refractory after 4 to 6 weeks of conservative management
  - Progressive neurologic defects
  - Disabling pain that is affecting daily activities
  - Associating spinal deformities
  - Cauda equine syndrome
- Chemonucleolysis is the only form of intradiscal therapy reportedly being used on children and adolescents. Many researchers suggest attempting this prior to surgery, as outcomes of failed chemonucleolysis followed by surgery are not significantly different than surgery alone. Chemonucleolysis has an 80% to 89% short-term success rate and a 64% midterm success rate. It is not recommended for severely extruded discs.[5]

6. How Do Compression Fractures Occur in Athletes? What Are the Best Imaging Tests? What Is the Best Way to Manage a Compression Fracture?

- Compression fractures in athletes occur via axial loading, hyperflexion, and hyperextension. The axial loading usually is precipitated by falls landing in the seated position often

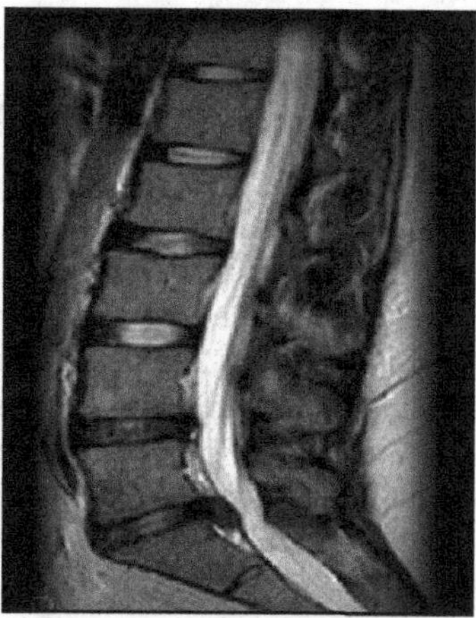

Figure 33-2. Magnetic resonance imaging showing a disc herniation at the L5 to S1 level with cord compression.

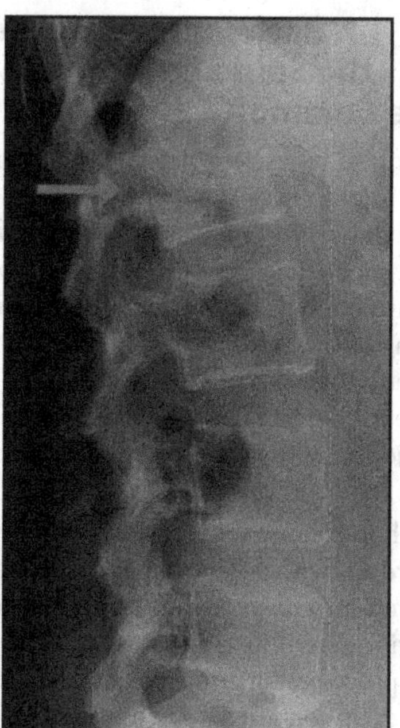

Figure 33-3. Lateral radiograph of a pediatric lumbar burst fracture.

combined with hyperflexion. The anterior spinal column fails in compression, while the middle column remains intact. This mechanism is common in gymnastics, diving, and jumping sports.

- Lateral spine radiographs are the imaging of choice. A typical compression fracture is seen as a wedge-shaped vertebra with a loss of the height of the anterior body and preservation of the height of the posterior body (Figure 33-3). Measurements should be made at the level of injury and on the vertebrae above and below the injury. Most of these fractures occur between T11 and L2. It is important to ensure that it is a wedge compression fracture and not a burst fracture. If in doubt, order a computed tomography (CT) scan. Using radiographs alone has an error rate of up to 25%.[5,7]
- Overall, compression fractures are generally stable and are rarely associated with neurologic compromise. Management is therefore typically conservative with bracing and physical therapy. If there is less than 40% vertebral body height loss and less than 20 degrees of local kyphosis, then analgesia and early mobilization are usually adequate. Patients in severe pain despite a stable fracture pattern may benefit from a hyperextension brace.
- If there is greater than 40% to 50% of vertebral body height loss, kyphosis greater than 20 degrees, or multiple adjacent compression fractures, the posterior column is subjected to significant tensile force injury and may fail. Progression of kyphosis, compensatory lumbar hyperlordosis, and low-back pain may ensue. It should be treated with either an extension brace or a molded body cast and regular observation for 3 months.
- Referral for operative treatment may be indicated for injuries that have documented progression of deformity despite nonoperative management or when neurologic stability is compromised because of the resultant deformity.[8]

7. Back Pain Associated With Extension of the Spine Is Common in Athletes. What Are the Common Causes of Extension-Based Back Pain?

- Spondylolysis refers to a defect in the pars interarticularis. The regions most commonly affected are L5 (in 85% to 95% of cases) and L4 (in 5% to 15% of cases). The prevalence of spondylolysis in the general population has been estimated to be between 3% and 6%. Bilateral spondylolysis at the same vertebral level can result in spondylolisthesis, the forward translation of one vertebra on the next caudal segment. Spondylolisthesis is graded according to the percentage of slip: grade I is a slip of 0% to 25%; grade II, a slip of 25% to 50%; grade III, a slip of 50% to 75%; and grade IV, a slip of > 75%. Family history, gender, and race all are implicated. Spondylolysis occurs in 15% to 70% of first-degree relatives of individuals with the disorder. Facet irritation may occur from repetitive extension and result in spondylolysis.[6]
- A tight thoracolumbar fascia may result from the rapid growth seen in puberty. A resulting hyperlordosis with a flat midback and thoracic kyphosis is characteristic, and several pain syndromes may result. Traction apophysitis may occur at the iliac crest, spinous process, or anterior vertebral ring apophysis. This also may cause an impingement of adjacent spinous processes forming a pseudarthrosis (Baastrup's syndrome). This is often is a diagnosis of exclusion after evaluation with a bone scan.[9,10]

8. Spondylolysis May Occur in Athletes Who Have a Certain Type of Repetitive Motion. What Imaging Tests Should Be Ordered to Diagnose Spondylolysis and Spondylolisthesis?

While the exact etiology of spondylolysis is not known, it is typically caused by a stress fracture due to the repetitive extension and torsion of the spine. Sports involving repetitive extension and rotation of the lumbar spine, such as dance, figure skating, and gymnastics, increase the risk of injury to the posterior elements of the spine. Forty percent recall a specific traumatic event.[1]

- Standing anteroposterior, lateral, and possibly bilateral oblique lumbar radiographs should be obtained in the athlete with low-back pain and suspected spondylolysis. A coned-down lateral radiograph of the lumbosacral junction produces a clearer image of the posterior bone structures than does a standard lateral radiograph, and nearly 90% of defects are appreciated in this view.[1] If obtained, left and right oblique radiographs will highlight the "Scotty dog." Spondylolysis is seen as a broken neck or a collar.
- When plain radiographs of a patient with persistent symptoms reveal negative findings, a single-photon emission computed tomography (SPECT) scan, CT scan, or MRI should be considered (Table 33-3).

9. What Are the Management Options for Spondylolysis and Spondylolisthesis, and When Can Athletes Return to Play?

- The majority of athletes with spondylolysis or pars stress reactions respond favorably to nonoperative treatment. This treatment includes a brief period of rest followed by physical rehabilitation. Therapeutic protocols may include the use of modalities for pain relief, bracing, exercise, ultrasonography, electrical stimulation, and activity modification. Physical therapy is recommended to reduce pain, to restore range of motion and function, and to strengthen and stabilize the spine. The role and best type of external immobilization continue to be debated. Athletes can return to play (RTP) when they are pain free, regardless of whether there is radiographic evidence of pars healing.

Table 33-3. Pros and Cons of Lumbosacral Magnetic Resonance Imaging, Single-Photon Emission Computed Tomography Scan, and Computed Tomography Scan

IMAGING TEST	*PROS*	*CONS*
Lumbosacral magnetic resonance imaging (coronal-oblique STIR sequence)	No radiation Soft tissue delineation Determine chronicity of fracture	Cost (expensive) Patient may be claustrophobic May miss early fractures or subtle fractures
Single-photon emission computed tomography scan	Accurate in determining location and chronicity	Radiation Duration of test (> 1 hr) Invasive (needs IV) Not readily available
Computed tomography scan	Fast Accessible (available in many locations) Accurate in determining location	Radiation

- A possible physical therapy protocol may consist of the following:
  - Visit one—Spondylolysis diagnosis finalized. Bracing may be used initially to limit hyperextension and to relieve pain at rest. Physical therapy initiates peripelvic flexibility and antilordotic strengthening. Activity restricted to physical therapy, stationary bike, and swimming, except butterfly and breast stroke.
  - Visit two (4 to 6 weeks later)—Clinical assessment determines no pain with activities and on lumbar hyperextension. If bracing was initiated, consider cessation of use. Begin spinal stabilization and strengthening with extensions to neutral, OR persistent pain at this visit initiates a search for a comorbid diagnosis.
  - Visit three (4 months after first visit)—May consider reimaging if still in pain. If lesion is nonunited and symptomatic, consider electrical stimulation with brace.

10. Is There a Place for Bone Stimulators in the Management of Spondylolysis or Spondylolistheses?

External electrical bone stimulation has been investigated as a possible adjunct to treatment for spondylolysis. Bone stimulators have been used with spinal fusions, nonunions, and fractures. However, there is no current indication for its use in spondylolysis. There have been several case reports using electrical bone stimulation to treat spondylolysis with good outcomes, but no current level I, II, or III study has been conducted showing a beneficial effect of bone stimulators. At this point, it is unclear what role bone stimulators will have in treatment, and more research needs to be done in this area.[9,10]

11. When Should I Refer My Patients With Spondylolysis or Spondylolistheses to an Orthopedist or Sports Medicine Specialist?

- Referral to a surgeon or sports medicine specialist should be made for patients who do not respond to nonoperative management at 3 months in the case of spondylolysis or spondylolisthesis. In the young athlete, surgical stabilization is indicated with a spondylolisthesis progression beyond 50%. If the patient remains symptomatic and has a persistent nonunion at 9 to 12 months, surgical posterolateral fusion is performed.

- Surgery should be considered in those with focal neurologic symptoms, a demonstration of slippage progression, persistent pain, or cosmetic deformity. RTP is allowed after there is demonstrated union, and the athlete is pain-free and manifests a full range of motion.[9,10]
- Consideration always should be given to atraumatic causes, such as discitis, osteomyelitis, and tumors. Warning symptoms include fevers, night pain, inordinate pain, age younger than 8, and any systemic symptoms. Inflammatory causes include reactive spondyloarthropathies, juvenile rheumatoid arthritis, and other collagen vascular diseases. Intra-abdominal causes also must be reviewed.

12. An Athlete Presents With Low-Back Pain. The History Provided Is Nonspecific, and the Physical Examination Is Unremarkable. What Could This Athlete Have?

Muscle strain has been reported to be the cause of up to 25% of all adolescent back pain. It may be associated with trauma or even just with carrying a heavy backpack. However, mechanical problems from computer use, physical activity, or heavy backpacks do not appear to be the etiology of back pain in school-aged children. Muscle strains are usually related to physical activity; they present as acute back pain without radiation. A herniated disc in children and adolescents presents similarly to that in adults and may be associated with pain radiating down one or both legs, pain with the Valsalva maneuver, or stiffness. Most patients will have a positive straight leg raise test result, although some may present with hamstring tightness and no radiculopathy.[11]

13. How Is Scoliosis Defined, and What X-rays Should Be Ordered? Is Scoliosis Associated With Back Pain? When Is Referral Necessary, and Can Physical Therapy Help?

- Scoliosis is defined as a lateral curvature of the spine greater than 10 degrees accompanied by vertebral rotation. Adolescent idiopathic scoliosis is present in 2% to 3% of children between 10 and 16 years of age.[8] Less common—but better defined—etiologies of the disorder include scoliosis of neuromuscular origin, congenital scoliosis, scoliosis in neurofibromatosis, and mesenchymal disorders such as Marfan's syndrome. Idiopathic scoliosis is typically not painful, but up to 25% of patients may report pain at some point.[8] Age of over 15 years, skeletal maturity (a Risser stage of 2 or more), postmenarchal status, and a history of injury were associated with pain on presentation. It may be identified by the Adam's forward bend test during physical examination. Severe pain, a left thoracic curve, or abnormal neurologic examination are red flags that point to a secondary cause for spinal deformity. Physical examination may reveal an obvious curve or spinal asymmetry, shoulder/scapular asymmetry, uneven waistline, oblique pelvis, trunk rotation, or unequal arm lengths with the Adam's forward bend test. The skin should be evaluated for possible signs of underlying spinal dysgraphism, such as café au lait spots, hairy patches, dimples, and spinal masses.[12]
- Abnormalities on physical examination require radiographic evaluation with a single-standing posteroanterior radiograph to allow the measurement of the curve using the Cobb angle and Risser staging of the iliac apophysis (Figure 33-4). MRI is indicated whenever there is a left thoracic curve, unusual pain, or abnormalities on neurologic examination, among other red flags, to evaluate for spondylolisthesis, tumors, or syringomyelia.
- Specialty consultation is needed if red flags are present or if there is a curve greater than 20 degrees, a progressive curve that has increased by more than 5 degrees, or if the patient is Risser stage 0 to 2. High thoracic or cervico-thoracic curves, or double curves, should also be evaluated by a surgeon. Referral should be made for patients if there is persistent back pain, and curves greater than 40 degrees may require surgical intervention and should also be evaluated.[13]

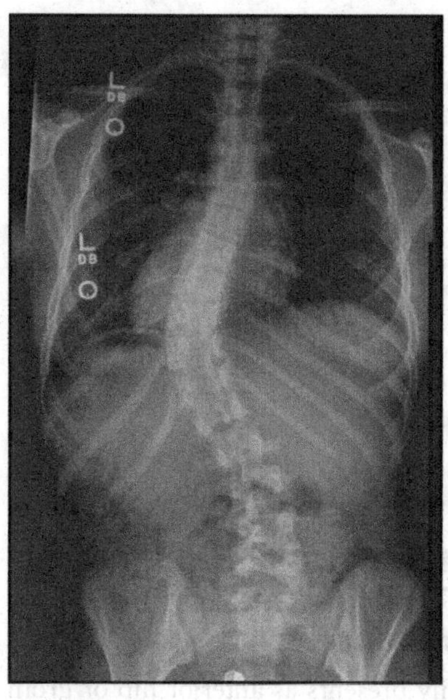

Figure 33-4. Anteroposterior radiograph of a patient with adolescent idiopathic scoliosis.

The aim of treatment is to prevent the progression of the curve. Of adolescents diagnosed with scoliosis, only 10% have curves that progress and require medical intervention.[8] The main risk factors for curve progression are a large curve magnitude (> 20 degrees), skeletal immaturity, and female sex. Physical therapy is generally not thought to be helpful in preventing the progression of the curvature. Bracing can be very effective in preventing curve progression, and is generally tolerated very well.[12]

References

1. Haidar R, Saad S, Khoury NJ, Musharrafieh U. Practical approach to the child presenting with back pain. *Eur J Pediatr.* 2011;170:149–156.
2. Hart ES, Merlin G, Harisiades J, Grottkau BE. Scheuermann's thoracic kyphosis in the adolescent patient. *Orthop Nurs.* 2010;29(6):365–371.
3. Papagelopoulos PJ, Mavrogenis AF, Savvidou OD, Mitsiokapa EA, Themistocleous GS, Soucacos PN. Current concepts in scheuermann's kyphosis. *Orthopedics.* 2008;31(1):52-58.
4. McIntosh AL, Sucato, DJ. Scheuermann's kyphosis. *Contemporary Spine Surgery.* 2008;9:1-8.
5. Dang L, Liu Z. A review of current treatment for lumbar disc herniation in children and adolescents. *Eur Spine J.* 2010;19:205–214.
6. Haidar R, Ghanem I, Saad S, Uthman I. Lumbar disc herniation in young children. *Acta Paediatr.* 2010;99(1):19–23.
7. Ballock RT, Mackersie R, Abitbol JJ, Cervilla V, Resnick D, Garfin SR. Can burst fractures be predicted from plain radiographs? *J Bone Joint Surg Br.* 1992;74:147-50.
8. Vaccaro AR, Kim DH, Brodke DS, et al. Diagnosis and management of thoracolumbar spine fractures. *Instr Course Lect.* 2004;53:359–373.
9. McCleary MD, Congeni JA. Current concepts in the diagnosis and treatment of spondylolysis in young athletes. *Curr Sports Med Rep.* 2007;6(1):62–66.
10. Hu SS, Tribus CB, Diab M, Ghanayem AJ. Spondylolisthesis and spondylolysis. *J Bone Joint Surg.* 2008;90(3):656–671.
11. Purcell L, Micheli L. Low back pain in young athletes. *Sports Health.* 2009;1(3):212–222.
12. Reamy BV. Adolescent idiopathic scoliosis: review and current concepts. *Am Fam Physician.* 2001;64(1):111–117.
13. Ramirez N, Johnston CE, Browne RH. The prevalence of back pain in children who have idiopathic scoliosis. *J Bone Joint Surg.* 1997;79:364–368.

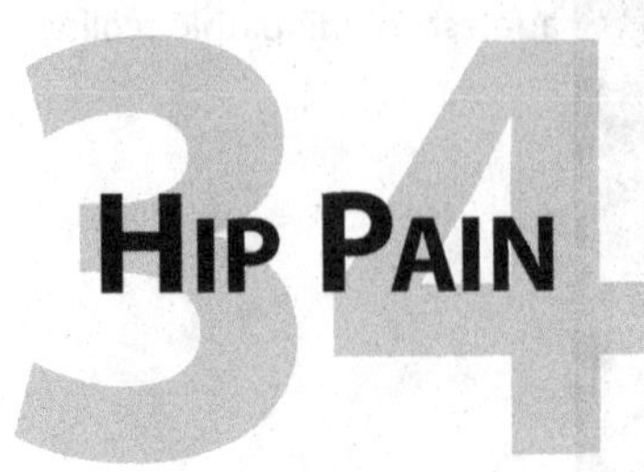

34 Hip Pain

Tracy L. Zaslow, MD, FAAP, CAQSM

1. Where Does Referred Pain From an Intra-articular Hip Injury Commonly Present, and How Should This Information Be Incorporated Into the Examination?

Referred pain from an intra-articular hip injury commonly presents as anterior hip or groin pain and as pain on the medial aspect of the thigh or knee. Thus, a complete hip and knee examination should be performed with presenting reports of pain in the groin or medial thigh or knee. Additionally, pain at the extremes of motion (especially internal rotation) or limited range of motion (ROM) signal a concern for intra-articular pathology.

2. A Patient Presents With a Fever, Limping, and Pain in the Hip Region. How Do You Differentiate Between Transient Synovitis and a Septic Hip?

Transient synovitis is the most common cause of hip pain in school-aged children (3 to 10 years-old)[1]; septic arthritis of the hip is rare. The delayed diagnosis of a septic hip can lead to devastating consequences.

- Patients with transient synovitis usually present with a 1- to 3-day history of limping, appearing uncomfortable, and a refusal to bear weight. Laboratory testing (including complete blood count, C-reactive protein [CRP], and erythrocyte sedimentation rate [ESR]) and hip ultrasonography are normal.
- Septic hip findings include a "sick" appearance and a fever. The fever rapidly worsens by the hour; fever (>38.5°C) is the best predictor of septic arthritis.[2] The patient will often refuse to bear weight on the involved limb; even just performing the simple log-rolling maneuver of the hip will elicit significant pain. CRP is commonly elevated early in the disease process while ESR may be normal in the first 24 hours; thus, a normal CRP and ESR do not rule out a septic hip.[3] Ultrasonography may be a useful tool to look for a hip joint effusion; however, ultrasonography may be falsely-negative if symptoms are present for less than 24 hours.[4] If the physical examination and laboratory results are suspicious for septic arthritis, then the gold-standard is aspiration. Surgical referral for irrigation and débridement is recommended when hip aspirate white cell counts are 50,000 or higher. Septic hip arthritis in the adolescent occasionally presents in a subacute form; one should consider hip aspiration in an adolescent with unusual hip pain and unimpressive but persistent laboratory findings that do not meet any other diagnostic criteria (Table 34-1).

Koutures C, Wong V.
Pediatric Sports Medicine: Essentials for Office Evaluation (pp 226-234)

TABLE 34-1. DIFFERENTIATING FEATURES OF TRANSIENT SYNOVITIS AND SEPTIC ARTHRITIS	
TRANSIENT SYNOVITIS	*SEPTIC ARTHRITIS*
Low-grade fever (<38.5°C)	Significant fever (>38.5°C)
Well-appearing	Ill-appearing; rapidly worsening
Normal WBC, CRP, and ESR	Elevated CRP early; later elevation of ESR
Normal hip ultrasonography	Hip effusion on ultrasonography, especially if symptoms >24 hours
WBC, white blood cell; CRP, C-reactive protein; ESR, erythrocyte sedimentation rate.	

TABLE 34-2. LEGG-CALVÉ-PERTHES VERSUS SLIPPED CAPITAL FEMORAL EPIPHYSIS		
	LEGG-CALVÉ-PERTHES	*SLIPPED CAPITAL FEMORAL EPIPHYSIS*
Typical age	• 4 to 8 years old (however, may be seen in all ages)	• Adolescent
Risk factors	• Male (4:1)	• Adolescent growth spurt • Obese (>95th percentile) • African American/Hispanic • Underlying illness: renal osteodystrophy, hypothyroidism, panhypopituitarism and hypogonadal conditions
Classic presentation	• Painless limp	• Limp +/– hip/knee pain • Obligate hip external rotation • Loss of internal rotation
Physical examination techniques	• Subtle asymmetry in hip motion (loss of hip abduction and/or internal rotation) • Positive Thomas test	• Obligate hip external rotation • Loss of internal rotation
Radiographic findings	• Avascular necrosis of the femoral head	• Posterior displacement of the metaphysis • Blurring of the metaphysis • Asymmetric physeal widening • Abnormal Klein's line

3. How Can a Health Care Provider Differentiate Between Legg-Calvé-Perthes Disease and Slipped Capital Femoral Epiphysis?

Please see Table 34-2 for a discussion on differentiating Legg-Calvé-Perthes disease from slipped capital femoral epiphysis (SCFE).

4. In Cases That Are Suspicious for a Slipped Capital Femoral Epiphysis, What Are Some Imaging, Initial Management, and Referral Recommendations?

Early diagnosis of SCFE is essential to prevent short- and long-term complications. Hip x-rays must be obtained in all patients suspicious for SCFE; key views include bilateral anteroposterior

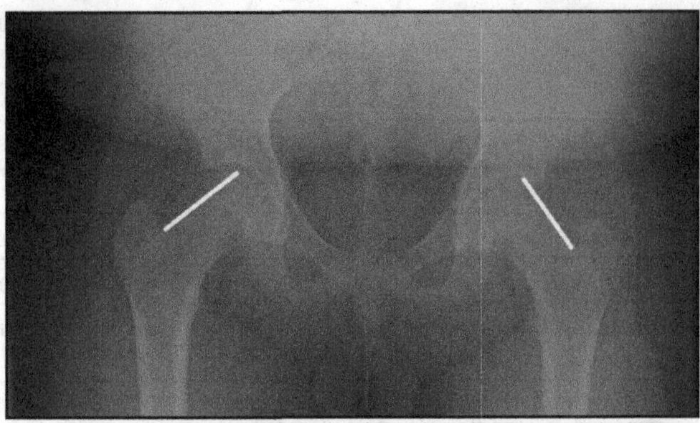

Figure 34-1. An anteroposterior view of the bilateral pelvis with abnormal Klein's line on the left side.

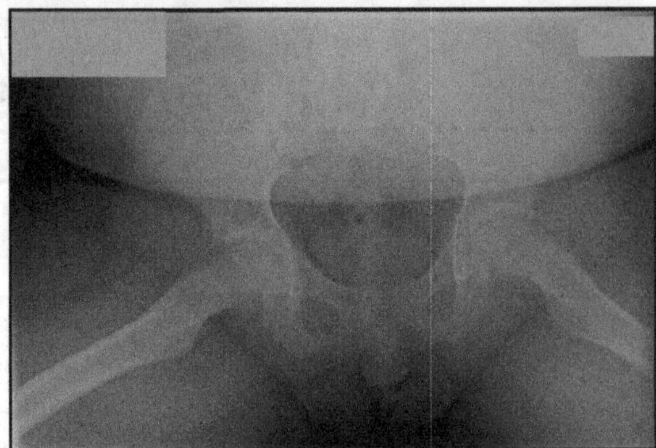

Figure 34-2. Slipped capital femoral epiphysis of the left hip (frog leg view).

(AP) and frog leg images. On a normal AP view, Klein's line drawn along the superior surface of the femoral neck should intersect a portion of the femoral head; on an AP view in a patient with SCFE, the line does not intersect the femoral head (Figure 34-1). Other notable findings include posterior displacement of the epiphysis compared with the metaphysis, blurring of the proximal metaphysis, asymmetric physeal widening, and a decrease in femoral epiphyseal height compared with the contralateral side (Figure 34-2).

When SCFE is suspected, the patient should not be allowed to bear weight. Even when going to x-ray, the patient should be sent by wheelchair. Weight bearing increases the risk of the slip worsening (stable becoming unstable or unstable worsening). Treatment involves emergent referral to orthopedic surgery for prompt in situ screw fixation.

5. Where Are the Labral and Chondral Surfaces of the Hip, and What Presentations May Suggest Tears of the Labrum or Damage to the Chondral Surfaces?

Articular cartilage covers the entire head of the femur, while cartilage over the acetabulum is composed of the labrum (a horseshoe rim of thickened fibrocartilage) and the central acetabular articular cartilage. The peripheral one-third of the labrum receives a rich blood supply, but the central two-thirds of the labrum has poor vascular supply and thus a low healing potential.

Articular cartilage injuries may present with anterior hip and groin pain, especially with internal rotation, flexion, and adduction, which compresses the articular surfaces. Labral tears are also often associated with painful catching, clicking, or snapping.

6. What Clinical Findings Suggest Femoral Acetabular Impingement?

Femoral acetabular impingement (FAI) refers to abnormal bony morphology of the hip joint that may alter biomechanics and force distribution, leading to chronic changes in the articular

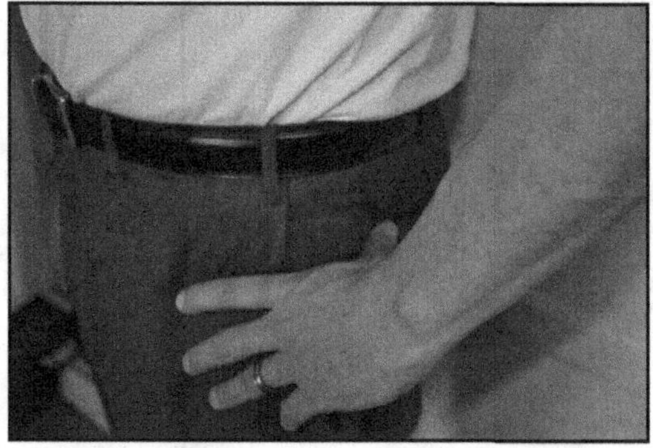

Figure 34-3. Photograph demonstrating C Sign.

cartilage and capsulolabral structure. The most common presentation of FAI is groin pain worsened by prolonged sitting (ie, prolonged hip flexion) and/or activity. Patients sometimes inadvertently perform the "C Sign" to indicate the location of the pain by gripping the lateral hip (just above the greater trochanter) between the abducted thumb and index finger (Figure 34-3). On physical examination, the patient's terminal hip motion may be limited, especially with internal rotation. Pain is often elicited by the "impingement sign" (the hip is flexed to 90 degrees and internally rotated).

AP pelvis radiographs are essential because an AP view of the hip limits the view of key bony landmarks. Additionally, frog-leg lateral radiographs can help to better visualize the femoral head-neck junction.[5] Further imaging with magnetic resonance arthrography of the hip with radial sequences can further elucidate the bony abnormalities and evaluate for labral tear and articular cartilage injury.

Two most common types of FAI on radiographs are pincer impingement (normal femoral head contacts an abnormally shaped acetabulum causing "pinching" of the labrum between the bony structures) and cam impingement (prominence at the femoral head-neck junction causing increased contact with a normal acetabulum during hip flexion and internal rotation). Figure 34-4 gives illustrations of pincer and cam forms of impingement.

7. How Is Femoral Acetabular Impingement Treated—From Both a Nonoperative and an Interventional Standpoint?

If no symptoms of painful clicking, catching, or locking are reported by a patient with FAI, first-line treatment includes rest, anti-inflammatory medication, and a physical therapy program emphasizing hip and lumbopelvic stabilization, correction of hip muscle imbalance, biomechanical control, and sport-specific functional progression. Additionally, in the skeletally mature athlete, an intra-articular hip injection with a corticosteroid and local anesthetic can be both therapeutic and diagnostic.

Surgery is indicated if there is painful clicking, catching, or locking, which indicate a labral tear and/or loose body, or if conservative management does not enable a pain-free return to full activity. The goal of surgery is to correct the cam and/or pincer deformities and repair any associated injury to the labrum or articular cartilage. Open or arthroscopic procedures have been shown to improve hip pain and function.

8. What Are the Common Sites, Involved Muscular Origins, and Mechanism of Injury of Pelvic Avulsion Fractures?

- Pelvic avulsion fractures tend to occur at the site of open apophyses (secondary ossification centers). Please see Figure 34-5.[6]
- Consider this type of fracture in all adolescents (aged 11 to 17 years) with "pulled muscles," as underlying associated fractures can be missed if no radiographic evaluation is performed.

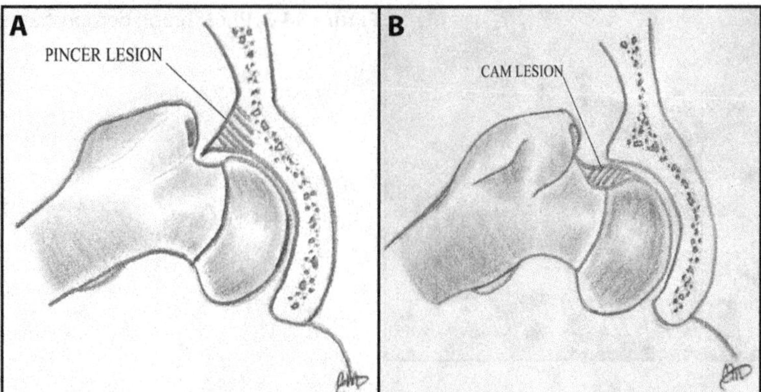

Figure 34-4. (A) Illustration of pincer impingement. (B) Illustration of cam impingement. (Graphite Pencil-Copyright © 2012 Cora Maglaya, PT, ATC, CSCS.)

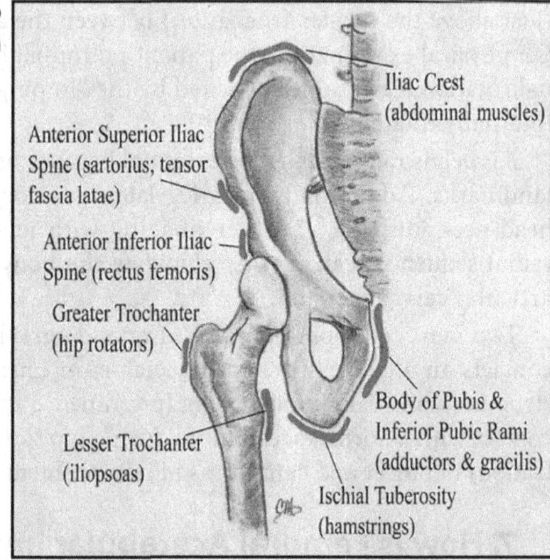

Figure 34-5. Apophyseal centers about the hip and pelvis. (Graphite Pencil-Copyright © 2012 Cora Maglaya, PT, ATC, CSCS.)

- The greatest susceptibility occurs at the time when the apophyses appear,[7-9] as they are the weakest link in the bone-tendon interface.

The mechanism of acute avulsion is either a sudden, violent, forceful muscle contraction (ie, kicking, running, jumping) or excessive passive lengthening (ie, gymnasts/cheerleaders performing the splits) with sudden shooting pain referred to the involved apophysis and decreased strength/loss of involved muscular function.

Chronic avulsions occur due to traction from repetitive trauma with ultimate displacement of the apophysis. These patients may present with more indolent symptoms and often do not recall an acute trauma, but rather a gradual increase in pain with activity and after activity. The physical examination also reveals tenderness to palpation over the affected apophysis and increased pain with resisted activation of the attached muscle group. When considering pelvic apophyseal avulsion, radiographs (AP and frog-leg lateral views) are the primary work-up modality (Figure 34-6). Bilateral comparison films can help to differentiate a true avulsion fracture from a normal adolescent variant.

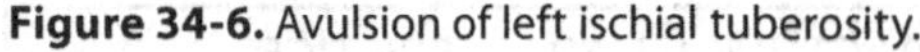

Figure 34-6. Avulsion of left ischial tuberosity.

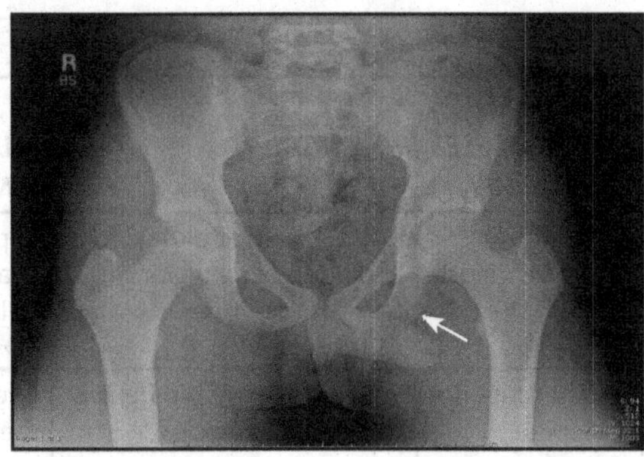

9. What Is the Usual Time Frame for Recovery in Nonoperative Cases of Pelvic Avulsion Fractures, and What Are the Usual Stages of Rehabilitation and Return to Usual Activities?

Treatment varies depending on the fracture site, the muscle forces across the physis, and the amount of displacement (Table 34-3). Most cases can be treated nonoperatively, observing a 5-stage rehabilitation protocol involving a gradual step-wise return to activity based on the resolution of pain and the improvement in radiographs (Table 34-4).[10]

10. What Are the Two Types of Femoral Neck Stress Fractures? What Are Their At-Risk Patient Populations, How Are They Identified on Examination/Imaging, What Are Some Activity Modification/Immobilization Recommendations, and Is There a Need for Urgent Referral?

- Inferior (low-tension) side of femoral neck (also known as compression type) is the most common type of femoral neck stress fracture and is considered low risk for a complete fracture.
- Superior (tension) side of the femoral neck is considered high risk because of the propensity to a complete fracture.

Females are most commonly affected. Historically, femoral neck stress fractures were specifically related to high-mileage running; however, more recently they have also been shown to be related to inexperienced runners running modest distances.

Patients with femoral neck stress fractures present with persistent groin pain that is worsened by activity and relieved by rest. There is usually no history of acute trauma or injury, but it is important to discuss any changes in the patient's recent training program. A report of the sudden worsening of pain may indicate that a stress fracture has become a complete and/or displaced fracture.

On physical examination, there is no significant swelling, ecchymosis, or deformity. An antalgic gait may be observed as the patient enters the examination room, but sometimes running or hopping activities are required to demonstrate the pain. Patients may have diffuse tenderness to palpation near the fracture site, but point tenderness is difficult to elicit. ROM may be limited by pain at the extremes of motion. Additionally, the straight leg raise may cause groin pain.

Work-up begins with AP and frog-leg lateral views of the hip. If they are negative, then magnetic resonance imaging of the hip is the best next step to evaluate for stress reaction changes (marrow edema) and/or more subtle evidence and localization of the fracture.

As compression fractures tend to be more mechanically stable, they are usually treated with 6 to 8 weeks of nonweight bearing to partial weight bearing as tolerated with pain as the guide. Tension-side fractures are potentially unstable with a high risk of nonunion, and thus are usually

TABLE 34-3. PELVIC APOPHYSEAL FRACTURE CHARACTERISTICS			
APOPHYSEAL SITE (MUSCLE ATTACHMENT)	*PHYSICAL FINDINGS*	*IMAGING FINDINGS*	*SURGICAL INDICATIONS*
Ischial tuberosity (Hamstrings)	Buttock pain at gluteal fold Radiation of pain along hamstrings Antalgic gait	Separation of crescent-shaped apophysis from ischial tuberosity	ORIF if > 2 cm displaced
Anterior superior iliac spine (Sartorius; Tensor fasciae latae)	Pain with active hip flexion or passive extension	Infero-lateral displacement of avulsion fragment	ORIF if > 2 cm displaced
Anterior inferior iliac spine (Rectus femoris)	Acute groin pain ↑pain with hyperextension or resisted hip flexion	Bilateral films to distinguish from os acetabuli Minimally displaced fragment because part of rectus femorus conjoined tendon remains intact	Encourage bed rest with hip/knee flexed for 1st few days ORIF if > 2 cm displaced
Iliac crest (Abdominal musculature)	Gluteus medius lurch	Avulsion fragment or apophyseal widening	ORIF if > 3 cm displaced
Lesser trochanter (Iliopsoas)	Hip in adduction/internal rotation Positive Ludloff sign (inability to flex hip while seated)		Bed rest with hip mildly flexed for first few days Surgery almost never indicated
Greater trochanter (Gluteus muscles)	Hip in slight flexion ↓hip abduction Positive Trendelenburg's sign	Avulsion fragment or apophyseal widening	ORIF if > 1 cm displacement
Symphysis pubis (Adductor longus)	↑pain with passive abduction or resisted hip adduction	May appear normal	Surgical intervention may be needed if unable to return to play

treated with surgical fixation to prevent displacement. After initial surgical/nonweight bearing management is complete, a rehabilitation program can facilitate return to full ROM and strength and also address underlying biomechanical gait abnormalities and/or core stability and lower-extremity weakness. Prior to a return to sports participation, patients must have radiographic evidence of bone healing, have pain-free full ROM, display a normal gait with walking and running, demonstrate symmetric muscle strength bilaterally, and complete a rehabilitation protocol.

11. What Is a Hip Pointer? Is There a Chronic Type of Injury to This Area? Who Is at the Highest Risk, and What Things Can Be Done to Prevent and Treat These Types of Injuries?

A "hip pointer" is a contusion of the iliac crest that occurs from a direct blow after a fall or collision. Patients usually present with acute pain that is often associated with swelling and significant ecchymoses, as well as tenderness to palpation over the iliac crest. Always remember to perform a

Table 34-4. Rehabilitation Program for Pelvic Avulsion Fractures

TREATMENT PHASE	*DAYS AFTER INJURY*	*SUBJECTIVE PAIN*	*X-RAY FINDINGS*	*RANGE OF MOTION*	*MUSCLE STRENGTH*	*LEVEL OF ACTIVITY*
I	0 to 7	Moderate	Visible avulsion	Limited	Poor	Protected weight bearing
II	7 to 14	Minimal	Visible avulsion	Improving with guided exercise	Fair	Protected weight bearing Guided exercise
III	15 to 30	Minimal with activity	Early callus	Improving with gentle stretch	Good	Guided exercise Resistance training
IV	31 to 60	None	Maturing callus	Normal	Good to Normal	Limited sport-specific activity
V	61 to Return	None	Bony remodelling	Normal	Normal	Gradual return to full activity

complete abdominal examination to rule out any significant intra-abdominal trauma. X-rays (AP/lateral views of the pelvis) can be performed if one is suspicious of an associated fracture or avulsion.

Chronic stress to the iliac crest, often seen in runners who rotate to the left and right during the running motion, can cause irritation known as iliac crest apophysitis. Pain is usually focal to one or often both of the iliac crests, and radiographs are usually unremarkable.

Treatment begins with ice and rest; as symptoms resolve, begin early ROM followed by hip/core strengthening. The prognosis is excellent with a gradual return to full activity, with pain as the limiting factor. Padding over the iliac crest can help prevent direct trauma to this area.

12. My Patient Reports That Her Hip "Snaps." What Are the Types of Snapping Hip, How Can They Be Identified, and What Are Some Treatment and Management Tips?

- "External" snapping hip ("coxa saltans externa"): iliotibial band rubbing or snapping over greater trochanteric prominence.
  - This type of snapping hip may occur from trauma or overuse; it is also noted as a painless incidental finding.
  - Lateral hip pain and/or the sensation of hip subluxation/snapping are often associated with running or with movement after prolonged sitting.
  - It is reproduced by passively maneuvering the hip through flexion and extension.
  - Tenderness may be about iliotibial band (ITB), especially over the greater trochanter prominence and bursa. Perform Ober test to assess ITB tightness (see Figure 35-6).
  - The history and examination are usually diagnostic, and no further studies are indicated unless the health care provider is concerned about other diagnoses.
  - Management includes rest, ice, local modalities to diminish inflammation, and exercise programs including ITB stretching and pelvis/core stabilization. In skeletally mature athletes, judicious corticosteroid injections into the greater trochanteric bursa can provide pain relief. While it is sometimes difficult to fully eradicate the snapping, conservative management usually eradicates pain.
  - In recalcitrant cases, the surgical relaxation of ITB may be considered.

- When the patient's pain is resolved, full return to play can occur. If the patient had surgical treatment, a gradual return to full activity is anticipated over 2 to 4 months after the procedure.

- "Internal" snapping hip ("coxa saltans interna"): iliopsoas tendon snaps across the iliopectineal bony prominence.
  - This type is often an incidental finding that is present in 10% of the active population.[11]
  - Pain aggravated by walking, running, and a variety of other athletic pursuits.
  - A classic examination maneuver involves the following: start with the hip in a position of abduction, flexion, and external rotation; then the hip is brought into extension with internal rotation, producing a snap that is usually at 30 degrees of hip flexion.
  - Palpation of the anterior hip elicits tenderness over the area just distal to the anterior superior iliac spine and medial to the sartorius muscle.
  - The diagnosis usually by history and examination; it can be confirmed by dynamic ultrasonogrpahy.
  - The management for nonpainful snapping hip solely necessitates reassurance.
  - The initial treatment for painful snapping is with relative rest and exercise program emphasizing stretching and core/pelvis stabilization.
  - If the patient is unable to return to his or her desired level of activity, surgical release/lengthening of the tendinous portion of the iliopsoas can be considered.
  - The athlete can return to play when his or her pain is resolved; however, if surgical intervention is performed, return to play usually occurs about 3 to 4 months postoperatively.
- Internal snapping hip: intra-articular labral tear.
  - Magnetic resonance arthrogram of the hip should be performed to evaluate for intra-articular pathology, and can be helpful to assess for associated inflammation.
  - If a labral tear is suspected or confirmed, a sports medicine specialist or orthopedic referral indicated.

References

1. Hart JJ. Transient synovitis of the hip in children. *Am Fam Physician.* 1996;54(5):1587–1591.
2. Caird MS, Flynn JM, Leung YL, et al. Factors distinguishing septic arthritis from transient synovitis of the hip in children: a prospective study. *J Bone Joint Surg Am.* 2006;88:1251–1257.
3. Kallio MJ, Unkila-Kallio L, Aalto K, et al. Serum C-reactive protein, erythrocyte sedimentation rate and white blood cell count in septic arthritis in children. *Pediatr Infect Dis J.* 1997;16(4):411–413.
4. Gordon JE, Huang M, Dobbs M, et al. Causes of false-negative ultrasound scans in the diagnosis of septic arthritis of the hip in children. *J Pediatr Orthop.* 2002;22(3):312–316.
5. Clohisy JC, Carlisle JC, Beaulé PE, et al. A systematic approach to plain radiographic evaluation of the young adult hip. *J Bone Joint Surg Am.* 2008;90(Suppl 4): 47–66.
6. Paletta GA Jr, Andrish JT. Injuries about the hip and pelvis in the young athlete. *Clin Sports Med.* 1995;14:591–628.
7. Femback SK, Wilkinson RH. Avulsion fractures of the pelvis and proximal femur. *AJR Am J Roentgenol.* 1981;137(3):581–584.
8. Metzmaker JN, Pappas AM. Avulsion fractures of the pelvis. *Am J Sports Med.* 1985;13(5):349–358.
9. Sundar M, Carty H. Avulsion fractures of the pelvis in children: a report of 32 fractures and their outcome. *Skeletal Radiol.* 1994;23(2):85–90.
10. Metzmaker JN, Pappas AM. Avulsion fractures of the pelvis. *Am J Sports Med.* 1985;13:349–358.
11. Byrd JW, Looney CG. Pelvis, hip and thigh injuries. In: Madden CC, Putukian M, Young CC, McCarty EC, eds. *Netter's Sports Medicine.* Philadelphia, PA: Saunders Elsevier. 2010:404-416.

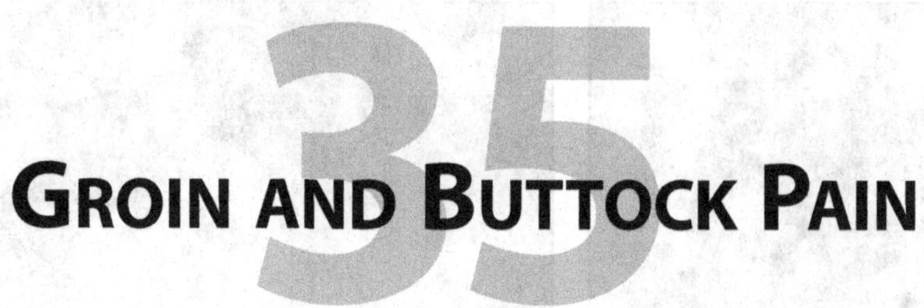

35 Groin and Buttock Pain

Christopher Lynch, MD and Chris Koutures, MD, FAAP

1. What Are Some Common Mechanical Dysfunctions, and How Can They Be Identified on Examination?

Abductor Dysfunction (Gluteus Medius and Iliotibial Band)

- The gluteus medius stabilizes the stance leg during normal stride and the single-leg stance by preventing the unsupported side from tilting or falling downward.
- Gluteus medius weakness will cause the overuse tightness and pain of the iliotibial (IT) band.
- Mild gluteus medius weakness will cause the opposite hip to drop to the downward position, resulting in an uncompensated Trendelenburg gait.
- More severe weakness results in a compensated Trendelenburg gait with excessive tilting or leaning toward the weak side to avoid dropping the opposite hip.
    - Standing Trendelenburg test: one leg is lifted off of the floor while the examiner observes the patient's hip levels from behind. Normal abductor strength of the stance leg is observed when the pelvis remains level on the raised knee side; it is considered abnormal if the pelvis sags on the raised knee side (Figure 35-1).

Buttock/Lumbar Extensor Dysfunction (Gluteus Maximus, Multifidus Spinae, and Hamstrings)

- Gluteus maximus weakness leads to an over reliance on the multifidus and hamstrings.
- Common examination findings include increased lumbar lordotic curve (overactivated multifidus) and forward pelvic thrust with active lumbar extension.
- Prone hip extension test: normal hip extension muscle activation is first the hamstrings, followed by the gluteus maximus, and finally, the multifidus. Common dysfunction is multifidus activated before or at the same time as the hamstrings, with gluteal activation occurring later (Figure 35-2).

Abnormal Pelvic Tilt

- The normal pelvic tilt results in the anterior superior iliac spine (ASIS) being in the same vertical plane as the symphysis pubis and in the same horizontal plane as the posterior superior iliac spine (PSIS).
- The anterior pelvic tilt (ASIS lower than PSIS) is often due to tight hip flexors, weak gluteus maximus/extensors, and weak transverse abdominis muscles (Figure 35-3).
- The posterior pelvic tilt (ASIS higher than PSIS) is often due to weak hip flexors and tight hamstring muscles.

Koutures C, Wong V.
Pediatric Sports Medicine: Essentials for Office Evaluation (pp 235-242)

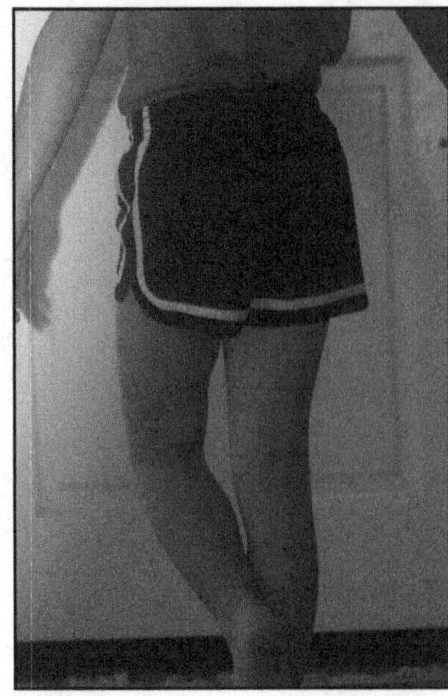

Figure 35-1. Abnormal Trendelenburg sign. The left buttock drops when the left knee is raised into flexion, which indicates weakness of the right gluteus medius (stance leg).

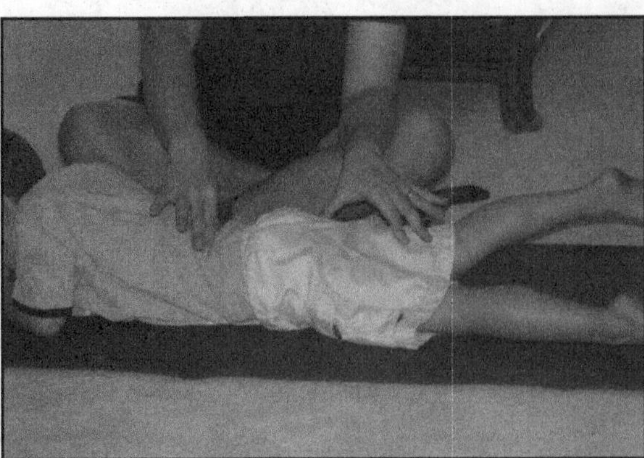

Figure 35-2. Prone hip extension. Place the thumb and the index finger of one hand on multifidi (parallel to lumber spine), the thumb of the other hand on the buttock and the index finger on the ipsilateral hamstring. Ask the patient to lift his or her entire leg—appropriate progression is the hamstring first, the gluteus maximus second, and the multifidi last.

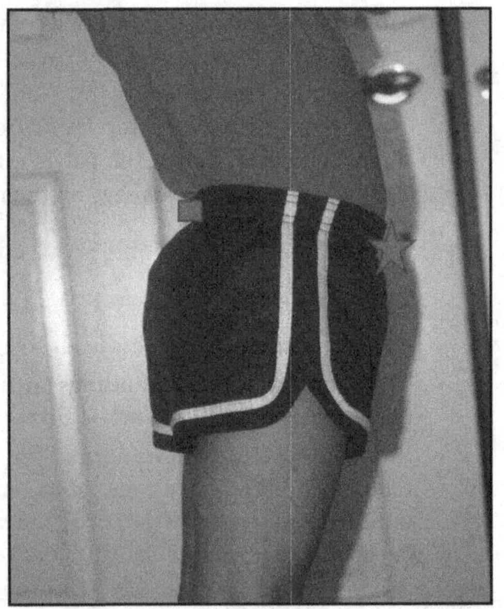

Figure 35-3. Anterior pelvic tilt. The anterior superior iliac spine (star) is lower than the posterior superior iliac spine (rectangle).

- The lowering of a hemipelvis (ASIS, PSIS, and iliac crest all lower on one side relative to the opposite side) may be due to an apparent leg length discrepancy or tight IT band.

Adductor Dysfunction (Adductor Longus/Brevis/Magnus, Gracilis, and Pectineus)

- Pubic symphysis pain manifests in hip extensor and transverse abdominis weakness.
- Supine active straight/bent leg adduction will result in pain and weakness.[1-3]

2. What Is a "Sportsman's Hernia," and Are There Any Reliable Imaging Studies to Help in the Diagnosis? Do All Cases Need Surgical Care?

A "sportsman's hernia" can present as vague, deep unilateral groin pain and may be due to disruptions in the conjoint tendon (internal oblique and tranverse abdominis aponeurosis) insertion into the pubic tubercle, with or without ilioinguinal nerve impingement or true abdominal herniation. Pain may be elicited superior to the pubic tubercle on single-finger examination of the groin and inguinal canal; a palpable defect is rarely found.

First-line management includes a 2- to 3-month rest from offending activities and a focus on adductor stretching and strengthening of the lower abdominal muscles. The need and utility of imaging is controversial. If it is indicated, pelvic ultrasonography or magnetic resonance imaging (MRI) are the most commonly utilized. Ultrasonography, if done in experienced hands, can act as a dynamic evaluation of soft-tissue structures, while MRI has increased sensitivity for underlying bony injury. Imaging is not necessary to confirm the diagnosis, as many athletes have undergone rehabilitation or surgical correction based on symptoms in the absence of an identified radiological anomaly.[4]

Generally, if surgery is being considered, one of the above imaging options will be utilized. Once a hernia has been identified, there is controversy regarding the indications for surgical correction.[5]

3. How Can an Adductor Strain ("Groin Pull") Be Identified and Managed?

Repetitive hip adduction (such as in skating or sudden cutting or twisting activities) can lead to strains of the adductor muscles (longus, brevis, and magnus) with pain, usually at the pubic tubercle origin or in the proximal muscle. The identification of the precise muscle can be difficult; the primary examination objectives are to identify tenderness in the adductor region and rule out other causes of medial groin pain (intra-articular hip injury, nerve entrapment, bone stress injury). Initial treatment includes avoiding aggravating activities and icing the identifiable points of tenderness. Emerging evidence suggests that nonsteroidal anti-inflammatory drugs should be avoided early after injury, as they may impair healing, perhaps by aggravating localized hemorrhage; acetaminophen may be an alternative for initial pain relief. Physical therapy should focus on abdominal muscle strengthening, stretching of the hip flexors, strengthening of adductors (initially static followed by dynamic exercises), and single-leg balance/functional work when the patient is pain-free.[6]

4. What Are Some Common Nerve Entrapments, and How Can They Be Found and Treated?

Please see Table 35-1 for a list of common groin and buttock region nerve entrapment syndromes.[1-3]

Dysthesia with percussion over the involved nerve (Tinel's sign) is a common diagnostic finding for both lateral cutaneous and cluneal nerve pathology, and the injection of lidocaine mixed with a steroid may be both diagnostic and therapeutic. Electromyography is difficult to perform, but does show sensory abnormalities in over 70% of cases. It may be difficult for physical examination alone to determine if the patient's pain is due to pudendal neuropathy versus perineal muscle spasm; referral to a urologist or gynecologist with expertise in this problem may be needed.[7]

Additional recommendations include oral anti-inflammatory medication, physical therapy focusing on the relaxation of the pelvic floor musculature, avoiding restrictive waist garments, and minimizing sitting and specific activities that exacerbate neuropathy (such as cycling or running with marked leg adduction). Attention to proper bicycle seat fit that focuses the athlete's weight directly on the ischial tuberosities can be helpful. Nerve decompression surgery can be performed in severe or prolonged cases.[8]

Table 35-1. Common Nerve Entrapments and Their Locations/Sensory Innervations and Mechanism of Injuries

NERVE	*LOCATION/SENSORY INNERVATION*	*MECHANISM OF INJURY*
Lateral cutaneous "Meralgia paresthetica"	Under the inguinal ligament and medial to the ASIS/ anterolateral thigh	Direct pressure, tight clothing/ belts, obesity, and ASIS avulsion fracture
Medial branch of the superior cluneal	Crosses the iliac crest laterally to the PSIS/fan-shape over the medial and lateral buttocks	Sudden forceful stretching of lower-back fascia with muscle contraction
Pudendal "Cyclist syndrome": symptoms include urinary frequency, dyspareunia, erectile dysfunction, pain aggravated by defecation, and foreign body sensation in the perineum, vagina, or rectum[1-3]	Multiple sites of entrapment: sacrospinous and sacrotuberous ligaments, obturator internus aponeurosis/perineum, penis or vaginal area	Trauma, surgery, childbirth, and prolonged sitting, especially in bicyclists with prolonged compression medial to the ischial tuberosities

5. Athletes in Certain Sports Such as Soccer and Ice Hockey Often Report Unilateral/Bilateral Midline Anterior Groin Pain. What Is Osteitis Pubis, What Is Usually Found on Examination and Imaging, and What Are Some Key Management Tips?

Osteitis pubis is traumatic long-standing irritation of the pubic symphysis and cartilage (joint between the iliac bones), along with aggravation of the associated adductor tendons and supporting ligaments. Clinical findings include tenderness and pain with supine bilateral straight leg resisted adduction testing (both legs raised 6 inches off of the table, while the examiner resists active adduction). Anteroposterior pelvis films may demonstrate irregularity of the pubic symphysis, which is suggestive of osteitis pubis, but generally they are not considered first line and they have a low specificity. Technetium-99m bone scan or MRI can depict increased pubic symphysis uptake, but are often only performed when other issues such as stress fractures, referred back pain, or osteomyelitis are considered.[9]

Initial management of osteitis pubis includes reducing all offending activity and beginning a focused 8- to 10-week rehabilitation program emphasizing adductor and core strengthening. Only when the patient is pain free is running allowed (first straight ahead, then with cutting/turning). Corticosteroid injection into the pubic symphysis (or a 3- to 5-day course of oral prednisone 1 mg/kg/dose) can be helpful in more symptomatic cases. If this focused program fails, surgical options range from simple curettage to a full arthrodesis (fusion of the pubic symphysis); curettage has been shown to be the best-tolerated procedure and the most successful in promoting full recovery.[2,3,5]

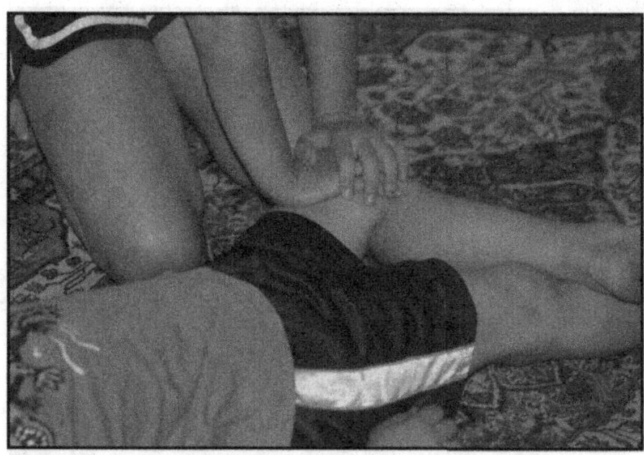

Figure 35-4. The FABER test, or Patrick test, for sacroiliac pain and dysfunction.

6. What Is the Sacroiliac Joint, and How Can Issues of Asymmetric Pelvic Rotation, Abnormal Pelvic Tilt, and Sacroiliac Dysfunction Be Identified on History and Physical Examination?

Physical Exam Assessment of the Sacroiliac Joint

The sacroiliac joint (SIJ) is a fibrous synovial joint at the connection of both pelvic iliac bones and the sacrum that has often underappreciated stability and mobility. The importance of normal SIJ mobility is demonstrated by the fact that treatments equalizing the symmetry of joint movement, including pelvic tilt exercises, often successfully resolve lower-back or buttock symptoms. Instability or limitations in mobility can cause pain during lumbar flexion or extension, or with lumbar or pelvic twisting or rotation. Leg length discrepancy or scoliosis with abnormal pelvic tilt can also place undue asymmetric SIJ stress, leading to pain. Inflammatory and connective tissue diseases (reactive arthritis, ankylosing spondylitis, infection, and gout) can also exacerbate SIJ pain.

Patients often present with a history of pain after repetitive bending or twisting activity or an asymmetric fall on the buttock, possibly with a popping sensation. Gait is usually normal, but range of motion to lower-back flexion and extension is limited. Right-left asymmetry in the heights of iliac crest, PSIS, and ASIS may suggest pelvic obliquity.

- Patrick test (also known as the Flexion Abduction External Rotation [FABER] test) stresses the SIJ by having the supine patient cross the affected side foot over the opposite knee ("figure-4" position) while the examiner gently pushes down on the flexed knee (Figure 35-4).
- Standing Gillette (or Stork) assesses SIJ motion by having the examiner place his or her thumbs on both PSIS dimples and then having the patient slowly raise one leg into 90 degrees of hip flexion (Figure 35-5). Normally, the PSIS will move slightly down when the leg is raised, but in SIJ dysfunction, the thumb on the affected side will not move or will ride upward.
- A diagnostic anesthetic joint injection is rarely needed.[1-3]

7. What Structures Are Commonly Involved in Greater Trochanteric Syndrome With Lateral Hip/Buttock Pain, and How Can These Issues Be Initially Managed?

The following are often involved in greater trochanteric syndrome (GTS) with lateral hip/buttock pain:

- Inflamed trochanteric bursa
- Overactivation of the IT tract

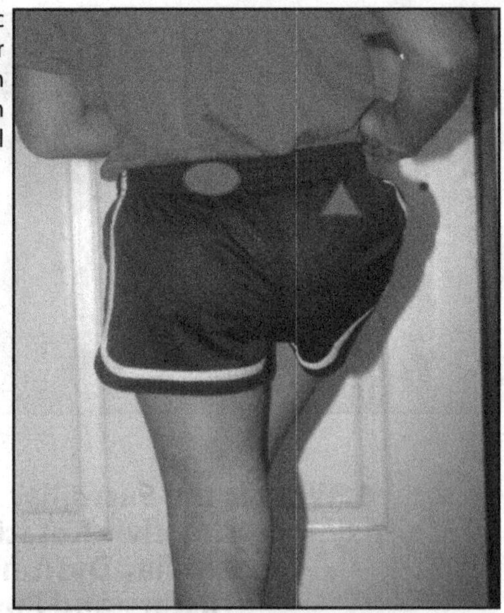

Figure 35-5. Normal Gillette or Stork test for sacroiliac mobility. With knee flexion, the ipsilateral posterior superior iliac spine (triangle) should be lower than the stance leg posterior superior iliac spine (oval). In restricted sacroiliac mobility, knee flexion leads to level or even raised ipsilateral PSIS.

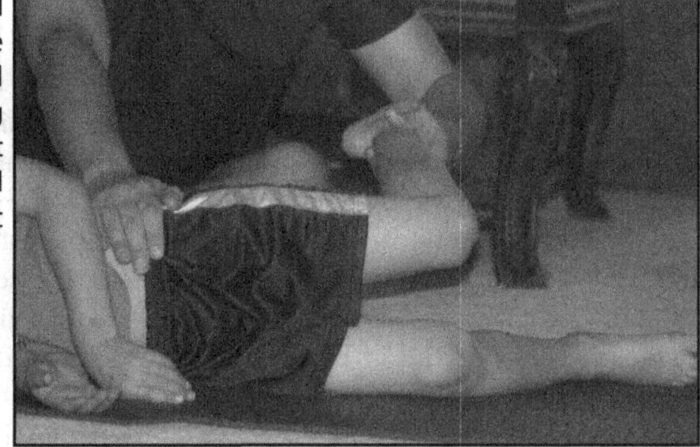

Figure 35-6. The Ober's test for iliotibial band tightness. Lateral decubitus position with the hips stacked on top of each other. Place a hand around the lower leg and put the upright leg into hip extension, then allow the upright knee to drop toward the lower knee. Limited to no upright knee movement indicates tight IT band on the upright leg.

- Strain of external hip rotators (obturator internus/externus, gemellus, piriformis, gluteus minimus, and quadratus femoris)

GTS is usually due to overuse of lateral/posterior muscle groups of the thigh. It may be more common in distance runners, particularly on the downhill side when training on uneven surfaces or those who adduct beyond the midline,[1] and in women due to their wider bony pelvis. Pain over the lateral hip, which may radiate down the lateral leg, is the hallmark. It may present as a lateral snapping hip as the IT band flips over the greater trochanter, possibly without any significant pain.

- Palpation over the lateral hip with the patient in the lateral decubitus position reveals point tenderness over the greater trochanter.
- A positive Ober's test (Figure 35-6) suggests a tight IT band as the released knee cannot adduct close to the examining table.

Although rarely needed, radiographs may show bony spurs over the greater trochanter. Activity modification, IT band stretching, and strengthening the gluteus medius muscle are key for initial rehabilitation, and corticosteroid injection into the trochanteric burse can be used for significant or persistent pain. Correcting an apparent leg-length inequality (usually due to pelvic obliquity and affects "shorter leg") is also essential.[1-3]

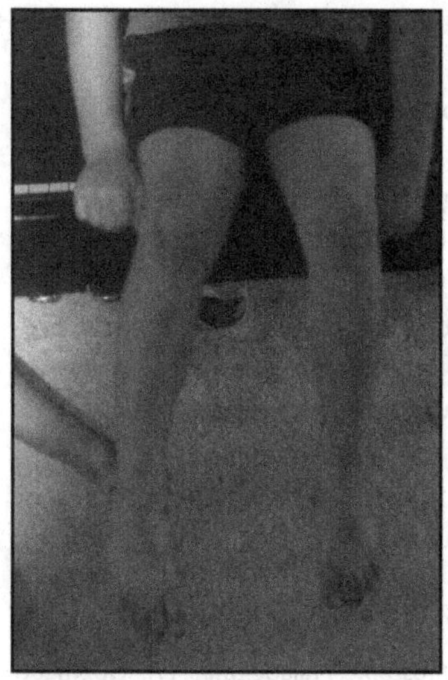

Figure 35-7. The Pace test for piriformis spasm. With the patient in the seated position, resist the abduction of the lower leg.

8. Pain in the Back of the Upper Leg Is Often Due to Piriformis Syndrome. What Is This Syndrome, and How Can It Be Identified and Treated?

The piriformis muscle originates from the anterior sacrum, exits the greater sciatic foramen, and inserts onto the greater trochanter. Irritation or swelling of the muscle or fascia can cause pain and may impinge on the nearby sciatic nerve, causing sciatica-type symptoms consisting of burning buttock pain that may radiate to the ipsilateral posterior thigh and down to the calf.[1] Pain may be induced by internal rotation and adduction of the hip, and also by prolonged sitting (particularly on hard surfaces). Pregnancy or a history of gluteal trauma are associated risk factors. Since the principal differential diagnosis includes radicular pain from a herniated intervertebral disc, a complete lumbar spine evaluation is also necessary.

Pertinent examination findings for piriformis syndrome include the following:

- Piriformis sign—Affected leg held in external rotation when in the supine position, resulting in pain relief.
- Pace test—Resisted abduction of the affected leg, eliciting pain by contracting the piriformis (Figure 35-7).
- Frieberg test—Internal rotation of the extended thigh to passively stretch muscle and cause pain.

Imaging studies are generally not helpful unless one is trying to rule out spinal pathology, and nerve conduction studies are occasionally helpful in evaluating for sciatic nerve dysfunction. Rest, anti-inflammatory medication, and muscle relaxants augmented by physical therapy (focused on adduction and flexion of the internally rotated hip and gluteal strengthening) reduce pain in most patients. Ultrasonography-guided piriformis injection with corticosteroids and local anesthetic or surgical release of the piriformis have been successfully used in refractory cases.[1-3]

9. What Are Some Common Medical Causes of Pelvic or Buttock Pain That Masquerade as Sports Injuries, and When Should the General Pediatric Provider Refer Cases of Pelvic/Buttock Pain to a Specialist?

- When an obvious source of musculoskeletal injury is not apparent, more insidious sources must be considered. Troubling signs include lingering neurologic changes, boney pain, fever, or changes in appetite or bowel and bladder function.

- In younger children, a refusal to crawl, sit, or walk may indicate back, pelvic, or gluteal pain.
- Unilateral sacroiliitis in children should raise the suspicion for an infection in the SIJ, and usually is associated with fever.
- Pelvic discomfort may be the presenting symptom of genitourinary infections, kidney stone disease, localized masses or hemorrhage, topical infections or rashes, pregnancy, or bowel inflammation.
- Inguinal or femoral hernias may be more noticeable after exercise and, while early presentations tend to be painless bulges, any failure for the bulge to reduce or the presence of significant pain suggests potential incarceration or strangulation of the hernia contents and is an indication for emergent surgical repair.

Any case of unexplained groin/buttock pain, especially associated with significant pain or dysfunction or fevers, should be referred for comprehensive evaluation.[2]

References

1. Johnson D, Pedowitz R. *Practical Orthopedic Sports Medicine and Arthroscopy.* Philadelphia, PA: Lippincott Williams & Wilkins; 2007.
2. Sarwark J, Labella C. *Pediatric Orthopedics and Sports injuries.* Elk Grove Village, IL: American Academy of Pediatrics; 2010.
3. Snider R. *Essentials of Musculoskeletal Care.* Rosemont, IL: American Association of Orthopedic Surgeons; 1997.
4. Robinson P, Bhat V, English B. Imaging in the assessment and management of athletic pubalgia. *Semin Musculoskelet Radiol.* 2011;15(1):14–26.
5. Ekstrand J, Ringborg S. Surgery versus conservative treatment in soccer players with chronic groin pain: a prospective randomized study in soccer players. *Eur J Sports Traumatol.* 2001;23(4):141–145.
6. Holmich P, Uhrskou P, Ulnits L, et al. Effectiveness of active physical training as treatment for long-standing adductor-related groin pain in athletes: randomized trial. *Lancet.* 1999;353:439–443.
7. Lu J, Ebraheim NA, Huntoon M, Heck BE, Yeasting RA. Anatomic considerations of superior cluneal nerve at posterior iliac crest region. *Clin Orthop Relat Res.* 1998;347:224–228.
8. Ramsden CE, McDaniel MC, Harmon RL, Renney KM, Faure A. Pudendal nerve entrapment as source of intractable perineal pain. *Am J Phys Med Rehabil.* 2003;82(6):479–484.
9. Nelson EN, Kassarjian A, Palmer WE. MR imaging of sports-related groin pain. *Magn Reson Imaging Clin N Am.* 2005;13(4):727–742.

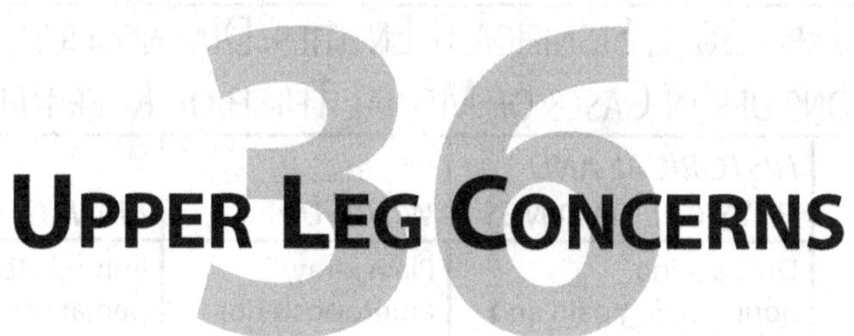

Upper Leg Concerns

T.J. Howell, MD and Valarie Wong, MD, FAAP

1. In Any Case of Medial Thigh or Knee Pain, What Structures and Significant Entities Must Be Considered and Evaluated?

The entities that must be considered when evaluating medial thigh or knee pain are discussed in Table 36-1.[1-9]

2. What Is the Mechanism of Injury for a Quadriceps Strain in an Adolescent Athlete? What Is the Best Way to Rehabilitate These Injuries? When Is a Referral Necessary?

- A quadriceps strain results from several different mechanisms, including excessive passive stretching of the muscle, activation of a maximally stretched muscle, or forceful eccentric contraction across the muscle tendon unit. The rectus femoris is the most commonly strained muscle of the quadriceps group. Activities that commonly result in quadriceps strains include kicking, jumping, and sudden changes in direction while running.[10-13] Strains are graded on the following scale, from 1 to 3:
  - Grade 1—Minor tear of muscle; mild pain, minimal loss of strength, no palpable defect
  - Grade 2—Severe damage to muscle; moderate pain, moderate loss of strength, muscle defect occasionally palpable
  - Grade 3—Complete tear of muscle; severe pain, complete loss of strength, muscle defect palpable
- Rehabilitation of a quadriceps strain is a stepwise process, beginning with the reduction of inflammation and pain, and progressing to increasing the patient's range of motion (ROM) and strength.[12] Return to play (RTP) can be several weeks from the acute injury, depending on the severity. Formal rehabilitation with a physical therapist can be beneficial. The following are the steps that take the patient from injury to RTP.
  - Step 1—Reduction of pain and inflammation (days 1 to 3)
    - Rest, ice, compression, elevation (RICE)
    - Ice + compression for 15 to 20 minutes, 3+ times a day, 30 to 60 minutes between sessions
    - Crutches as needed (usually for grades 2 or 3)
    - Nonsteroidal anti-inflammatory drugs (NSAIDs) as needed for the first 3 to 7 days
  - Step 2—Increase ROM (days 3 to 7)
    - Passive ROM exercises; stretching (never to pain, no ballistic stretching); heat, ultrasonography, and/or electrical stimulation

Koutures C, Wong V.
Pediatric Sports Medicine: Essentials for Office Evaluation (pp 243-250)

Table 36-1. Significant Entities/Diagnoses to Consider in Cases of Medial Thigh or Knee Pain			
DIAGNOSIS	*HISTORICAL AND PHYSICAL FINDINGS*	*WORK-UP*	*MANAGEMENT*
Slipped capital femoral epiphysis	Dull, aching, nonradiating pain and altered gait Pain may present in hip, groin, thigh, or knee. Worse with physical activity, no history of trauma[1,7]	Plain x-ray, anteroposterior and lateral/frog-leg views	Immediate referral to pediatric orthopedic surgeon Acute/unstable slips should be admitted Unilateral chronic slips should be evaluated immediately by pediatric orthopedist Nonweight bearing until evaluated[1,2,7]
Legg-Calvé-Perthes disease (avascular necrosis of the hip)	Acute or insidious onset of hip pain and/or limp, no history of trauma Higher risk in children with underlying disease such as lupus, renal failure, or steroid use[3,7]	Plain x-rays usually negative initially, bone scans show decreased perfusion, MRI will show marrow changes[3,4]	Nonweight bearing, referral to pediatric orthopedist Splinting or surgery may be required[3,4]
Septic arthritis	Pain with weight bearing or motion of affected joint, typically febrile and ill-appearing In infants or neonates, fever may be absent May present with irritability and pseudoparalysis of affected limb[5,7]	Labs may show WBC > 12,000 cells/μL, ESR > 40 mm/h, CRP > 2 mg/L confirmed by aspiration and culture[5]	Urgent drainage and administration of IV antibiotics[5]
Gonococcal arthritis	Similar presentation to septic arthritis in sexually active patients May present with monoarthritis or oligoarthritis[6]	Aspiration and culture for *Neisseria gonorrhoeae* (chocolate agar or Thayer-Martin medium)	Drainage of fluid, IV ceftriaxone; oral cefixime may be considered in mild cases where close follow-up can be arranged, but first dose should be parenteral Treatment duration of at least 7 days, with possible switch to oral therapy 24 to 48 hours after symptoms improve Should also receive treatment for chlamydia infection, with either single-dose of azithromycin or 7-day course of doxycycline[6]

(continued)

Table 36-1 (continued). Significant Entities/Diagnoses to Consider in Cases of Medial Thigh or Knee Pain

DIAGNOSIS	*HISTORICAL AND PHYSICAL FINDINGS*	*WORK-UP*	*MANAGEMENT*
Fractures	History of trauma, pain, limp or refusal to bear weight, tenderness	Plain x-rays typically sufficient	Referral to orthopedic specialist for further management (eg, casting and reduction)
Osteosarcoma	Localized pain, typically chronic, may begin following an injury Systemic symptoms generally absent Palpable, tender soft-tissue mass in metaphyseal regions of long bones, most commonly distal femur, proximal tibia, and middle/proximal femur[8,9]	Labs may show elevated alkaline phosphatase, lactate dehydrogenase, and/or ESR Plain x-ray will show characteristic "sunburst" lesion Diagnosis confirmed by biopsy[8,9]	Referral to oncology
Ewing's sarcoma	Localized pain and/or swelling, typically chronic, worsening over time May be aggravated by exercise and worse at night Soft-tissue mass may be palpable, and will typically be tender Fever, fatigue, weight loss in about 10% to 20% of cases[9]	Plain x-ray will show poorly marginated destructive ("onion peel" or "moth-eaten") lesion and soft-tissue mass[9]	Referral to oncology

CRP, C-reactive protein; ESR, erythrocyte sedimentation rate; IV, intravenous; MRI, magnetic resonance imaging; WBC, white blood cell

- Step 3—Increase strength, endurance, and flexibility (1 to 3 weeks)
  - Isometric exercises done through pain-free ROM
  - Light cardiovascular exercises
- Step 4—Continued increase of strength and coordination
  - Isotonic and isokinetic exercises
  - Continued cardiovascular exercise
  - Proprioceptive exercises
- Step 5—RTP
  - Sport-specific conditioning and drills
  - RTP is considered when there is normal ROM, freedom from pain, near normal strength compared with the unaffected leg, and good performance is demonstrated on sport-specific drills[10]

- While the diagnosis of a quadriceps strain is mostly based on history and physical examination, imaging may be considered in cases where the diagnosis is unclear or if additional information is needed to define the type and location of the strain. Subspecialty referral should be considered in severe injuries, where there is significant tearing of the muscle seen on MRI.[10,11]

3. What Are the Signs and Symptoms That an Athlete Has Sustained a Quadriceps Contusion? What Is Myositis Ossificans and Its Association With a Quadriceps Contusion? Is It Preventable?

- Signs and symptoms of a quadriceps contusion include the following[10]:
  - History of trauma
  - Localized tenderness, swelling, and bruising that may or may not be visible
  - Loss of knee flexion and/or knee effusion
- A quadriceps contusion usually is a result of direct impact to the anterior thigh. Athletes in contact sports or sports where collision with other players is common are at highest risk. The patient's history and physical examination are sufficient for diagnosis. The athlete typically reports a history of impact and severe anterior thigh pain with exquisite tenderness.
- Myositis ossificans is heterotopic ossification within the quadriceps muscle. It is typically associated with more severe quadriceps contusions. Ossification usually occurs over the anterior aspect of the femur. Therapies such as early ROM and bisphosphonates have been proposed for prevention, but these are somewhat controversial.[10-12] Most cases resolve with conservative management, but surgical excision may be considered if ossification is causing functional limitation >6 months after the inciting injury.

4. If an Acute Quadriceps Contusion Presents Within the First 24 Hours After Sustaining an Injury, What Is the Best Position to Brace the Leg? After the First 24 hours, How Is It Best Rehabilitated?

- First 1 to 2 days
  - Brace at 120 degrees of knee flexion with an ace or plastic wrap
  - Crutches should be prescribed
  - Rest, ice, compression
- After the first 1 to 2 days
  - Begin with flexion exercises
  - Sport-specific noncontact drills once pain-free ROM is achieved
- RTP
  - Only after muscle is no longer tender to palpation
  - Thigh pad should be worn to prevent recurrence
- Referral may be necessary in severe cases or when pain or weakness persist[10]

5. Are There any Objective Findings to Help Grade a Hamstring Strain, and What Are Some Treatment Recommendations?

- Hamstring strains occur in sports that involve running at high speed or rapid deceleration and acceleration.[13] Football and soccer players, as well as track and field runners and hurdlers, are at higher risk for this type of injury. Additional risk factors for hamstring strain include the following[14]:
  - Inadequate warm-up
  - Increased training volume
  - Muscle fatigue

- Hamstring inflexibility or weakness (may be weakness relative to quadriceps)
- Cross-pelvic posture (eg, lumbar lordosis with anterior pelvic tilt)
- Lumbar-pelvic weakness
- Poor biomechanics (eg, running or change of direction)

- Patients with hamstring strains typically present with a history of sudden onset of pain in the posterior thigh during running or other high-risk activities. A limp or other gait abnormalities may be present. The physical examination typically reveals decreased ROM and strength. Hip flexion and extension are typically diminished. Concentric strength may be tested with the patient in the prone position and his or her knee flexed to 90 degrees. Eccentric strength can be assessed with the knee flexed at 15 to 30 degrees. External rotation of the leg during strength testing emphasizes the biceps femoris, while internal rotation assesses the semimembranosus and semitendinosus muscles.[13] Ecchymosis, swelling, and/or a palpable defect may be present.
- The grading of strains are as follows[13]:
  - Grade I—Mild swelling and pain, mild or no loss of strength
  - Grade II—Moderate to severe pain, moderate loss of strength
  - Grade III—Severe pain, complete loss of strength, large hematoma
- Diffuse ecchymosis, palpable defects, and extensive swelling are indicative of more severe injury. Referral should be made to an orthopedic specialist in these cases, or in cases of grades II to III distal hamstring injuries, grade III proximal injuries, or severe avulsion injuries. Initial management of mild injuries involves RICE. NSAIDs may be used for pain control. Rehabilitation should then be initiated, and may be done under the guidance of a physical therapist. Functional rehabilitation programs typically incorporate multiplanar movements, trunk stability and proprioception exercises, agility training, and eccentric hamstring strengthening.[15,16]

6. In the Setting of an Acute Posterior Leg/Hamstring Injury, How Can the Primary Care Provider Differentiate Between an Ischial Tuberosity Injury Versus a Mid-Belly Hamstring Injury?

Ischial tuberosity injuries and mid-belly hamstring injuries can typically be differentiated through a thorough history and physical examination, including imaging. The patient's description and localization of the pain will help narrow the type of injury (Table 36-2).[11,12]

7. What Should the Pediatric Provider Consider in Cases of Chronic or Recurrent Hamstring Strains/Posterior Leg Pain, and How Can They Be Differentiated and Treated?

- As previously stated, risk factors for hamstring strains include inadequate warm-up and muscle fatigue (see discussion in question 5). If any of the issues mentioned in the list in question 5 are not corrected, recurrent injury can occur. Additionally, previous injury increases the risk of recurrent strain, especially if the rehabilitation was incomplete.
- RTP too soon after a previous injury puts athletes at a higher risk of a recurrent strain. This is especially true in adolescent and preadolescent athletes, where growth spurts result in decreased flexibility.[11,14] In the setting of previous injury with poor rehabilitation and resulting fibrous tissue formation, decreased flexibility becomes an even greater risk factor.
- Strength imbalances between muscle groups can predispose athletes to injury as well.
- Injuries to other areas of the lower extremities such as the knee or ankle can put patients at a higher risk for hamstring strain by disrupting the kinetic chain and causing increased loading or strain on the hamstring.[14-16]

Table 36-2. Ischial Tuberosity Injuries Versus Mid-Belly Hamstring Injuries		
	ISCHIAL TUBEROSITY INJURY	*MID-BELLY HAMSTRING INJURY*
History	Proximal posterior thigh pain experienced typically after activities involving running/jumping and sudden acceleration/deceleration; typical in skeletally immature athletes undergoing growth spurts	More diffuse pain or pain localizing to mid-hamstring; acute onset during running/jumping, may also be caused by direct trauma/impact
Physical Examination	Point tenderness to palpation over ischial tuberosity, localized swelling, decreased range of motion and strength	Tenderness to palpation over mid-hamstring, localized swelling, decreased range of motion and strength
Imaging	Plain x-ray may be diagnostic	Plain x-ray typically negative; abnormalities may be seen on ultrasonography or magnetic resonance imaging

- An evaluation with a physical therapist or athletic trainer can help to identify some of these issues. Discussing proper warm-up and reasonable training schedules with athletes can be beneficial as well. Old injuries may require rehabilitation and the retraining of proprioception and coordination.[15,16]
- Several different entities can cause chronic posterior thigh pain. Proximal hamstring syndrome can occur after an acute hamstring injury, and is caused by the inflammation and constriction of the sciatic nerve. Patients typically describe localized pain in the buttocks, with radiation to the thigh. Pain is worse with hamstring stretching or running and sitting, and may be relieved when the patient is supine. The diagnosis is most often made clinically, but imaging can play a role in ruling out other causes of pain. MRI may show proximal hamstring inflammation, but can be negative. Conservative treatment is sufficient in most cases. NSAIDs may be used for pain relief, and activities should be modified. Surgery may be required in chronic cases to release the lateral part of the proximal hamstring tendon.[17]
    - **Piriformis syndrome** is another cause of posterior thigh pain. Swelling or inflammation of the piriformis muscle can cause the compression and irritation of the sciatic nerve, with resultant buttock and posterior proximal thigh pain. The pain is typically worsened by lifting or bending over, and may radiate from the low back to the posterior thigh.[11] There is occasionally a history of trauma to the gluteal or sacroiliac region. On examination, there may be a palpable mass, and hip flexion, internal rotation, and adduction typically cause pain in the buttock. Although it is a clinical diagnosis, imaging with MRI can be helpful in ruling out other causes of radicular pain. Treatment typically includes NSAIDs and physical therapy. Stretching of the piriformis muscle and local pain reduction modalities are commonly used.[11]
    - **Lumbar radiculitis** (inflammation of the nerve root) may also present with posterior leg pain. Children and adolescents may develop a radiculitis after a traumatic injury (eg, football helmet to the back) a disc herniation (see Chapter 33, question 5), or a pathologic process such as a tumor.

TABLE 36-3. TYPES OF BENIGN BONY TUMORS BY CLASSIFICATION	
CLASSIFICATION	*DIFFERENTIAL DIAGNOSIS*
Bone forming	Osteoid osteoma, osteoblastoma
Cartilage forming	Osteochondroma, enchondroma, periosteal chondroma, chondroblastoma, chondromyxoid fibroma
Fibrous	Fibrous dysplasia, ossifying fibroma, nonossifying fibroma
Cystic	Unicameral bone cyst, aneurysmal bone cyst
Other	Langerhans cell histiocytosis of bone, giant cell tumor

8. How Does an Athlete Get an Ischial Apophysitis? What Is the Best Way to Rehabilitate These Injuries and to Prevent Them in the Future?

Ischial apophysitis is an overuse injury. Similar to other types of apophysitis (eg, Osgood-Schlatter disease), it is caused by repetitive microtrauma, in this case at the insertion of the hamstring to the ischium. It is most common in sports that involve sprinting, running, and jumping. Athletes are particularly vulnerable to this type of injury during growth spurts, due to the acute loss of flexibility that accompanies rapid growth. Patients with ischial apophysitis typically present with proximal posterior thigh pain in the absence of trauma, with gradual onset.[11] Management consists of rest, icing, and NSAIDs for pain control. Prevention involves activity modification or reduction and proper warm-up and stretching.[11]

9. What "Mimickers" Should Be Considered in Young Athletes Who Have Upper Leg Pain?

- As seen in Table 36-1, several entities can cause thigh pain that mimics injuries or strain. In fact, some of these may be diagnosed incidentally on imaging that is obtained due to an acute injury. These lesions include benign bony tumors, osteosarcoma, and Ewing's sarcoma.
- Benign bone tumors may be discovered incidentally or may present with localized pain and swelling. In some cases, a pathologic fracture may be the presenting finding. There are many different types of benign bony tumors, and they can be classified as bone forming, cartilage forming, fibrous, cystic, and other (Table 36-3).[18]
- History can narrow the differential diagnosis.
  - Age of presentation can be helpful, as most benign tumors present in the second decade of life.[18] Ossifying fibromas usually present in the first 5 years of life, while Langerhans cell histiocytosis of bone presents in the first decade.
  - The pattern of pain, if present, can also be useful, and can help differentiate benign lesions from malignant lesions. Osteoid osteoma typically causes pain that resolves within 25 minutes of taking NSAIDs or aspirin. Tumors such as unicameral cysts and nonossifying fibromas, which tend to be nonaggressive, are usually asymptomatic. Pain may be caused by pathologic fracture, local mass effect, or compression. Aneurysmal cysts, chondroblastomas, and chondromyxoid fibromas are typically more aggressive, and are associated with dull, slowly progressive pain that is often worse at night.[18] Malignant tumors usually cause rapidly progressive pain that wakes the patient from sleep.
  - A thorough physical examination is key and may show signs of underlying syndromes associated with benign bony tumors (eg, café au lait macules in McCune-Albright syndrome).

- Plain radiography is the imaging modality of choice. Features of benign lesions include the following[18]:
    - Well-defined borders (intact cortex) that do not extend into the soft tissue
    - Lesions that do not cross other structures such as the cortex or growth plate
    - Multiple lesions
    - Small size
- Malignant lesions of bone include osteosarcoma and Ewing's sarcoma. Osteosarcoma typically presents with chronic localized pain that may begin after injury and may be intermittent. Constitutional symptoms are typically absent. A tender, large palpable mass may be felt on examination. Long bones are the most commonly involved, usually in the metaphyseal region. In the lower extremities, the distal femur is the most common site, followed by the proximal tibia and middle or proximal femur.[8] See Table 36-1 for information on work-up.
- Ewing's sarcoma presents similarly to osteosarcoma, with a gradual onset of localized pain and swelling, often preceded by a minor trauma. The pain is typically worse with activity and at night. A mass may be palpated on examination, and erythema and swelling is common. Systemic symptoms (eg, fever, malaise, weight loss) is present in 10% to 20% of patients. Ewing's sarcoma affects long bones predominantly, and occurs distally and proximally with equal frequency.[9] See Table 36-1 for x-ray findings.
- Most benign tumors can be monitored with serial x-rays. Referral for excision should be considered for symptomatic or aggressive lesions. Patients with malignant tumors should be referred to pediatric oncology.

References

1. Guzzanti V, Falciglia F, Stanitski CL. Slipped capital femoral epiphysis in skeletally immature patients. *J Bone Joint Surg Br.* 2004;86(5):731–736.
2. Bishop JA, Hresko MT, Kasser JR, et al. Delay in diagnosis of slipped capital femoral epiphysis. *Pediatrics.* 2004;113(4):e322–e325.
3. Dillman JR, Hernandez RJ. MRI of Legg-Calve-Perthes disease. *Am J Roentgenol.* 2009;193(5):1394–1407.
4. Herring JA, Kim HT, Browne R. Legg-Calve-Perthes disease. Part II: prospective multicenter study of the effect of treatment on outcome. *J Bone Joint Surg Am.* 2004;86-A(10):2121–2134.
5. Del Beccaro MA, Champoux AN, Bockers T, Mendelman PM. Septic arthritis versus transient synovitis of the hip: the value of screening laboratory tests. *Ann Emerg Med.* 1992;21(12):1418–1422.
6. Workowski KA, Berman SM. Sexually transmitted diseases treatment guidelines, 2006. *MMWR Recomm Rep.* 2006;55(RR-11):1–94.
7. Nigrovic PA. Overview of hip pain in childhood. In: Basow DS, ed. *UpToDate.* Waltham, MA: 2012
8. Meyers PA, Gorlick R. Osteosarcoma. *Pediatr Clin North Am.* 1997;44(4):973–989.
9. Widhe B, Widhe T. Initial symptoms and clinical features in osteosarcoma and Ewing sarcoma. *J Bone Joint Surg Am.* 2000;82(5):667–674.
10. Kary JM. Diagnosis and management of quadriceps strains and contusions. *Curr Rev Musculoskelet Med.* 2010;3:26–31.
11. Nielson JH, ed. Pelvic, Hip, and Thigh Injuries. In: *The Adolescent Athlete.* New York, NY: Springer; 2007.
12. Nuccion S, Hunter D, Finerman G. Hip and pelvis: adult. In: DeLee J, Drez D, Miller M, eds. *Orthopaedic Sports Medicine: Principles and Practice.* 2nd ed. Philadelphia, PA: WB Saunders; 1994:1449.
13. Fields KB, Copland ST, Tipton JS. Hamstring injuries. In: Basow DS, ed. *UpToDate.* Waltham, MA: 2012.
14. Croisier JL. Factors associated with recurrent hamstring injuries. *Sports Med.* 2004;34(10):681–695.
15. Drezner JA. Practical management: hamstring muscle injuries. *Clin J Sport Med.* 2003;13(1):48-52.
16. Heiderscheit BC, Sherry MA, Silder A, Chumanov ES, Thelen DG. Hamstring strain injuries: recommendations for diagnosis, rehabilitation, and injury prevention. *J Orthop Sports Phys Ther.* 2010;40(2):67-81.
17. Young IJ, van Riet RP, Bell SN. Surgical release for proximal hamstring syndrome. *Am J Sports Med.* 2008;36(12):2372.
18. Tis JE. Overview of benign bone tumors in children and adolescents. In: Basow DS, ed. *UpToDate.* Waltham, MA: 2012.

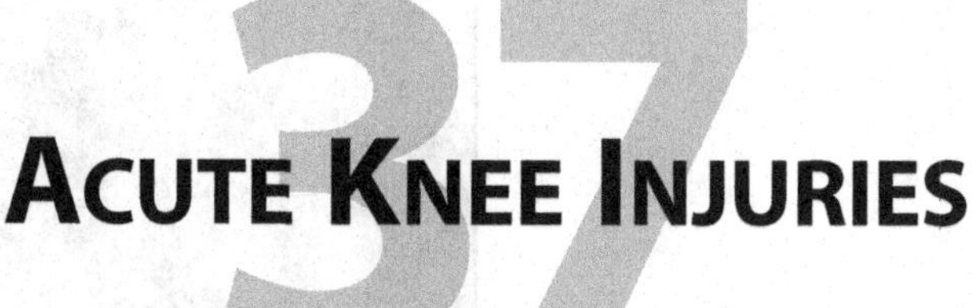

Acute Knee Injuries

Chris Koutures, MD, FAAP

1. What Is the Difference Between a "Suprapatellar Effusion" and Localized Swelling of the Knee, and Why Is the Differentiation Important?

A suprapatellar effusion is diffuse swelling which often obliterates the superior aspect of the patella and infers serious intra-articular injury (Figure 37-1).

Some common causes of a suprapatellar effusion are as follows:

- Intra-articular ligament sprain (anterior or posterior cruciate ligament)
- Osteochondral fracture
- Patellar dislocation/subluxation
- Tibial plateau or tibial tubercle fracture
- Meniscal tear
- Septic joint/infectious process
- Rheumatologic process

Any suprapatellar effusion must be evaluated for signs of a septic joint (fever/chills, warmth, red skin streaks, tense joint with significant pain); positive findings warrant emergent orthopedic referral.

Localized swelling often can be identified with a fingertip,and tends to represent a focal process such as the following:

- Fat pad contusion
- Tibial tubercle swelling (Osgood-Schlatter disease)
- Baker's cyst (popliteal fossa)
- Inflammation of pes anseurine or distal iliotibial band bursa

Most cases of localized swelling can initially be managed by the general health care provider.

2. How Does Knowing the Mechanism of Injury Help the Health Care Provider to Figure Out What Knee Structure May Be Injured?

Hearing the exact mechanism of injury is essential in making a proper diagnosis or referral. Often, the physical examination confirms what is heard in the history, and in cases where pain or swelling make the examination difficult, the history alone may dictate further management (Table 37-1).

Koutures C, Wong V.
Pediatric Sports Medicine: Essentials for Office Evaluation (pp 251-258)

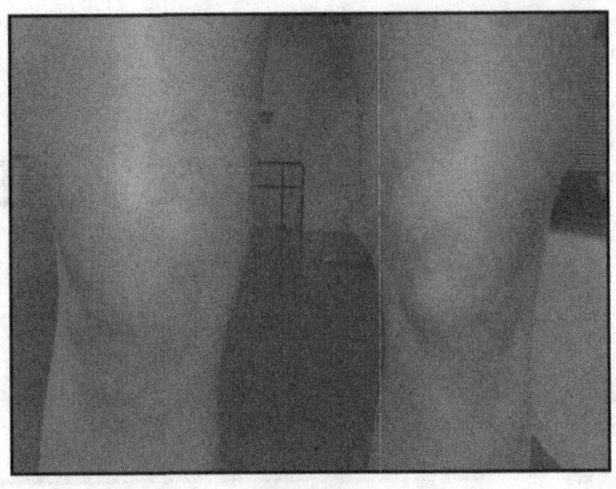

Figure 37-1. Right knee demonstrating suprapatellar effusion.

Table 37-1. Correlation of History and Injured Region	
MECHANISM OF INJURY	*INJURED STRUCTURE*
Landing from a jump or twist/cutting on a straight knee with a buckling sensation and immediate "pop"	Anterior cruciate ligament tear
Direct impact to the outside of the knee (valgus stress)	Medial collateral ligament tear or physeal fracture (in skeletally immature patient)
Direct impact to the shin with the knee bent about 90 degrees (dashboard injury in car accident)	Posterior cruciate ligament tear
Rotation or twist about the knee, pain often going downstairs	Medial or lateral meniscus tear
Knee "dislocated" or completely gave way	Patellar dislocation or anterior cruciate ligament tear (true knee dislocation is extremely rare)
Direct impact to inside of the knee (varus stress)	Lateral collateral ligament sprain (rare)

3. What Examination Techniques Can Help to Determine Some of the Above Injuries?

Table 37-2 discusses the proper examination techniques for some of the injuries discussed above.

4. When Should I Image the Knee?

Imaging of the knee should always begin with routine x-rays. Common indications for x-ray include the following:

- Suprapatellar effusion
- Inability to bear weight
- Inability to fully straighten knee
- Ligament laxity in skeletally immature patient to look for potential avulsion or physeal injury
- History of frank patellar subluxation or dislocation
- Focal tenderness of patella, femoral condyles, or fibular head

Computed tomography scan or magnetic resonance imaging should be done only after x-rays and often with a sports medicine specialist consultation.

Table 37-2. Proper Examination Techniques	
STRUCTURE OF CONCERN	*EXAMINATION TECHNIQUES*
Anterior cruciate ligament tear	**Lachman Test** (Figure 37-2) Knee bent to 30 to 45 degrees with relaxed hamstrings Pull tibia forward relative to femur, assess end point Lack of firm end point suggests incompetent anterior cruciate ligament **Anterior Drawer** Knee bent to 90 degrees Sit on foot Pull tibia forward relative to femur, assess anterior motion
Meniscal tear	**Duck Walk** (Figure 37-3) Patient squats (like catcher in baseball) Takes 5 steps forward (walks like a duck) Catch, click, or focal pain implies meniscal tear **Joint Line Tenderness** Run finger along medial and lateral space between femur and tibia Pain suggests tear **McMurray Test** (Figures 37-4 and 37-5) With patient supine, place finger on lateral or medial joint line Rotate knee into flexion with varus/valgus stress with finger on joint line Pain and click implies meniscal tear **Apley Test** Patient lies on stomach with knee bent 90 degrees Examiner places hand on heel to push tibia against femur Internally and externally rotate heel Pain or click implies meniscal tear
Patellar instability (dislocation or subluxation)	**Visual Examination** Dislocated patella located adjacent to lateral femoral condyle **Apprehension Test** (see Figure 38-2) Patient supine, knee bent 30 degrees Place thumbs on medial border of patella Push patella laterally Patient pain or apprehension indicates patellar instability
Medial collateral ligament tear	With patient supine and knee extended Apply valgus stress test (pull lower leg away from other leg) at full extension and 30 degrees of flexion, compare laxity with noninjured knee (Figure 37-6) Laxity in full extension implies injury (not just to medial collateral ligament, but also to other medial or posteromedial structures [indicates immediate referral]) Laxity only at 30 degrees of flexion implies isolated medial collateral ligament injury

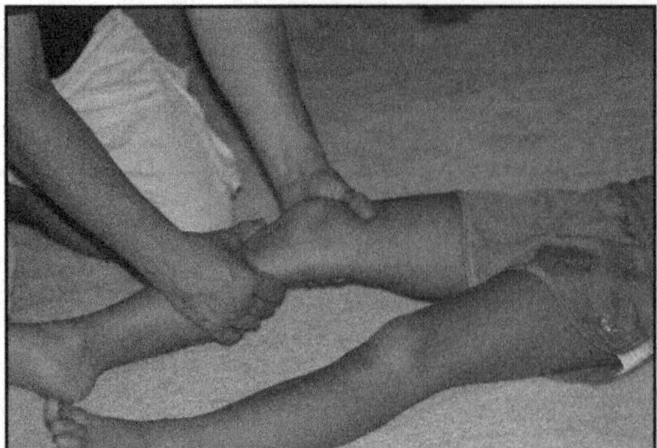

Figure 37-2. Lachman test.

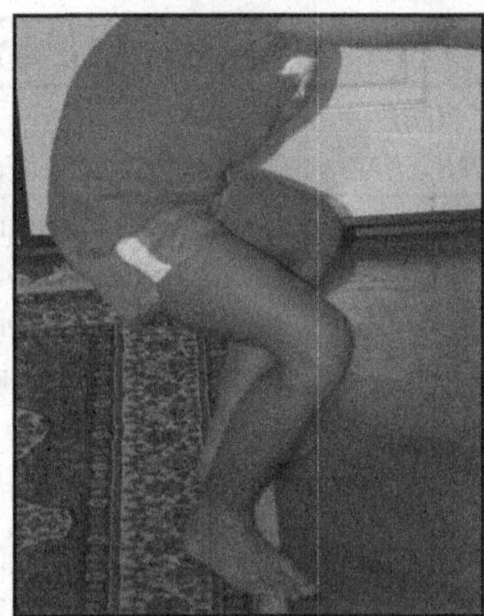

Figure 37-3. Side view of a patient doing the "duck walk."

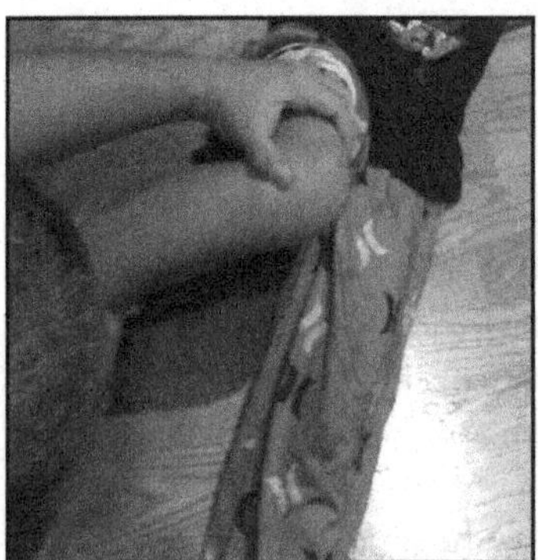

Figure 37-4. McMurray test for a lateral meniscal injury.

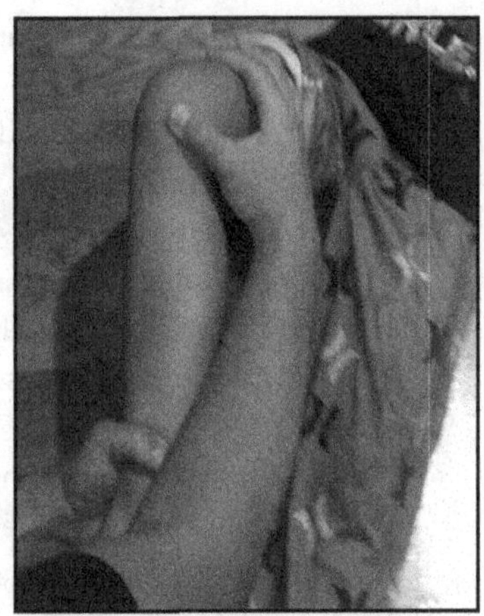

Figure 37-5. McMurray test for a medial meniscal injury.

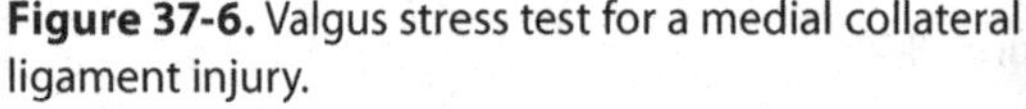

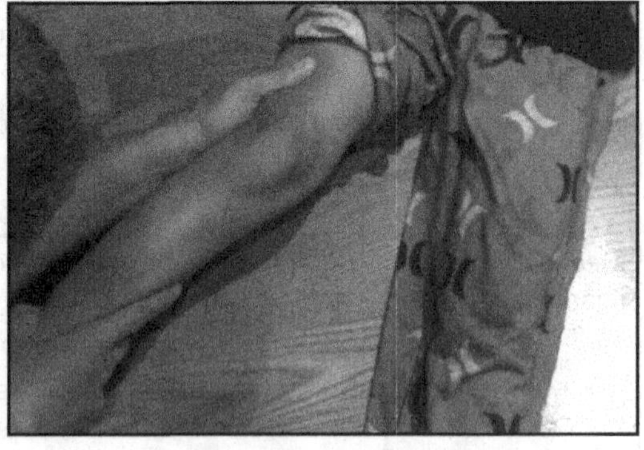

Figure 37-6. Valgus stress test for a medial collateral ligament injury.

5. What X-Ray Views Should I Order for an Acute Knee Injury?

The four commonly recommended x-ray views of the knee are as follows:

1. Anteroposterior (AP)
2. Lateral

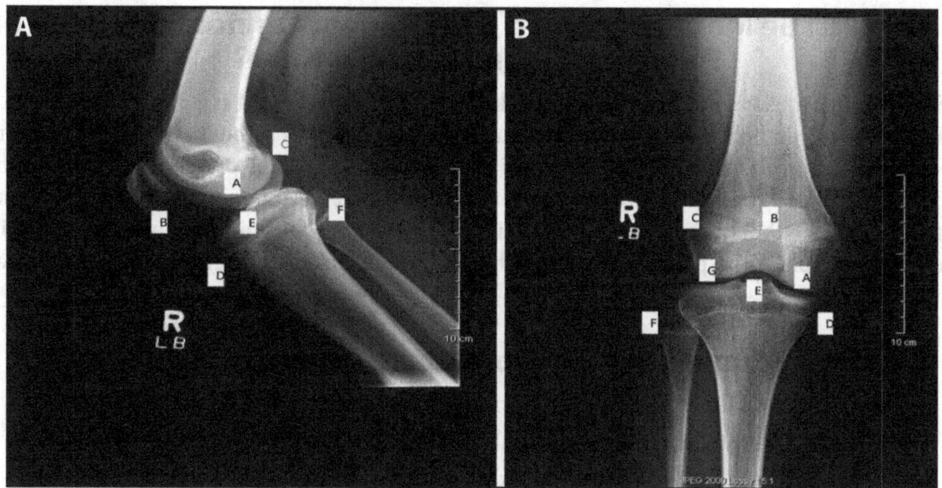

Figure 37-7. (A) Lateral and (B) anteroposterior x-ray views of the knee.

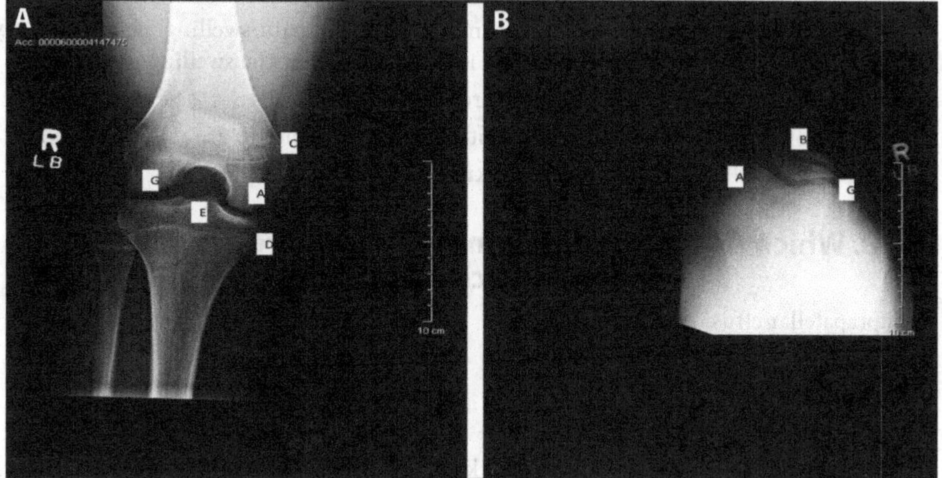

Figure 37-8. (A) Tunnel and (B) sunrise x-ray views of the knee.

3. Tunnel (also known as notch view)
4. Sunrise

Examples of each view and key anatomic sites/locations of potential abnormalities are referenced below and illustrated in Figures 37-7 and 37-8.

- A-Medial femoral condyle (osteochondral lesion; best seen on tunnel view)
- B-Patella (fracture or osteochondral lesion; best seen on lateral or sunrise views)
- C-Distal femoral physis
- D-Proximal tibial physis
- E-Tibial spines/insertion of anterior cruciate ligament (ACL) or posterior cruciate ligament (PCL); best seen on lateral or tunnel views
- F-Fibular head
- G-Lateral femoral condyle (osteochondral lesion; best seen on tunnel view)

6. Should I Be More Concerned if My Patient Cannot Fully Bend or Fully Straighten His or Her Knee?

The inability to straighten the knee (also known as "locked knee") is a bigger concern. One possible issue would be a meniscus tear with a flap (also known as a "bucket handle tear") stuck between the femur and tibia, often causing significant pain. Another possibility is a disruption of the knee extensor mechanism (patellar sleeve fracture, patellar tendon rupture, or avulsion of the tibial tubercle). Full knee extension is crucial for proper walking gait, so in any case of limited knee extension, place the patient nonweight bearing on crutches and refer for urgent specialty evaluation.

7. What Should I Initially Do With an Acute, Swollen Knee?

- Long-leg immobilizer in extension or near-full extension.
  - Usually indicated only for the initial 3 to 5 days to provide support and comfort.
  - Prolonged use may result in a stiff knee with significant quadriceps atrophy.
- Crutches (if needed for ambulation).
- Protection, rest, ice, compression, and elevation (see Chapter 24, question 1).
- If it is difficult to perform the initial examination due to pain/swelling, obtain an x-ray at the first visit and re-examine the patient in 3 to 5 days after the swelling goes down.
- Physical therapy referral or office-based rehabilitation.
  - Focus on maintaining quadriceps, gluteal, and core strength.
  - Decrease swelling to help regain full knee range of motion (ROM).

8. Which Acute Injuries/Symptoms Require a Visit With a Sports Medicine Specialist?

- Suprapatellar effusion.
- Locked knee/inability to fully extend.
- Concern over ligament injury.
- Any fracture or osteochondral lesion.
- Patient unable to bear weight on injured knee.
- Strong patient/family emphasis on immediate return to play (RTP).
- Any health care provider concern that merits specialty evaluation.

9. Why Should One Be Concerned About the Physis if an Athlete Gets a Lateral Blow Causing Valgus Stress to the Knee? Has the Athlete Injured the Medial Collateral Ligament?

- A lateral blow stretches the medial structures, most often causing a midsubstance medial collateral ligament (MCL) tear.
- In a skeletally immature patient, the distal femoral or proximal tibial physis might be the weakest link, especially during an adolescent growth spurt.
- Growth plate injuries will have primary tenderness at the distal femur or proximal tibia.
- An MCL sprain will have pain along the ligament course on the medial knee.
- Scrutinize x-rays for physeal widening or Salter-Harris fracture lines; use comparison views of noninjured knee or stress x-rays (AP view taken with the knee placed in a valgus stress position).

- If physeal injuries are a concern, place the patient nonweight bearing on crutches in either a posterior splint or a long leg immobilizer in extension while awaiting immediate specialty referral.

10. What Is Osteochondritis Dissecans, and Why Should I Be Concerned?

- Osteochondritis dissecans (OCD) disrupts the articular cartilage and underlying bone either from acute or chronic stress.
- Please see Chapter 38, question 12, for further discussion of OCD lesions.

11. What Are Some Important Factors to Consider With an Acute Anterior Cruciate Ligament Tear?

- An intact ACL is generally essential for knee stability in sports that require twisting, cutting, landing, and other quick movements.
- The classic office presentation is a swollen knee that had a "pop" after an abrupt landing, turn, or twist on a straight knee.
- Concurrent injuries include meniscus or collateral ligament tears and osteochondral lesions.
- X-ray evaluation should be obtained at the patient's first visit to assess the growth plates, evaluate for osteochondral lesions, and identify an avulsion of the ACL insertion onto the tibial spine (a finding that mandates immediate orthopedic surgical evaluation).
- Once an ACL rupture is diagnosed, early physical therapy is recommended to reduce swelling, assist in return of full ROM, and maintain quadriceps strength.
- All patients with a suspected or confirmed ACL tear should have orthopedic surgical consultation; many patients need ACL reconstruction to return to high-risk sports. The goal of repair is to increase knee stability and attempt to reduce ongoing damage to the articular cartilage and menisci.
- For athletes with an unstable knee who choose to defer surgical reconstruction, absolute avoidance of high-risk activities has been shown to be far superior to physical therapy and bracing in reducing the risk of future knee instability and further soft-tissue damage.
- Regardless of operative versus nonoperative care, the act of rupturing an ACL increases risk for early onset degenerative joint disease often within 20 years of the injury.
- The ruptured ACL cannot be sutured; reconstruction is done by grafting either part of a patellar tendon, distal hamstring muscle, or cadaver graft.
- The skeletally immature patient presents a unique challenge in that standard reconstruction techniques may cross open physes and potentially cause growth alterations. Newer operative techniques that do not involve the physes have been developed,[1] so referral to a pediatric orthopedic surgeon who is well versed in the latest surgical techniques is highly recommended.
- Postoperative care includes the immobilization in knee extension to allow bone plug healing for several weeks followed by several months of intense physical therapy. Many patients are able to return to their sport of choice in 6 to 12 months; the use of knee derotational braces during the postoperative return is surgeon-dependent, as the literature does not have strong evidence supporting the need.

12. Will a Brace Help an Athlete With an Acute Knee Injury Return to Play Sooner?

For the majority of injuries, braces will not play a significant role in expediting a RTP. The most important factors will include an accurate diagnosis followed by diligent rehabilitation to rebuild support muscle strength (quads, gluts, hamstrings), maintain full knee ROM, and regain balance and postural stability. The practitioner can use office-based functional testing to help with RTP decisions. Particular injuries that may benefit from bracing include a MCL sprain (functional hinged knee brace) or patellar instability (lateral buttress knee support).

Reference

1. Kocher MS, Smith JT, Zoric BJ, et al. Transphyseal anterior cruciate ligament reconstruction in skeletally immature pubescent adolescents. *J Bone Joint Surg Am*. 2007;89(12):2632-2639.

38 Chronic and Overuse Knee Injuries

Rebecca A. Demorest, MD, FAAP

1. What Are the Common Structures Involved in Chronic Knee Pain?

Figure 38-1 illustrates several common structures and landmarks that will be discussed throughout this chapter, such as the iliotibial band (ITB), the medial plica, and the medial collateral ligament (MCL).

2. What Are the General Principles Regarding the Rehabilitation of Chronic Knee Pain?

Appropriate rehabilitation for chronic knee pain focuses on the following long-term goals:

- Pain cessation
- Physical improvement
- Return to sport

Avoiding offending activities and participating in cross training can help to keep an athlete active and healthy, while focusing on rehabilitation. An athlete can typically play as long as he or she is not limping or not experiencing a significant increase in pain. Ice to the affected area after activity (20 minutes on/20 minutes off) should become routine with chronic knee pain. There is usually no role for heat unless to warm up prior to activity. Nonsteroidal anti-inflammatory drugs (NSAIDs) should be used very sparingly after activity. If their use is required on a daily basis, then the athlete is doing too much activity.

Physical therapy (PT) with a qualified physical therapist and a step-wise home exercise program (HEP) should focus on stretching and strengthening the structures surrounding the knee. The focus is not purely on the quadriceps and hamstrings, as the core body (abdominal, hip, gluteal and back muscles) is of the utmost importance and if ignored, symptoms tend not to improve. The one-legged squat test is a good office test to assess for core body strength. If the patient's knee buckles into valgus, the core body is not able to stabilize the knee during activity and is a likely contributor to the chronic issue (Figure 38-2).

PT programs should be advanced to functional activities once the patient's muscle strength and flexibility have improved. A HEP must be performed 5 to 6 days per week to improve symptoms. Giving exercises in the office is usually not successful for multiple reasons (limited physician knowledge base, time, ability to advance and teach exercises properly), so a complete 6 to 8 weeks of a structured rehabilitation program and HEP are needed to see improvements. Many athletes get frustrated before getting to this point, so a complete discussion regarding what to expect should be undertaken before PT referral.

A gait and running analysis are also typically helpful in pinpointing deficits and preventing recurrence, as proper form cannot be overemphasized. Reviewing what can be done and what should not

Koutures C, Wong V.
Pediatric Sports Medicine: Essentials for Office Evaluation (pp 259-268)

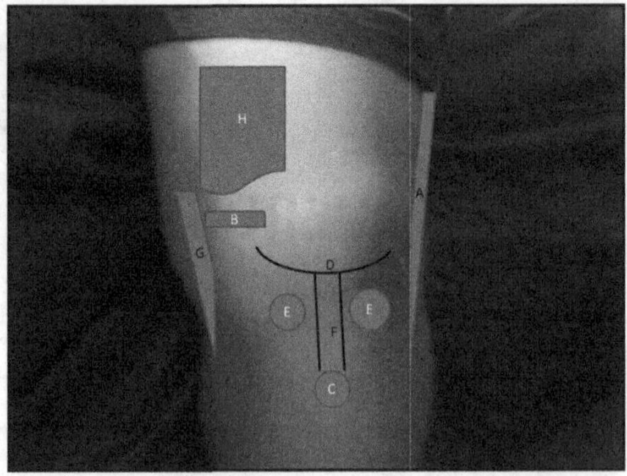

Figure 38-1. Useful knee landmarks. (A) iliotibial band, (B) medial plica, (C) tibial tuberosity, (D) inferior pole of patella, (E) fat pad, (F) patellar tendon, (G) medial collateral ligament, and (H) vastus medialis oblique muscle.

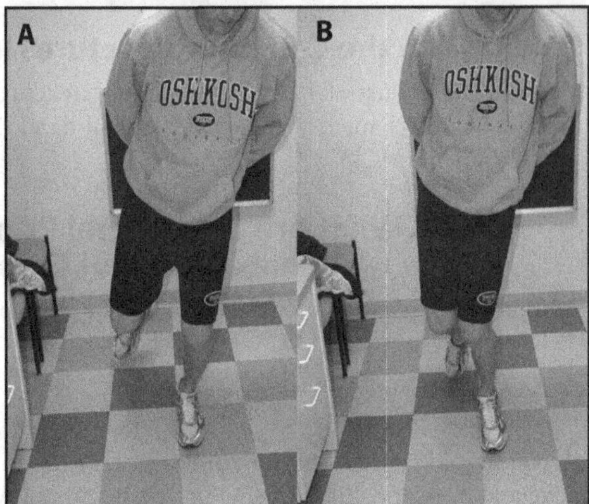

Figure 38-2. (A) Proper single leg squat form. (B) Improper single leg squat form with knee buckling into valgus.

be done in terms of sports activity and exercise should also be thoroughly discussed. If the pediatrician is not familiar or comfortable with this, a referral to a sports medicine specialist is advised.

3. What Is Patellofemoral Stress Syndrome? How Is It Diagnosed and Treated, and When Is Referral Necessary?

Patellofemoral stress syndrome (PFSS) is one of the most common injuries in general sports medicine clinics and is an overall common diagnosis for chronic anterior knee pain. Contributing factors include the following:

- Increased Q angle (Figure 38-3)
- Femoral anteversion
- Foot hyperpronation
- Gluteal/hip weakness
- Tight hamstrings
- Patellar malalignment

Described as chronic unilateral or bilateral pain around and behind the patella with walking, running, jumping, and weight bearing activity, PFSS typically presents in those aged 8 years and older. Other characteristics include the following:

- Pain with stair climbing (especially downstairs)

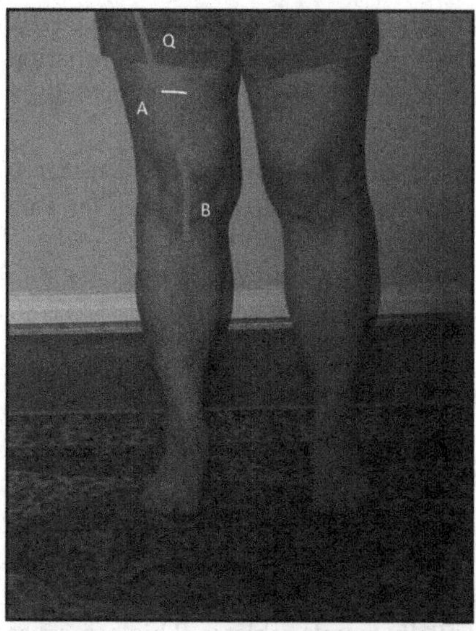

Figure 38-3. Q angle (Q) made from line running from ASIS to patella (A) and extension of line running from patellar to tibial tubercle (B).

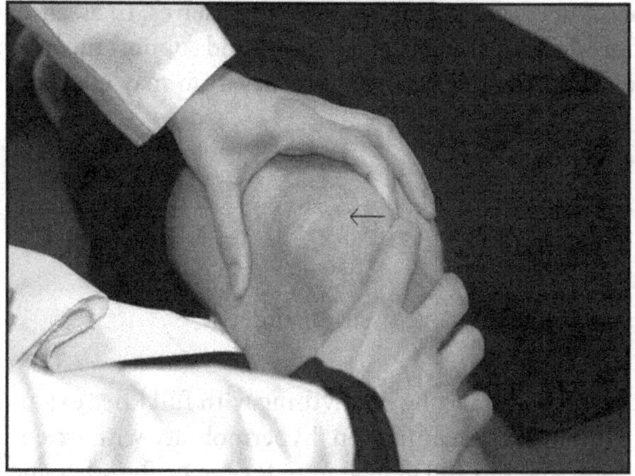

Figure 38-4. Apprehension test for patellar instability. Placing your knee underneath the patient's knee to allow 30 degrees of relaxed flexion, gently try to laterally sublux the patella. A look of apprehension or pain is a positive finding. Instability/laxity may be noted. Be careful not to displace too aggressively, as one could dislocate the patella. (Reprinted with permission from Demorest RA. Adolescents with joint pain: a sports medicine perspective. In: McDonagh JE, White PH, eds. *Adolescent Rheumatology*. London, England: Informa Healthcare; 2008:238.)

- Prolonged sitting (theater sign)
- Prolonged standing (especially if the knees are "locked")

Patients with PFSS typically have no pain at rest or at night, no effusion, and no true catching or locking of the knee. Activities are generally limited secondary to pain.

On physical examination, the patient can typically weight bear with no limp, and there may be hyperpronation and/or genu recurvatum upon gait evaluation. No effusion is typically present (if it is, one should consider another diagnosis). Medial or lateral facet tenderness is common, as is pain with compression or apprehension testing (Figure 38-4) with or without patellar hypermobility, malalignment, or maltracking.[3] Ligament testing is normal. Quadriceps atrophy (especially the vastus medialis oblique [VMO]) is common. Full range of motion (ROM) is present, with some pain possible upon full knee flexion. Tight hamstrings and a problematic one-legged squat are also common.

Radiographic studies are generally normal and include 4 views (anteroposterior [AP], lateral, tunnel, and sunrise [see Figures 37-7 and 37-8]). There may be a slight lateral tilt or a shallow femoral groove on sunrise. A magnetic resonance imaging (MRI) is not typically helpful in making the diagnosis.

Treatment of PFSS includes a rehabilitation program focusing on lower-extremity flexibility (hamstrings, hip flexors, IT band) and core strengthening (see question 2). Chronic pain can continue if athletes are noncompliant with rehabilitation and the HEP; thus, a maintenance HEP must be kept up for the life of the sport, as PFSS pain can persist into adulthood. If hyperpronation is present, over-the-counter orthotics may be useful. Patellar bracing or McConnell taping may be helpful if the patient has patellar instability.

Running, jumping, and landing mechanics also need to be closely evaluated; more research is needed, but flexibility and good core strength combined with proper running/jump/landing mechanics may decrease the risk for injury and help with prevention.

Patients with a history or physical examination that does not fit with PFSS and those who do not improve with PT/HEP should be referred to a sports medicine specialist.

4. There Are Patients, Commonly Dancers, Who Have Hypermobile Joints and Tend to "Lock Out" Their Knees. Can This Be a Cause of Chronic Pain? Are X-rays Necessary? What Is the Best Management, and When Is Referral Necessary?

Usual knee ROM is from 0 degrees (full extension) to approximately 120 to 135 degrees (full flexion). The ability to "lock the knees" and hyperextend to (–)5 or (–)10 degrees is known as genu recurvatum, and can be seen in growing children and especially female athletes. This can cause pain in athletes, especially those who lock their knees to stand and support themselves. In essence, one is "hanging on the ligaments" instead of properly training the stabilizing and support muscles (quadriceps, hamstrings, gluteal and hip muscles). Athletes with genu recurvatum may also lack appropriate proprioceptive feedback.[1]

Genu recurvatum can be caused by the following:

- Ligamentous laxity
- Knee instability due to prior injury
- Malalignment of the tibia and femur
- Disease (cerebral palsy, muscular dystrophy, connective tissue disorder)
- Congenital defect

Pain may be experienced, especially with prolonged standing or anything with full knee extension (rowing, dancing, ice skating, cutting). On physical examination, hypermobility with extension and weakness of the quadriceps, hamstrings, and hip and gluteal muscles can be found. Some athletes may have excessive hip or tibial rotation. A full history and physical examination should be performed to evaluate for concomitant or previous injury causing the defect. A gait, standing, and running evaluation can be helpful in assessing the stationary and dynamic movements of the athlete that can be contributing to chronic pain. Imaging studies are typically not used to make this diagnosis; however, if other causes are suspected, appropriate imaging should be pursued.

Treatment usually consists of trying to teach the athlete to not "lock the knees" into full extension with standing or sports activity. If chronic pain continues, PT to help train the supporting muscle groups to function properly and ice after activity may help. Bracing has no role in the management for sports, although a brace to help prevent hyperextension may provide a temporary relief of symptoms. Those with continued difficulties should be referred to pediatric orthopedics, as surgical management may be warranted, especially if prior trauma or injury is the cause.

5. A Patient Reports That His or Her Knee Frequently "Gives Out." What Is Patellar Subluxation/Laxity?

- In an extended and relaxed knee, the patella typically moves half its diameter in either direction with gentle manipulation.
- Those with instability have excessive movement, especially when the knee is engaged (weight bearing and flexed).

- Patellar subluxation occurs with transient partial lateral dislocation.
- Frank patellar dislocations can occur, especially with trauma.

- Previous trauma or generalized instability can cause the patella to recurrently sublux, then it usually relocates on its own. Recurrent subluxations increase the risk of future subluxations as the medial retinacular tissue gets stretched.

Athletes may twist or turn and feel the knee "give way." Instability may also be felt with walking, stair climbing, running, and cutting. There is usually minimal to no swelling, but an effusion may present with traumatic subluxation. On physical examination, discomfort is often felt along the medial retinaculum, medial and/or lateral facets, and with compression and apprehension testing. Apprehension testing may reveal patellar hypermobility with the ability to dislocate the patella. The examiner needs to be careful not to traumatically dislocate the patella during the examination causing undue patient pain. Patients may also have quadriceps atrophy and may have an inability to fire the VMO. Imaging should include the usual four radiographic views of the knee; the sunrise view may show a tilt or subluxation of the patella. MRI is typically not necessary unless there is acute trauma.

Rehabilitation focuses on ROM, flexibility (hamstrings, hip flexors), strengthening of the core body and quadriceps, and eventually functional activity to alleviate the patient's symptoms and decrease the risk of recurrent subluxations. A patellar stabilizing brace with a lateral buttress or McConnell taping may help to stabilize the patella during sports activity and decrease discomfort. Ice for 20 minutes after activity along with occasional NSAID use after activity may help as well. Continued activity depends on the individual's pain and function, and cross training may be advised if weight-bearing impact activity is bothersome.

Incomplete rehabilitation may result in recurrent instability or dislocation, and may lead to surgical intervention (lateral release, distal osteotomy). Surgery may be considered if there are anatomic factors causing continued problems and a failure of rehabilitation after 6 months of a dedicated PT/HEP program. The patient and his or her family should be informed that surgery may not completely alleviate the issue, as this is a difficult problem to fix.

6. Skeletally Immature Patients Often Present With Focal Pain at Either the Inferior Tip of the Patella or at the Tibial Tubercle That Worsens With Activity and Improves With Rest. What Are the Most Likely Diagnoses, and What Clinical Findings Might Suggest More Serious Alterations to the Extensor Mechanism?

Chronic traction apophysitis can occur in growing children and teenagers, as bone is more vulnerable to injury than the surrounding patellar tendon.

- Sinding-Larsen-Johansson (SLJ) syndrome occurs in individuals who are 9 to 14 years of age at the inferior patellar pole.
- Osgood-Schlatter (OS) disease occurs in persons aged 11 to 17 years at the tibial tuberosity.
- Skeletally mature children typically experience patellar tendinopathies.

Focal pain ("finger-tip diagnosis") is insidious in onset, may be unilateral or bilateral, and occurs with running, jumping, and kneeling. Pain usually lessens at rest and does not occur at night. Soft-tissue swelling may be present over the tibial tuberosity or inferior pole of the patella. Most patients will have tight hamstrings and feel anterior knee discomfort with full flexion of the knee as the area of discomfort is being stretched. The noticeable "bump" of the tibial tuberosity in patients with OS disease may also persist into adulthood.

Radiographs are not typically necessary for diagnosis, but AP and lateral views of the knee may show a fragmentation of the tibial tuberosity or inferior pole of the patella. This is considered normal in growing children, but abnormal in skeletally mature adults. The fragments seen on childhood x-rays may persist into adulthood.

Rehabilitation should focus on the flexibility of the quadriceps, hamstrings, and hip flexors, along with core body strengthening. Stretches (each held for 30 seconds) should be done at least 10 to 20 times per day. Icing after activity can help to alleviate pain. NSAIDs on an as-needed basis after activity may also help.

A patellar tendon strap (hook and loop fastener strap placed across the patellar tendon) may also alleviate pain by changing the tension to the patellar tendon. Athletes may usually continue to play as long as they are not limping or having a significant increase in pain. Cross training on the bike, elliptical, or in the pool may keep these individuals active during times of decreased activity. Rest alone will not treat this problem, as the pain will likely recur once activity is commenced. Rarely, immobilization or casting may be used to treat OS disease or SLJ syndrome if the patient's pain cannot be controlled with conservative management. Immobilization/casting will cause extensive quadriceps atrophy and the patient will be at greater risk for further injury if proper PT is not performed afterward.

Beware of the "acute" OS disease or SLJ syndrome. Acute injuries to the tibial tuberosity and inferior pole of the patella must be evaluated for a Salter-Harris type III fracture of the proximal tibia/tibial avulsion or a patellar sleeve injury.

If an athlete cannot perform a straight leg raise without an extensor lag, then he or she needs to be immediately evaluated for a more serious injury (fracture, patellar tendon rupture) that may require surgery.

Patients not responding to typical treatment and those with concerning acute issues should be referred to a sports medicine specialist. Skeletally mature or almost-skeletally mature patients should also be referred, as these diagnoses do not occur once the apophyses have closed.

7. Swimmers Often Present With Medial Knee Pain Without Experiencing Trauma. What Is "Breaststroker's Knee?"

Breaststroker's knee is a general term used for pain experienced along the medial knee caused by the stretching of the MCL and medial capsule/structures due to valgus stress during breaststroke kicking. This does not typically cause discomfort during flutter or butterfly kicks, weight training, or cross training unless the athletes place undue valgus stress on the knee or increased resistance in the water (using fins). The physical examination shows medial knee pain without effusion or MCL instability. Quadriceps atrophy may be recognized, and weak one-legged squats are also typical. Imaging is not usually necessary, as this is a clinical diagnosis.

Treatment consists of stopping breaststroke kicking and any offending activities for a minimum of 3 to 4 weeks. PT focusing on strengthening the core (hip and gluteal) musculature and quadriceps is extremely important. Stretching the hip and hamstrings is also mandatory. Use of ice and NSAIDs (sparingly) after activity may help with pain. When the athlete is pain free and returns to activity, his or her kicking form must be thoroughly evaluated and modified. A correct breaststroke kick form includes the following[2]:

- Keeping the legs together during the recovery and thrust phases
- Keeping the knee and hip centers aligned during the initiation of the stroke
- Avoiding excessive leg external rotation

Avoiding excessive drag (fins, etc) is also suggested. Most athletes can continue to swim other strokes, but some may choose to stop breaststroke if their pain returns.

Referral to a sports medicine specialist is necessary if there is injury, swelling, or ligamentous instability, or if the pain does not get better with typical rehabilitation.

8. How Does Medial Plica Syndrome Cause Knee Pain in Runners?

Plicas are remnant bands of embryologic tissue that divide the knee medially, laterally, and superiorly that typically resorb. The medial plica is a rubber band-like structure between the medial patellar facet and the MCL that can become irritated and cause chronic pain during running, jumping, squatting, cutting, and pivoting. Athletes typically present with atraumatic medial knee pain during impact or repetitive flexion/extension activities.

The physical examination may show some medial swelling, although usually not a true effusion. Pain is elicited with palpation of the medial compartment between the facet and MCL; the rubber band-like structure may be palpated or a "pop" elicited with repetitive flexion and extension. Ligamentous examination is normal. Quadriceps atrophy, tight hamstrings, and a weak core body are also typical.

Imaging is not typically necessary. Occasionally, an MRI can define a medial plica if surgery is anticipated.

Treatment consists of ceasing the offending activities and beginning a structured PT/HEP similar to that of PFSS. Running and sports activity form should be evaluated and corrected if they are contributing to the patient's pain. Ice and NSAID use (sparingly) after activity may help with pain. If conservative rehabilitation is not successful, surgical removal may be considered.

Referral to a sports medicine specialist is recommended if there is a more concerning history or physical examination, or if the patient does not respond to typical conservative treatment.

9. What Other Conditions Can Cause Pain on Terminal Extension of the Knee?

Fat pad impingement occurs when the medial or lateral fat pads become painfully impinged by the patellar tendon upon full extension of the knee. Patients may have pain with rapid terminal extension (bounce test), but no effusion occurs. Imaging is not particularly helpful, although an MRI may show the inflammation of the fat pads.

Treatment consists of ice after activity and the sparing use of NSAIDs. PT and a HEP consisting of core body strengthening and hamstring flexibility is of the utmost importance. Injections (cortisone) into the fat pads may help to alleviate pain, but if this is not followed by an intensive PT course, pain tends to recur. If the diagnosis is not clear or the patient does not respond to conservative treatment, he or she should be referred to a sports medicine specialist.

10. How Does Distal Iliotibial Band Syndrome Cause Lateral Knee Pain in Running Sports?

The ITB is an important lateral-stabilizing structure that originates at the supracondylar tubercle of the femur and inserts on Gerdy's tubercle of the proximal tibia. It can become directly irritated during sports activity such as running, jumping, and cutting from rubbing over bony prominences. Athletes typically present with lateral-sided pain at either the proximal hip or the distal knee. (Please see Chapter 35, question 7, for further discussion of proximal ITB issues.)

In distal ITB syndrome, a lateral click may be felt or heard with repetitive flexion and extension of the knee. Descending stairs, cutting, and running are especially painful for the individual.

Physical examination will elicit pain upon palpation of the distal ITB with occasional clicking palpated with repetitive knee flexion and extension. A positive Ober's test is also found in many cases (see Figure 35-6). There is no knee effusion and ligaments are intact. Tight hamstrings and quadriceps, along with weak one-legged squats, are common.

Radiographs are not usually helpful. An MRI can help to evaluate the ITB; however, this is usually a clinical diagnosis.

Treatment consists of ceasing the offending activities and beginning a structured PT/HEP similar to that of PFSS, with a particular focus on ITB stretching and hip strengthening. Weak hips can cause the knee to buckle into valgus and continue to irritate the ITB. Running and sports activity form should be evaluated and corrected if they are contributing to the patient's pain. Ice and NSAID use (sparingly) after activity may help with pain. A countertension band around the ITB may help to alleviate discomfort during sports activities.

A running, gait, or sports functional evaluation is crucial to recovering from ITB syndrome. The proper shoe (cushioned, motion controlled, or stability) based upon foot type and gait, along with replacing shoes every 300 to 500 miles, can help as well. One should avoid running in the road against traffic, as the bevel of the road makes the left leg functionally longer and can contribute to left-leg ITB (most common in runners).

Chronic ITB that is ignored and allowed to get worse is extremely difficult to treat and can end running careers. Cortisone injections into the lateral bursa may help to reduce acute pain, and rarely, ITB surgical release may be suggested. Referral to a sports medicine specialist is recommended if the patient's history and physical examination do not fit with ITB or if he or she is not recovering with conservative management.

11. How Can a Discoid Meniscus Cause Chronic Knee Pain?

Typical menisci are C-shaped shock absorbers that sit between the tibia and femur, but approximately 3% of the population has a congenital discoid meniscus (usually laterally) that is shaped like a disc instead of a C.[3] Menisci can be injured with twisting and flexion maneuvers of the knee, and there is an increased risk for damage with a discoid meniscus secondary to pressure on the larger, misshaped meniscus. Isolated meniscal injuries without significant trauma are rare in children, unless they have a discoid meniscus.

A common nonacute presentation of discoid meniscus is localized non- or minimally painful prominence or popping usually at the lateral joint line. These findings may also be incidentally identified on routine knee examinations.

In the setting of an acute trauma to the meniscus, patients typically present with a twisting, cutting, or squatting mechanism that causes pain or a "pop" along the posteriormedial or posteriorlateal joint line. A mild to moderate effusion is usually present and an inability to bear weight, a limp, and decreased ROM (inability to fully flex or extend knee) are found, along with posteromedial/posterolateral joint line tenderness and a positive McMurray test (see Figures 37-4 and 37-5). Concomitant injuries (anterior cruciate ligament, MCL) can also occur after an acute trauma.

- True knee catching or locking (knee stuck in flexion for at least a few minutes without instantaneous relief) with relief after wiggling it around to get it to unlock is characteristic and may suggest a bucket handle tear or flipped meniscus.
- The inability to fully straighten the knee (extension) is considered a surgical emergency due to the possibility of a flipped meniscus being present. If this is the case, it is extremely important to make the patient nonweight bearing on crutches as he or she can damage the articular surface of the knee by walking on a partially bent knee.

Imaging studies including standard knee radiographs are typically normal except for shadows showing the joint effusion (if present). An MRI is extremely helpful in assessing for a discoid meniscus, meniscal damage, or other injury.

Otherwise asymptomatic, discoid menisci require no particular treatment other than observation and the acceptance of the potential higher risk of future meniscus tear due to the larger and misshapen discoid meniscus. There is no role for prophylactic removal of an asymptomatic discoid meniscus.

For a symptomatic, acute meniscal tear, treatment is typically surgical, as meniscal tears do not tend to heal. Surgical repair versus removal depends on the location and extent of the injury. Meniscal repair is preferred when possible, although immobilization and healing post-surgery is typically longer than with meniscal removal. PT is an important part of the recovery process. Return to play is based upon surgical findings and recovery. Once they are fully functional, patients may return to play. Complications include a risk for arthritis if the meniscus is removed ("bone on bone"). Continued damage to a nonrepaired meniscal injury can create a bigger injury and more damage.

Any patient with a suspected discoid meniscus should be referred to a sports medicine specialist for further evaluation.

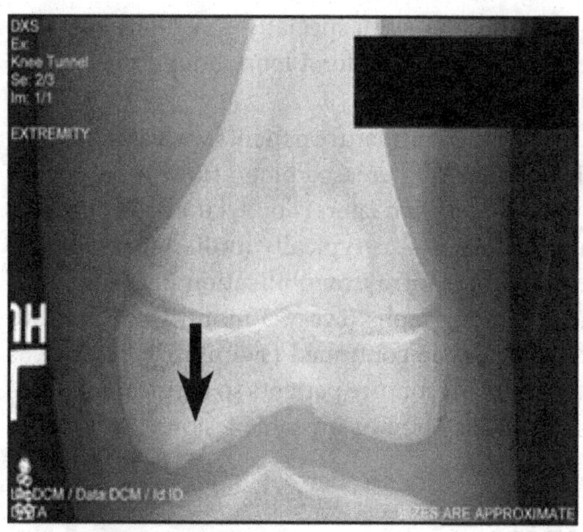

Figure 38-5. Tunnel view knee radiograph depicting OCD injury. (Reprinted with permission from Demorest RA. Adolescents with joint pain: a sports medicine perspective. In: McDonagh JE, White PH, eds. *Adolescent Rheumatology*. London, England: Informa Healthcare; 2008:247.)

12. What Is a Baker's Cyst, and Can It Cause Chronic Knee Pain?

A Baker's cyst is a collection of physiologic fluid trapped in a cyst located in the posterior popliteal compartment of the knee. Sometimes, Baker's cysts can occur due to meniscal pathology (tears). An athlete typically experiences a fullness or cyst/marble structure in the back of his or her knee. Pain can occur with full flexion or activity. Activity can cause the cyst to burst, which can cause an effusion and typically some pain relief. If a meniscal tear is present, typical examination findings of joint line tenderness and clicking/catching may be present.

Radiographs are not usually helpful, although an MRI may show meniscal pathology or visualize the cyst.

Treatment is typically benign neglect. If a patient presents with significant discomfort, PT similar to that for PFSS can help. Aspiration may be done; however, cyst recurrence is very common. Underlying issues such as meniscal pathology should be treated. Surgical cyst removal can be curative. Patients with an unclear history, examination, and meniscal pathology or those not responding to conservative care should be referred to a sports medicine specialist.

13. An Athlete Who Has Sustained an Injury to His Knee Is Not Improving With Proper Conservative Management. What Else Should Be in the Differential?

Osteochondritis dissecans (OCD) is a subchondral lesion to the bone that is common among growing teenagers. In the knee, OCD most commonly occurs on the lateral portion of the medial femoral condyle, but it can also occur on the lateral femoral condyle and the patella. The true etiology of OCD is unknown, but different mechanisms have been suggested (viral, trauma, avascular necrosis).

OCD can mimic PFSS, and is frequently missed and misdiagnosed. Episodic knee pain and swelling (a true effusion) with catching and locking of the knee can also occur. The inability to bear weight and a limp are common. Patients may also have atraumatic quadriceps atrophy and the inability to fully extend or flex the knee, especially if they have a loosening OCD fragment casing it to act like a loose body. If they cannot fully extend the knee they need to be placed nonweight bearing on crutches. Medial facet tenderness, pain over the medical femoral condyle, and pain with full flexion of the knee or squatting is also common.

Imaging is very helpful in diagnosing OCD. Knee films should include the usual four views; if the posterior femoral condyles are involved (most common location), the tunnel view is extremely helpful and essential to obtain (Figure 38-5.[3]) Patellar OCDs are best viewed on lateral and sunrise views, but they can be difficult to see and so they can be missed. An MRI can be extremely helpful in localizing and visualizing the lesion, and it is often ordered with specialty consultation. MRIs are also used for determining the stability of the lesion, evaluating for a loose body or loosening fragment, and assessing the cartilage and articular surfaces.

Conservative management is usually followed in skeletally immature patients with small, stable lesions who have a good potential to heal on their own due to increased blood flow to areas near the physis. Medial femoral condylar lesions tend to do better than lateral condylar or retropatellar lesions. Impact activity (running, jumping, competitive sports) is typically limited for 3 to over 12 months to allow the lesion to heal, and some patients require immobilization or crutch use/nonweight bearing status to assist in healing. Repeat radiographs (every 3 months) are used to assess how the patient is healing. Nonimpact activity may be continued (swimming, biking) as long as it does not elicit pain. OCDs will not heal in skeletally mature patients so surgical management is recommended. Readily refer any cases of OCD, as large or unstable lesions benefit best from surgical consultation.

References

1. Loudon JK, Goist HL, Loudon KL. Genu recurvatum syndrome. *J Orthop Sports Phys Ther.* 1998;27(5):361-367.
2. McMaster WC. Swimming and diving. In: Ireland ML, Nuttiv A, eds. *The Female Athlete.* Philadelphia, PA: Elsevier Science; 2002:744.
3. Demorest RA. Adolescents with joint pain: a sports medicine perspective [figure 9]. In: McDonagh JE, White PH, eds. *Adolescent Rheumatology.* London, England: Informa Healthcare; 2008:247.

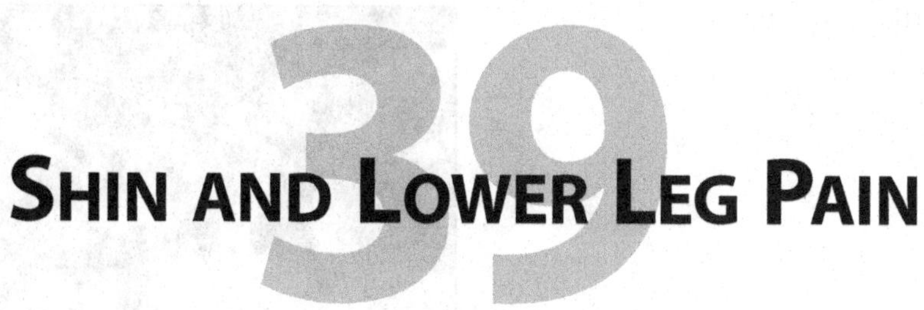

39 SHIN AND LOWER LEG PAIN

Jeremy Ng, MD and Matthew Grady, MD, FAAP

1. What Is the Significance of Genu Valgum (Knock Knees) and Genu Varum (Bowlegs), and What Is Their Relationship to Blount's Disease?

Genu valgum and genu varum are part of normal knee alignment development.

- Birth—Knee alignment starts with genu varum of 10 to 15 degrees
- 12 to 14 months—Femoral-tibial alignment is at neutral.
- 3 to 4 years—Alignment progresses to a maximum valgus alignment of 10 to 15 degrees.
- 5 to 9 years—Gradual correction of the alignment, with most individuals maintaining a small amount of physiological genu valgum.

Bracing is not required and does not affect the natural progression from genu varum to genu valgum.

Blount's disease is a growth disorder causing medial angulation and internal rotation of the proximal tibia. Clinically, it can appear to resemble genu varum, but standing anteroposterior (AP) x-rays demonstrate the tibia deformity. It can present at ages 2 to 4 (infantile Blount's disease) or after age 8 (adolescent Blount's disease).

- Infantile Blount's disease is often bilateral and presents in children who are in the lower percentiles for height and weight. The cause is unknown.
- Adolescent Blount's disease is thought to occur as the result of repetitive microtrauma that impairs growth of the proximal medial tibial physis, causing an angular varus deformity that can be unilateral or bilateral and occurs almost exclusively in obese children, especially those of African descent.

2. Are Calf Muscle Injuries Common in the Pediatric Population?

In the absence of direct trauma, calf muscle injuries are uncommon in the pediatric population. Bone pain (shin splints, stress fractures of the tibia and fibula, tumor) or vascular etiology (popliteal artery [PA] entrapment, chronic exertional compartment syndrome) are much more common.

3. Are Ruptures of the Achilles Tendon Common in the Pediatric/Adolescent Populations? What Examination Findings Can Reassure the Health Care Provider That the Achilles Is Intact?

- Acute Achilles tendon rupture in the pediatric population is extremely rare.
- Spontaneous Achilles tendon rupture may occur in any patient with underlying medical conditions such as inflammatory and autoimmune diseases, infections, collagen abnormalities, and certain neurologic conditions.

Koutures C, Wong V.
Pediatric Sports Medicine: Essentials for Office Evaluation (pp 269-277)

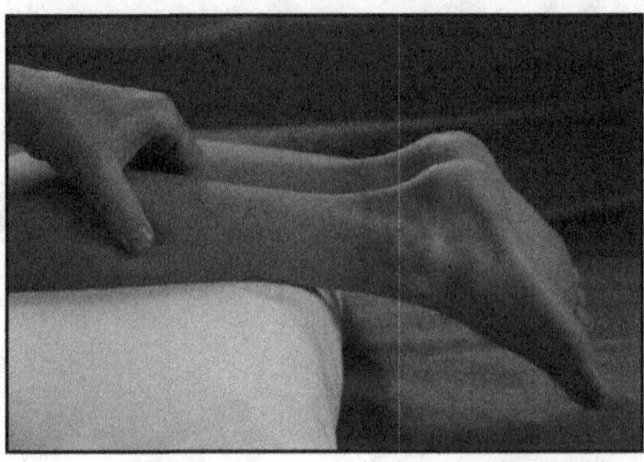

Figure 39-1. Thompson's test.

- Medications such as corticosteroids and fluoroquinolones have been cited for spontaneous injury, mostly in adults.[1]
- The ability to do a series of symmetric single leg heal lifts is reassuring that the Achilles is intact.
- Special Testing—Compare all findings with the contralateral leg.
    - Calf squeeze test (Thompson's test)—The patient lays prone on the table (or kneeling on a chair), with his or her ankles hanging over the edge. The calf muscles are then squeezed between the examiner's thumb and forefingers in the middle third (the musculotendinous junction) below the place of the widest girth (Figure 39-1). The test is presumed normal if passive plantar movement of the foot is observed. The test is presumed positive (Achilles rupture) if no plantar movement of the foot is observed. (Note: the test may be "positive" with a torn gastrocnemius aponeurosis and an intact Achilles tendon.)
    - Knee-flexion test (Matles test)—The patient lays prone and actively flexes his or her knee to 90 degrees. The test is positive if the ankle falls to neutral or dorsiflexion, indicating a likely Achilles rupture.

4. Does Every Athlete With Lower-Leg Pain Have to Stop Activity?

No. If the pain does not impair function (alter gait, decrease performance, etc) then stopping the activity is not necessary. Formal evaluation is needed if function is impaired. If evaluation is ongoing, general guides include the following ABC's of management:

- Activity modification
    - Modified or reduced volume or intensity of normal training; consider low or nonimpact alternate activities (Table 39-1) if significant pain with usual training activities.
- Bracing
    - The patient may use a controlled ankle motion (CAM) walker fracture boot, taping, ace wrapping, and pneumatic compression splints while undertaking modified activity.
- Continued rehabilitation (can be home or formal physical therapy, and focuses on the following:)
    - Increasing range of motion (first active then passive).
    - Strengthening (starting with isometric exercises) and proprioception exercises.
    - Progression back to sport-specific activities.
    - "Prehabilitation": while recovering from one injury, perform exercises to prevent second injury.

Table 39-1. Examples of Modified Training Activities for Lower-Leg Pain		
• Swimming • Cycling • Elliptical • Antigravity treadmills	• Deep water running • Shallow water training (pain tolerance determines water depth)	• Speed bands • In-place circuit training • Upper body

Table 39-2. Comparison of Medial Tibial Stress Syndrome and Tibial Stress Fracture[2-7]	
MEDIAL TIBIAL STRESS SYNDROME	*TIBIAL STRESS FRACTURE*
History Symptoms present when starting activity; subside with continued exercise As symptoms progress, pain may be present for longer periods during activity and then eventually, throughout activity Further progression leads to pain after activity	**History** Insidious onset (2 to 3 weeks) of localized exertional pain (dull ache) at end of activity As symptoms progress, pain occurs earlier in activity; does not abate as quickly postactivity Later occurs in nonsports-related activities that involve weight bearing (walking up stairs)
Physical Examination Pain on distal 1/3 of tibia; may extend proximally 5-cm area of tenderness along the bone Pain along the posterior medial border of tibia (curl finger around and under tibia to find area of maximal tenderness)	**Physical Examination** Focal bony tenderness proximal, anterior, or posterior medial mid-tibia + Hop test: hop on one leg (should reproduce pain in the bone) + Tuning fork test: hit fork and place on the bone (vibration will reproduce pain)
Imaging AP and lateral tibia x-rays: normal Bone scan: diffuse uptake distal medial tibia MRI: edema along periosteum of posterior medial tibia without cortical/bone marrow edema CT: normal	**Imaging** AP and lateral tibia x-rays: normal for first 2 to 4 weeks; bone healing may be visible later as periosteal reaction (Figure 39-2A), usually the posterior or medial border Bone scan: focal uptake in affected bone MRI: bone marrow edema +/– cortical break CT: may show fracture line but CT not usually needed to make diagnosis and will miss early stress fractures
AP, anteroposterior; CT, computed tomography; MRI, magnetic resonance imaging.	

5. How Can Medial Tibial Stress Syndrome (ie, "Shin Splints") and Tibial Stress Fractures Be Differentiated on History, Examination, and Imaging?

Table 39-2 provides information on the physical examination, history, and imaging options for medial tibial stress syndrome and tibial stress fractures.[2-7]

TABLE 39-3. THE "SOUZA STEPS"
• Begin with 2 sets of 10 ankle circles in both directions. • Exercises are performed on soft surfaces (grass, field turf, beach, etc). • All exercises should stress the head forward, straight stick (straight line from head to ankle, hips tall [anterior pelvis facing up]), and ankle steps over opposite mid calf. • Entire activity takes approximately 5 minutes.
EXERCISES
1. Walk on toes: maintain plantarflexion on touch down. Do not let the heel sink back toward the ground. Work on stabilizing the lower leg with the posterior leg muscles. 2. Walk on heels: do not let the upper body lean forward to offset the center of gravity. Maintain straight body posture through an emphasis on using anterior lower-leg muscles and core. Keep hyperdorsiflexion throughout the stride, and do not let the forefoot sink into the soft surface at ground contact. 3. Plantarflexion/internal rotation: the forefoot steps in front of the opposite foot in "uni-track" style. (If walking in snow, the patient would not see 2 footprints side by side, but rather 1 footprint where each foot is placed directly in front of the other.) 4. Plantarflexion/external rotation: same as above, but the heel steps over the opposite heel in a straight line. 5. Inversion: walk on lateral aspect of foot. Do not let the patient look bowlegged. The knee should remain facing straight ahead. Make the lower leg (posterior tibial muscle) do the work. 6. Eversion: walk on the medial aspect of foot, ankle dorsiflexed. Do not let the knees sink inward, making them look knock-kneed. Make the lower leg (peroneal muscles) do the work. 7. Repeat step 1 going backwards. 8. Pick up the grass (intrinsic foot muscles): walk using same described posture and mechanics with ankle in dorsiflexion, but curl the toes at ground contact and try to grab the grass blades and pull them out of the ground during the heel recovery phase.

6. Are There any Recommendations/Pearls for Both Prevention and Treatment of Medial Tibial Stress Syndrome? How Important Is Shoe Type and Arch Support/Orthotic Treatment in the Prevention of Lower-Leg Pain?

- Shin splints occur as the end result of excessive overloading of the bone often due to poor biomechanics, a flawed training program (too much, too soon), and insufficient muscle strength for the running demands.
- Shoe type and arch support/orthotic treatment do not address the underlying biomechanical flaws or muscle insufficiency associated with shin splints, but they can help as a temporizing measure.

Prevention and Treatment

- Prevention and treatment address common biomechanical flaws including excessive pronation secondary to tight gastrocnemius muscles and overstriding (landing with the foot in front of the body). We recommend gastrocnemius stretching and promoting a running form that stresses dorsiflexing the ankle thus allowing the foot to make contact with the ground directly underneath the body (eg, under the center of mass).
- Strengthening intrinsic foot and ankle muscles is also important. A series of exercises developed by Paul Souza known as the "Souza Steps" has been highly successful in preventing shin splints (Table 39-3).

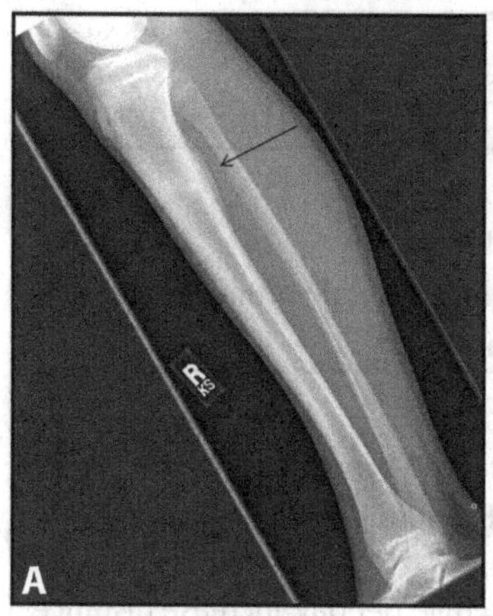

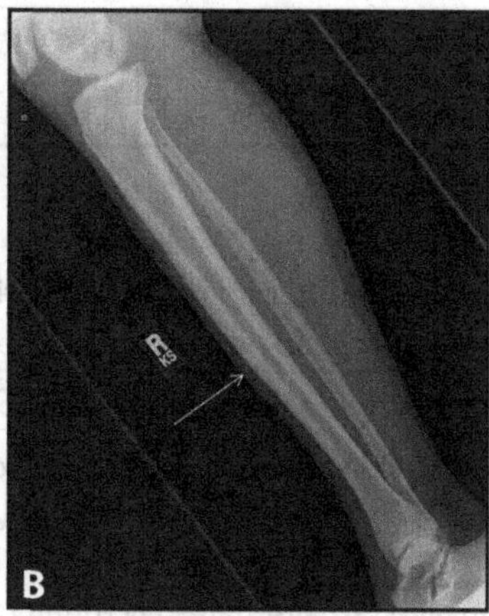

Figure 39-2. (A) X-ray of a proximal tibial stress fracture. (B) X-ray of an anterior tibial stress fracture.

7. What Are the Lower-Risk Types of Tibial Stress Fractures, and What Are the Higher-Risk Types of Tibial Stress Fractures? How Are the Treatments Different, and Which Ones Warrant Specialty Referral?

- Tibial stress fractures account for approximately 50% of stress fractures in athletes, and risk is location specific.[4]
- Referral to an orthopedic surgeon or a sports medicine specialist should be made for patients with high-risk stress fractures or low-risk fractures that fail conservative management.

Lower-Risk Tibial Stress Fractures

These are stress fractures on the compression side (posterior medial border).

- Can be either distal tibia or proximal tibia (slightly longer healing; Figure 39-2A).
- One should attempt to identify and correct any mechanical or training program flaws.
- Usual healing time is 4 to 8 weeks. The athlete should avoid nonsteroidal anti-inflammatory drugs since they decrease fracture healing.
- Treatment is rest until the patient is pain-free, then a gradual bone-loading program, progressing back to full play. There is no consensus for return-to-running programs, but a full sample program is listed in Table 39-4.

Higher-Risk Tibial Stress Fractures

Higher-risk fractures include medial malleolus stress fractures and anterior tibial cortex (tension-sided) stress fractures (Figure 39-2B). Patients with these types of fracture are at risk for nonunion, complete cortical fracture, and avascular necrosis. Table 39-5 provides information on treatment options for these types of fracture.

8. What Are the Different Compartments of the Lower Leg, and What Are Some Common Presentations of Both Acute and Chronic Exertional Compartment Syndrome in Athletes?

See Figure 39-3 for an illustration of the cross section of muscles, nerves, and vessels of the four compartments of the lower leg. Table 39-6 describes the common presenting symptoms of concern for acute/chronic exertional compartment syndromes.

- Acute compartment syndrome (ACS) in athletes is rare and most often occurs in the setting of trauma (tibial or fibula fracture, muscle contusion with significant bleeding) or ischemic

Table 39-4. Sample Return to Running Program for Low Risk Tibial Stress Fractures

REST PHASE (1 TO 4 WEEKS)

- Full weight bearing as tolerated; crutches if walking is painful
- No running; allow cross training without bone loading (swimming, weight lifting, stretching)
- When able to hop pain free, patient can progress to next phase

GRADUAL LOADING OF THE BONE PHASE (2 TO 4 WEEKS)

- Start with bicycle and elliptical for at least 1 week before restarting running
- Around 4-week mark, restart a running phase; athlete should continue to do alternate exercises for cardio
- Restart running very gradually; start alternate-day running, ¼ mile per day. Increase distance by ¼ mile mile every other day
- After 2 weeks, start running every day; restart at ¼ mile and increase by ¼ mile each day for 1 week; fully cleared after 1 week of daily, pain-free running

Table 39-5. Treatment Options for Higher-Risk Tibial Stress Fractures

MEDIAL MALLEOLUS STRESS FRACTURES: POSITIVE BONE SCAN AND NEGATIVE PLAIN FILMS OR INCOMPLETE FRACTURE ON MRI

Conservative Management

- Nonweight bearing or pain-free weight bearing with immobilization (aircast brace, CAM walker fracture boot, cast)
- Bone stimulator may be helpful
- Healing time, 4 to 5 months

Orthopedic Referral if Earlier RTP Is Needed

- Percutaneous drilling and immobilization or internal fixation
- Healing time, 2 to 4 months

Complete Fracture on Plain Films

- Orthopedic referral for internal fixation with malleolar screws (union in 10 weeks)

Nonunion or Displaced Fracture

- Orthopedic referral for ORIF (union in 10 weeks) +/– bone grafting

ANTERIOR TIBIAL CORTEX STRESS FRACTURE TREATMENT OPTIONS

Conservative Management

Trial of extended period of nonweight bearing

- Bone stimulator may be helpful
- Healing time, 8 to 12 months

Intramedullary Nailing

- Allows immediate weight bearing and start of PT
- Pain relief by nail stabilization may allow RTP before complete bone healing
- Healing time, 9 to 16 weeks

Anterior Tension Band Plating

- Downside is soft-tissue stripping to place plate
- Healing time, minimum 10 weeks

CAM, controlled ankle movement; MRI, magnetic resonance imaging; ORIF, open reduction internal fixation; PT, physical therapy; RTP, return to play.

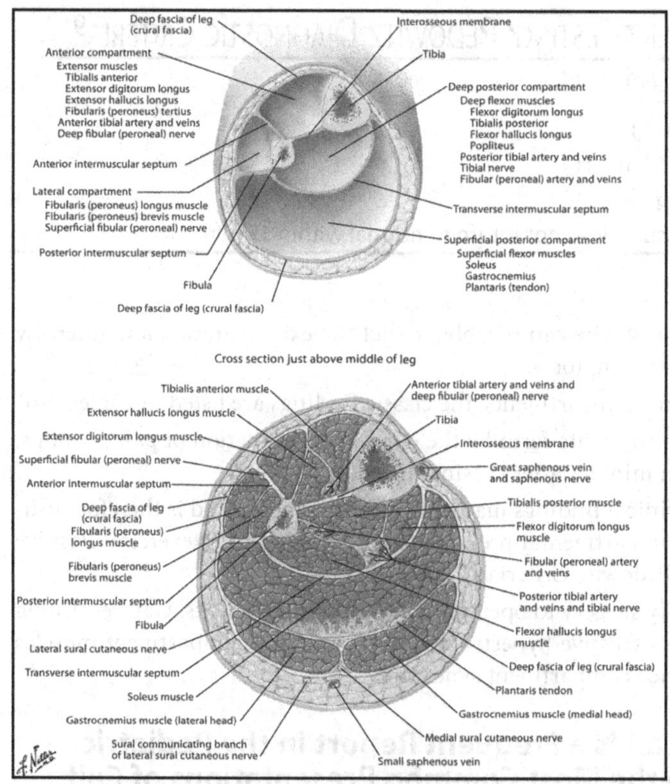

Figure 39-3. Illustration of a cross section of muscles, nerves, and vessels of the four compartments of the lower leg. (Reprinted with permission of Elsevier, Inc. www.netterimages.com/image/4820.htm)

TABLE 39-6. FOUR COMPARTMENTS OF LOWER LEG WITH COMMON PRESENTING SYMPTOMS OF CONCERN FOR ACUTE/CHRONIC EXERTIONAL COMPARTMENT SYNDROMES

DEEP POSTERIOR (40% OF CECS)	*SUPERFICIAL POSTERIOR (5% OF CECS)*
Weakness +/– pain plantarflexing great toe and foot, inverting foot	Weakness +/– pain plantarflex foot or pain with passive dorsiflexion
Paresthesias plantar aspect of foot	Hypothesia posterolateral lower leg or foot
LATERAL (10% OF CECS)	*ANTERIOR (45% OF CECS)*
Weakness +/– pain everting foot	Weakness +/– pain dorseflex or inverting foot
Decreased sensation distal-lateral 2/3 of lower leg and dorsum of foot excluding first web space	Decreased sensation first web space
	Transient/persisting foot drop

CECS, chronic exertional compartment syndrome.

event (sickle cell crisis). Occlusive dressings (splint/cast/ski boot) that do not allow the soft tissues to swell after injury have also caused ACS.

- Presentation of ACS is deep, poorly localized, burning pain that is out of proportion to the examination. As ischemia progresses, muscle dysfunction of the affected compartment will be present. Pain with passive muscle stretching is the most sensitive finding early in the process. The classic five P's of ischemia (pain, paraesthesias, pallor, pulselessness, and paralysis) are more consistent with arterial disruption and are not reliable indicators for ACS.
- ACS is a medical emergency that requires immediate open fasciotomy/compartment release.
- CECS is a reversible ischemia secondary to a noncompliant compartment that is unresponsive to the up to 20% expansion of muscle volume that occurs with exercise.[8] At rest there

Table 39-7. Compartment Testing: Pedowitz Diagnostic Criteria[9]
HISTORY PLUS ONE OF THE FOLLOWING:
• Pre-exercise pressure ≥ 15 mm Hg
• 1 min postexercise pressure ≥ 30 mm Hg
• 5 min postexercise ≥ 20 mm Hg
Suspicious but not diagnostic: pressure does not return to normal within 15 min

is no pain; with exercise, the athlete can reliably predict the exact duration and intensity of exercise needed to provoke symptoms.

- CECS may affect one or more compartments; the classic findings are listed in Table 39-6.
- CECS is differentiated from the acute form by the complete elimination of pain, cramps, and muscle tightness within minutes after ceasing the activity.
- Diagnosis made solely on clinical findings may lead to misdiagnosis, and is therefore usually confirmed with intracompartmental pressure testing pre- and postexercise. Positive tests are determined using Pedowitz Criteria (Table 39-7).[9]
- Treatment of CECS is usually surgery to open the affected compartments. Gait retraining to reduce the inappropriate excessive hypertrophy of the anterior compartment muscles has been used to treat anterior compartment syndrome.

9. Cramping of the Calf Is a Frequent Report in the Pediatric Population. What are the Most Common Presentations of Calf Cramping, and What Are Some Uncommon Presentations That Should Be Considered in Difficult Cases?

Calf muscle cramping can be either exercise-associated muscle cramping (EAMC) or can be cramping at rest. Significant cramping at rest is associated with an extensive list of neuromuscular disorders that are best evaluated by a neurologist.

- EAMC is primarily caused by muscle fatigue. Dehydration and electrolyte abnormalities can contribute to EAMC, but they are not the primary causes. Training intensity, duration of exercise, and prior level of fitness are the primary determinates of muscle fatigue.[10]
- In a small percentage of individuals, the cause of leg pain is an anatomic variation involving the medial gastrocnemius and popliteal artery (PA) causing impaired arterial blood flow (see Figure 39-4). Collectively, these anatomic variants are called popliteal artery entrapment syndrome (PAES). The presentation of pain is very similar to CECS. Symptoms start with exertion, and the severity of the symptoms correlates more with the intensity of exercise rather than volume. Since CECS is more common than PAES, adolescent evaluation of ischemia-type pain usually starts with compartment testing for CECS. If testing is normal, then investigation for PAES with arteriogram or magnetic resonance angiogram is indicated.
- Causes of PAES include the following[11]:
    - Type I—Medial head gastrocnemius (MHG) is normal, PA is deviated medially and has an aberrant course.
    - Type II—MHG is located laterally, no deviation of PA.
    - Type III—Abnormal muscle bundle from MHG surrounding the PA.
    - Type IV—PA is located deeply and entrapped by the popliteus muscle or a fibrous band.
    - Type V—Popliteal vein is also entrapped with any type of PA.

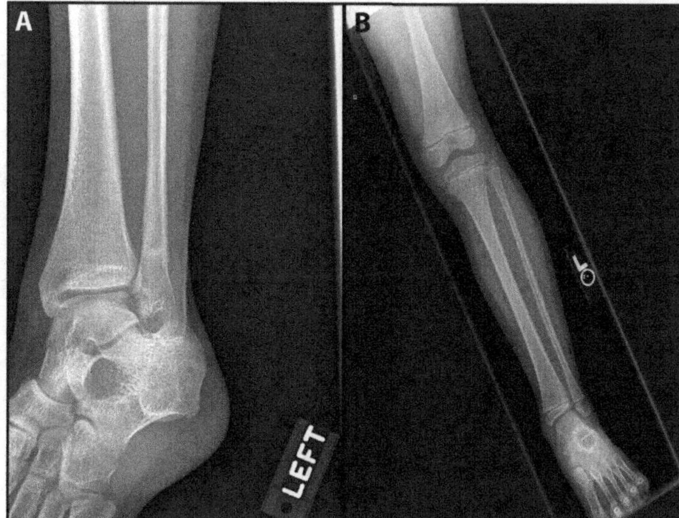

Figure 39-4. Fibula stress fractures in (A) a 15-year-old track runner and (B) a 6-year-old child who was jumping on a trampoline.

10. What Sports/Activities Create the Highest Risk for Fibular Stress Injuries, Where Are They Usually Found on Examination/Imaging, and How Are They Best Initially Treated?

- Most fibular stress fractures in young athletes occur in the metaphyseal-diaphyseal junction of the distal fibula, about 5 to 6 cm from the tip of the lateral malleolus (Figure 39-4A).
- Since the fibula is a minimal weight bearing bone, most of the force that causes the stress fracture comes from muscular forces and poor mechanics. With running, strong contraction of ankle plantar flexors pull the fibula toward the tibia, causing bone stress at the site of common fibula stress fractures. Running or jumping mechanics that cause the foot to evert/pronate place a valgus stress on the ankle joint and contribute to fibula stress.
- Fibula stress fractures are mostly commonly seen in distance runners and athletes who land and jump with the foot everted (long jump/triple jump; Figure 39-4A) and have been diagnosed after repetitive trampoline jumping (Figure 39-4B)
- Generally, treatment is rest for 2 to 6 weeks followed by low-impact exercise and a gradual return to running. Pneumatic bracing is an effective adjunct treatment. Occasionally, CAM walker fracture boot immobilization is necessary early in treatment, but prolonged immobilization should be avoided to prevent secondary muscle atrophy.

References

1. Sode J, Obel N, Hallas J, et al. Use of fluroquinolone and risk of Achilles tendon rupture: a population-based cohort study. *Eur J Clin Pharmacol.* 2007; 63: 499–503.
2. Bederka B, Amendola A. Leg pain and exertional compartment syndromes. In: Delee J, Drez D, Miller M, eds. *Delee and Drez's Orthopaedic Sports Medicine.* 3rd Ed. Orlando, FL: W.B. Saunders; 2009:1849-1856.
3. Dixon S, Newton J, Teh J. Stress fractures in the young athlete: a pictorial review. *Curr Probl Diagn Radiol.* 2011;40(1): 29-44.
4. Harrast MA, Colonno D. Stress fractures in runners. *Clin Sports Med.* 2010; 29(3): 399–416.
5. Moen MA, Tol JL, Weir A, et al. Medial tibial stress syndrome: a critical review. *Sports Med.* 2009; 39(7): 523-546.
6. Patel D, RothM, Kapil N. Stress fractures: diagnosis, treatment, and prevention. *Am Fam Physician.* 2011; 83(1): 39-46.
7. Reshef N, Guelich DR. Medial tibial stress syndrome. *Clin Sports Med.* 2012;31(2):273-290.
8. Wilder RP, Magrum E. Exertional compartment syndrome. *Clin Sports Med.* 2010; 29: 429–435.
9. Pedowitz RA, Hargens AR, Mubarak SJ, Gershuni DH. Modified criteria for the objective diagnosis of chronic compartment syndrome of the leg. *Am J Sports Med.*1990;18(1):35-40.
10. Schwellnus MP, Drew N, Collins M. Muscle cramping in athletes- risk factors, clinical assessment and management. *Clin Sports Med.* 2008;27(1):183-194.
11. Rich NM, Collins GJ, McDonald PT, et al. Popliteal vascular entrapment. *Arch Surg.* 1989;114:1377-1384.

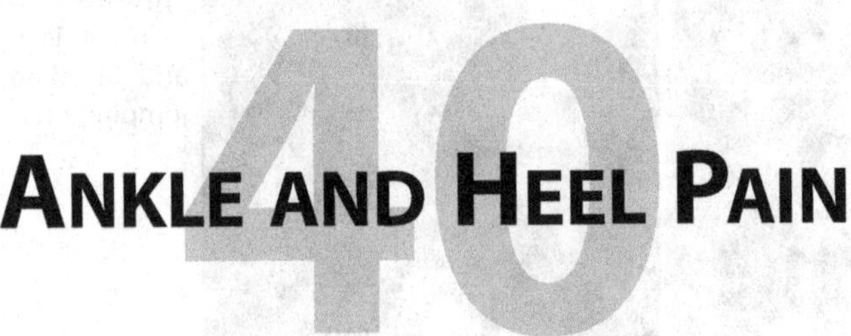

Ankle and Heel Pain

Tho Brian Hang, MD and Cynthia R. LaBella, MD

1. Lateral Pain After Inversion of the Foot and Ankle Is a Common Office Presentation. What Structures Must Be Evaluated in a Patient With Such an Injury?

- Please see Figure 40-1, which details key anatomy structures of the lateral ankle that are vital in making an accurate diagnosis.
- When evaluating an ankle inversion injury, one must consider the skeletal maturity of the athlete, as fractures are more common than sprains in skeletally immature patients.

2. What Tests Can Be Performed to Assess Stability and Determine the Severity (Grade) of an Ankle Sprain?

- The anterior drawer test can determine the degree of injury to the anterior talofibular ligament (Figure 40-2). It is performed with the patient seated, knee flexed to 90 degrees, and ankle plantarflexed slightly to relax the gastrocnemius muscles. The examiner then stabilizes the distal tibia with one hand while the other hand cups the heel and pulls it briskly forward, assessing the laxity of the ankle by comparing it with the uninjured ankle.
- The talar tilt test evaluates for laxity in the calcaneofibular ligament, and is performed with examiner's hands in the same position as for the anterior drawer test (Figure 40-3). The examiner then briskly inverts the injured ankle, assessing its laxity by comparing it with the uninjured ankle.
- Please see Table 40-1 for a classification of ligament sprains.

3. How Is a Salter-Harris Type I Fracture of the Distal Fibula Physis (Growth Plate) Identified, and What Are Some Key Management Tips?

- The majority of radiographs will be normal when dealing with fractures through the growth plate, although there may be some widening of the growth plate and overlying soft-tissue swelling compared with the opposite extremity.
- The key to diagnosis is identifying focal tenderness to palpation directly over the distal fibular physis, which is approximately 1 to 2 cm proximal to the tip of the lateral malleolus (Figure 40-4).
- Repeat imaging at 1 week after injury may show callus formation around the physis, confirming a fracture.

Koutures C, Wong V.
Pediatric Sports Medicine: Essentials for Office Evaluation (pp 278-286)

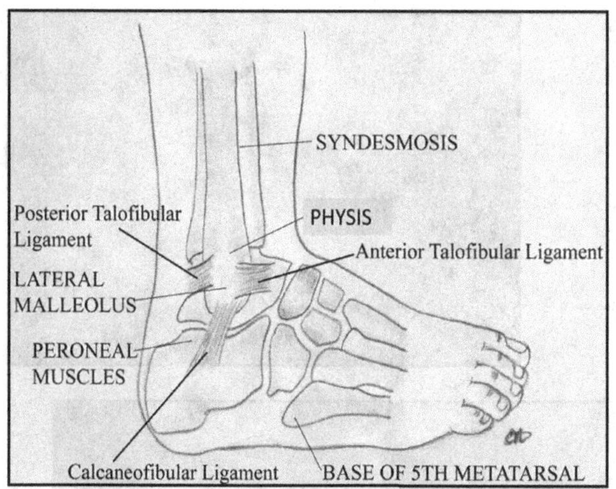

Figure 40-1. Lateral ankle structures. (Graphite Pencil-Copyright © 2012 Cora Maglaya, PT, ATC, CSCS.)

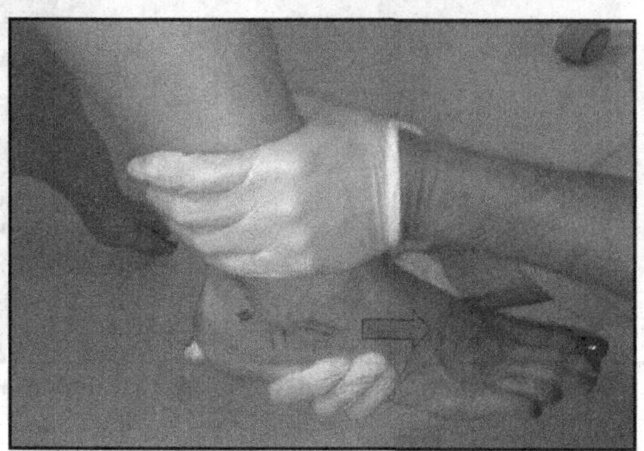

Figure 40-2. The anterior drawer test.

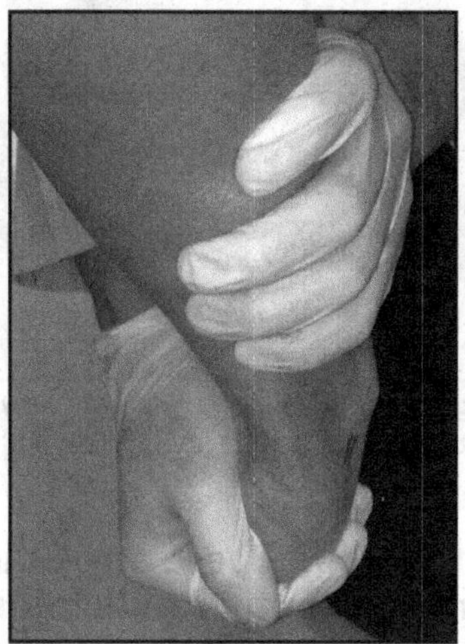

Figure 40-3. The talar tilt test.

TABLE 40-1. CLASSIFICATION OF LIGAMENT SPRAINS		
GRADE 1	*GRADE 2*	*GRADE 3*
Stretch	Partial tear	Complete tear
No laxity	Mild laxity with firm end point	Significant laxity with no end point

- Treatment includes an air stirrup or short-leg walking cast. If the pain is severe, crutches may be necessary for the first few days until weight bearing is more comfortable. Rest from high-impact activities (running and jumping) is required for healing, which usually takes about 4 to 6 weeks, at which time it will be safe for the athlete to return to sports and other physical activities. Formal physical therapy is usually not necessary.
- It is very rare for Salter-Harris type I fractures of the distal fibula to cause problems with bone growth.[1]

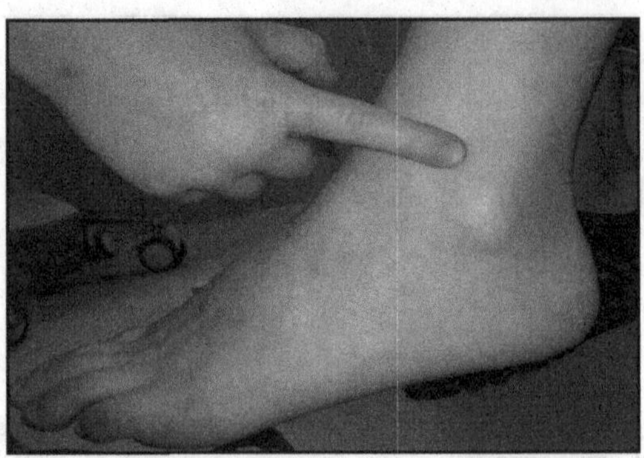

Figure 40-4. Location of distal fibula physis.

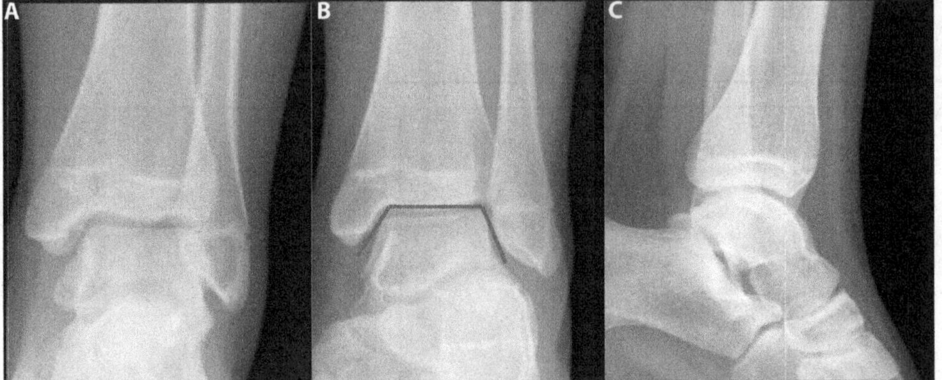

Figure 40-5. Ankle radiograph views. (A) Anteroposterior (AP) view, (B) mortise (internally rotated) view, and (C) lateral view.

4. Are There any Guidelines to Determine Who Needs X-rays After an Ankle Injury? If They Are Necessary, Which Views Are Ordered, and What Are the Key Findings?

- The Ottawa ankle rules are published guidelines to help determine who needs radiographs after an ankle injury. These guidelines can be applied to children older than 6 years.[2,3] With these guidelines, radiographs should be obtained if any of the following exist:
  - Inability to bear weight (for 4 steps) on the injured ankle immediately after sustaining an injury or in the emergency department/site of evaluation.
  - Point tenderness over the posterior edge of the distal 6 cm of either malleolus.
  - Point tenderness over base of the fifth metatarsal.
  - Point tenderness over the navicular bone.
  - Age > 55 years.
- Three views of the ankle should be obtained: anteroposterior (AP), mortise, and lateral (Figure 40-5).
  - The mortise view is an AP view but with the ankle slightly internally rotated, which provides a better view of the mortise (the upside down "U" space between the talar dome and medial and lateral malleoli) and talar dome, and is helpful in identifying syndesmotic injury.
  - Any asymmetry in the mortise indicates a significant ligament injury, occult fracture, or syndesmotic sprain, which may require surgery.

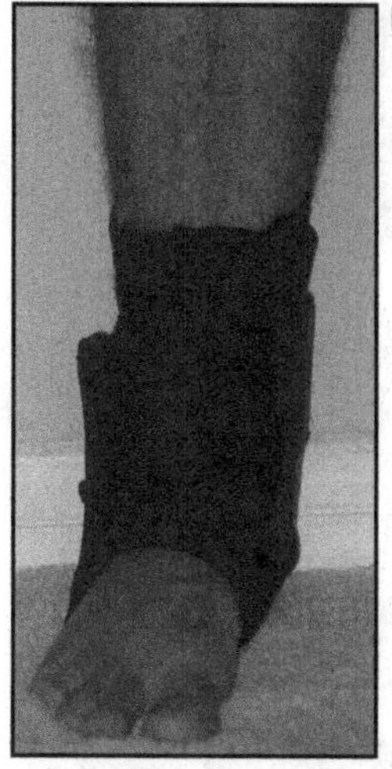

Figure 40-6. Semi-rigid lace-up and hook and loop fastener strap ankle brace.

5. Should Ankle Sprains Be Immobilized in a Cast or Brace? Which Injuries Need Crutches, and if So, for How Long? Are There Exercises That Can Be Started Soon Afterward?

- Ankle sprains should be supported in an air stirrup or a lace-up ankle brace, and the patient should be allowed to bear weight as tolerated.
- With severe pain, crutches and a CAM (controlled ankle motion) walker boot or posterior mold splint may be necessary for the first few days until weight bearing is more comfortable.
- Casting is generally not recommended because it can cause stiffness and delay the recovery of motion and strength.

Early ankle rehabilitation exercises prevent stiffness and muscle atrophy, and promote earlier recovery. They should be started within 24 to 48 hours of the injury or as soon as the patient can tolerate them. These include range of motion (ROM) exercises such as writing the alphabet in the air with the big toe, nonweight bearing calf stretches, and isometric strengthening exercises.

6. Who Needs Physical Therapy After an Ankle Sprain? What Are Some Key Elements to a Comprehensive Ankle Rehabilitation Program?

- Simple rehabilitation exercises, as described above, are usually sufficient for first-time ankle injuries in nonathletes.
- Formal physical therapy can facilitate return to sport or functional activities and reduce the risk of reinjury, and thus is beneficial for all athletes and nonathletes with repetitive injuries or chronic pain after an ankle sprain.
- Comprehensive ankle physical therapy consists of the following 3 phases:
  - Regain ROM and reduce pain and swelling.
  - Core and lower-extremity strengthening.
  - Proprioception exercises and injury prevention education.

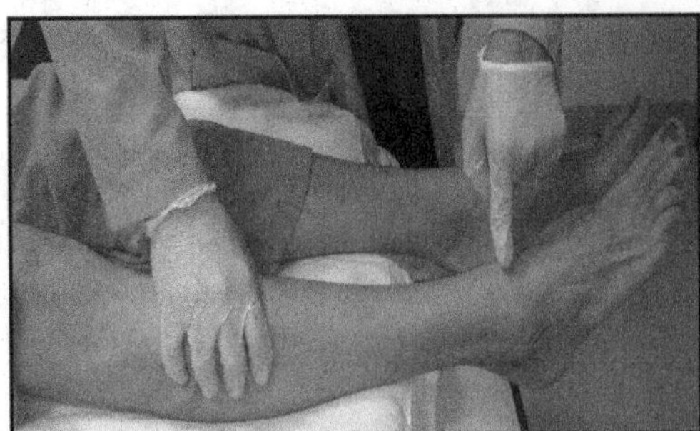

Figure 40-7. Syndesmotic squeeze test.

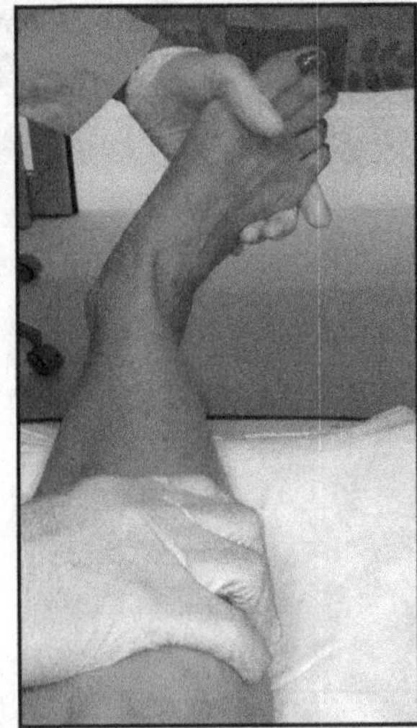

Figure 40-8. External rotation stress test.

7. What Is the Role of Taping or Bracing for the Prevention of an Initial Ankle Sprain and the Reduction of the Risk of Future Ankle Sprains?

- Semi-rigid ankle braces have been shown to reduce the risk of first-time and recurrent ankle sprains (Figure 40-6).
- Ankle taping appears to be equally effective in reducing reinjury.
- Thus, taping or bracing is recommended for athletes returning to sports involving running and jumping.

8. What Is a "High" Ankle Sprain, and How Might Its Management Differ From That of a "Usual" Ankle Sprain?

- "High" ankle sprains occur at the tibiofibular joint, just above the true ankle (tibiotalar) joint and involve diastasis (separation) of the syndesmosis (one or more of the five ligaments that connect the tibia to the fibula).
- The classic mechanism is a twisting injury to the ankle while it is dorsiflexed with the foot externally rotated. Compared with lateral ankle sprains, "high" ankle sprains are much less common.
- "High" ankle sprains do not typically have soft-tissue tenderness and often have minimal swelling, thus, these injuries are sometimes overlooked.
- Physical examination findings for "high" ankle sprains are as follows:
  - The squeeze test is performed by squeezing the proximal tibia and fibula together (Figure 40-7). If a syndesmotic tear is present, the squeeze test will cause a separation of the distal tibia and fibula and will cause pain distally at the ankle and syndesmosis.
  - The external rotation test is performed with the knee extended and the ankle in the neutral position; one hand stabilizes the proximal tibia and the other hand externally rotates and dorsiflexes the foot and ankle (Figure 40-8). Pain or instability at the syndesmosis is highly suggestive of "high" ankle sprain.

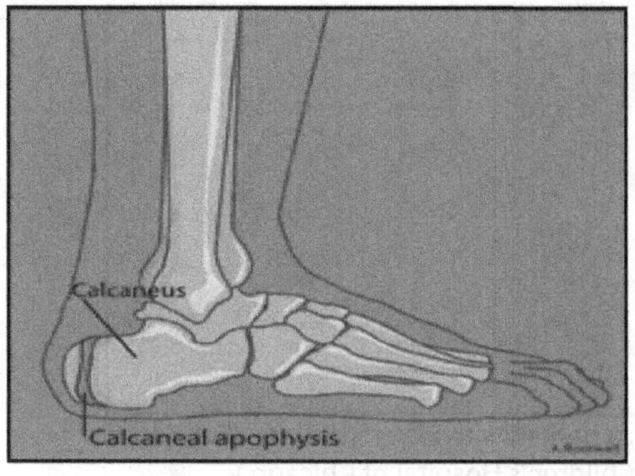

Figure 40-9. Location of calcaneal apophysis. (Reprinted with permission of Ann & Robert H. Lurie Children's Hospital of Chicago.)

- In "high" ankle sprains, ankle radiographs may show some widening of the ankle mortise. Stress radiographs with external rotation of ankle or magnetic resonance imaging (MRI) can be helpful if the diagnosis is still uncertain.
- "High" ankle sprains typically take longer to heal than lateral ankle sprains—often 6 weeks or longer until the athlete is able to resume athletic activities. Most patients can be treated nonoperatively with a period of nonweight bearing or a CAM walker boot until ambulating is nonpainful, followed by formal rehabilitation. More severe injuries and those associated with medial (deltoid) ligament injury or a fibular fracture may require surgical stabilization. The RTP after surgery can take several months.

9. A Patient Presents With Medial Ankle Pain After an Eversion Injury. Besides Evaluating the Medial Ankle, Why Is It Crucial to Palpate the Proximal Fibular Region?

- Medial ankle sprains are more likely to be associated with fractures, especially of the proximal or distal fibula. When the ankle is forcefully everted and externally rotated, the force can be transmitted proximally through the interosseous membrane to exit through the proximal fibula as a fracture (Maisonneuve fracture). Patients with these fractures should be referred to an orthopedic specialist. An examination under anesthesia may be necessary to evaluate the stability of the ankle.

10. What Is Sever's Disease of the Heel? What Are the Main Causes? Who Is at Highest Risk, and What Can Be Done for Treatment? Does Every Case Need X-rays, and Can a Child Play Sports With This Type of Heel Pain?

- Sever's disease is painful irritation and inflammation of the sides and back of the calcaneal apophysis at the Achilles tendon insertion (Figure 40-9). It is caused by repetitive tension and/or pressure on the apophysis, which is much less resistant to such forces than the surrounding bone.
- Running and jumping generate large compression forces on the heels, and tight heel cords add tensile force at their insertion near the apophysis.
- Sever's disease is most often seen in physically active children between 8 and 13 years old, and is the most common cause of heel pain in this age group, especially in athletes who play sports that require repetitive jumping, cleated shoes, or bare feet.
- Many cases are bilateral.
- The diagnosis is clinical, but when pain is severe or occurs at rest, radiographs can be ordered to evaluate for other causes of heel pain (calcaneal fractures, bone cysts). In Sever's disease, x-rays are normal.

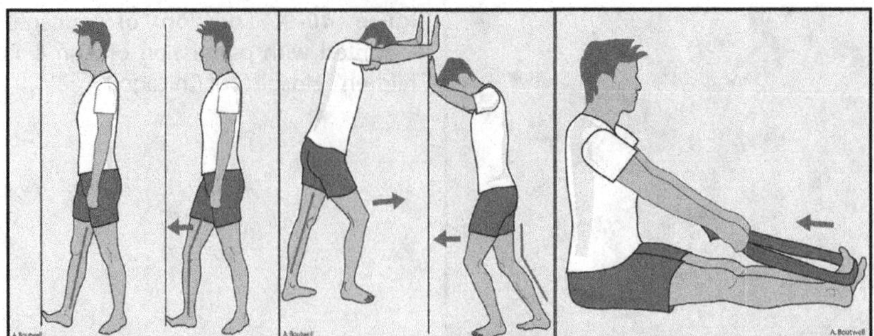

Figure 40-10. Recommended stretches for a patient with Sever's disease. (Reprinted with permission of Ann & Robert H. Lurie Children's Hospital of Chicago.)

- Treatment involves a short period of rest from painful activities to take pressure off of the apophysis and to allow the inflammation to resolve. Athletes may participate in sports activity if there is no limp or severe pain during/after activity.
  - Ice can reduce pain and inflammation.
  - Stretching of calf muscles should be done several times per day to relieve tension on the growth center (Figure 40-10).
  - Heel cups can absorb shock and good arch supports may decrease pain.
  - Anti-inflammatory medications may be used when pain persists despite rest, ice, stretching, and proper shoe supports.

11. What Are Some Other Fairly Common Causes of Pain in the Heel/Posterior Ankle, and How Can They Be Identified and Managed?

- Os trigonum—An accessory bone that sits in the posterior ankle.
  - It is usually round, oval, or triangular, and varies in size. During growth, it may eventually fuse with the talus, or it may remain as a separate small bone connected to the talus by a fibrous band. Os trigonum syndrome is a painful inflammation after a traumatic ankle sprain, or more commonly, when the patient is subjected to repetitive plantarflexion such as from dancing en pointe or jumping while playing basketball.
  - Radiographs can confirm the presence of the accessory bone. An MRI demonstrating edema within the os and surrounding soft tissues can confirm the diagnosis of os trigonum syndrome.
  - Treatment includes rest, ice, nonsteroidal anti-inflammatory medications, physical therapy, and ankle taping. A CAM walking boot may be used to restrict painful ankle movement. Cortisone injections to the area are sometimes helpful for severe inflammation. Rarely, surgery is recommended for cases that do not resolve with any of these treatments, although this is not usually necessary in children.
- Achilles tendinopathy—An overuse injury due to excessive stress, such as from repetitive running or jumping, leading to swelling and small tears in the tendon that cause pain, stiffness, and weakness.
  - If the injury is not treated properly and the stress continues, the weakened tendon is at risk for rupture or progression to tendinosis, a condition in which the tendon become thickened and irregular, leading to chronic pain and stiffness.
  - Achilles tendinopathy is most common in activities that require repetitive running, jumping, or leaping. Poor flexibility of the calf muscles and pes planus (flat feet) increase the risk. Other contributing factors include inadequate rest between training sessions, training on hard surfaces such as cement, and poor-fitting or worn-out shoes.

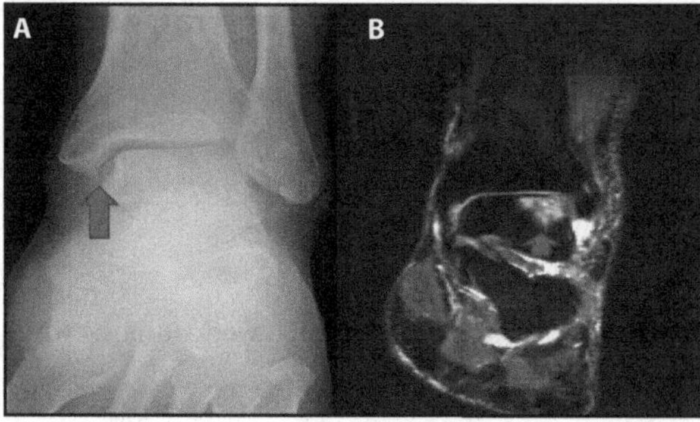

Figure 40-11. Osteochondral lesion of talus. (A) Radiograph of medial talar dome lesion, left ankle. (B) MRI of medial talus, right ankle, demonstrating bone edema with articular cartilage loss.

  - Treatment includes avoiding painful activities, ice, and anti-inflammatory medications. Physical therapy will address imbalances in muscle strength and flexibility, and can speed recovery and prevent reinjury. Specifically, eccentric strengthening exercises for the calf muscles may strengthen the tendon and reduce the risk for recurrent injury. Shoe inserts can also be helpful.
- Achilles tendon rupture most frequently affects men in their 40s and 50s.
  - A painful pop in the back of the ankle followed by the inability to bear weight are the hallmarks of the injury. On physical examination, the Thompson's test confirms the injury (see Figure 39-1). These injuries may be successfully treated operatively or nonoperatively with functional bracing and rehabilitation. Benefits of operative repair might be a speedier return to activity, while risks include infection and wound breakdown. While risk of rerupture was generally thought to be higher with nonoperative care, a recent meta-analysis found no significant difference in rerupture rate with operative versus nonoperative care.[4]
- Retrocalcaneal bursitis occurs when the bursa between the Achilles and calcaneus becomes inflamed. There may be swelling and redness on either side of the tendon. Treatment is similar to that for Achilles tendinopathy.
- Calcaneal stress fractures should be considered when heel pain persists despite adequate rest and activity modification. An ankle MRI will confirm the diagnosis, and treatment consists of a CAM walker boot or crutches until ambulation is pain free.

12. What Are Osteochondral Lesions of the Talar Dome? When Should They Be Suspected on History or Examination, and What Radiologic Findings are Common?

- Osteochondral lesions result from acute trauma or repetitive microtrauma, and should be considered when there is persistent pain and/or swelling after an ankle sprain, despite adequate rest and rehabilitation.
- Athletes may also report locking, catching, or instability of the ankle.
- Radiographs often reveal the lesion in the anterolateral or anteromedial talar dome. MRI is then performed to grade the lesion (Figure 40-11).
  - Grade 1: edema in the subchondral bone with intact articular cartilage.
  - Grade 2: irregular or fissured cartilage.
  - Grade 3: full thickness cartilage injury with joint fluid tracking into subchondral bone.
  - Grade 4: loose ostechondral fragments within the joint.
    - Grade 1 and 2 injuries typically respond well to rest from impact activities for 3 to 6 months. Grade 3 and 4 injuries usually require surgical fixation.

13. Which Ankle/Heel Injuries Require Specialty Referral, and Which Are More Urgent?

The following injuries should be referred to an orthopedic surgeon:

- Achilles tendon rupture.
- Disruptions of mortise or syndesmosis.
- Maisonneuve fracture.
- Osteochondral fractures.

The first 3 injuries should be referred on an urgent basis (seen within a week at most) while osteochondral lesions can be referred on a more routine basis.

References

1. Spiegel PG, Cooperman DR, Laros GS. Epiphyseal fractures of the distal ends of the tibia and fibula: a retrospective study of 237 cases in children. *J Bone Joint Surg*. 1978;60A:1046–1050.
2. Stiell I, Wells G, Laupacis A, et al. Multicentre trial to introduce the Ottawa ankle rules for use of radiography in acute ankle injuries. Multicentre Ankle Rule Study Group. *BMJ*. 1995;311(7005):594–597.
3. Dowling S, Spooner CH, Liang Y, et al. Accuracy of Ottawa ankle rules to exclude fractures of the ankle and mid-foot in children: a meta-analysis. *Acad Emerg Med*. 2009;16(4):277–287.
4. Soroceanu, A, Sidhwa F, Aarabi, S, et al. Surgical versus nonsurgical treatment of acute achilles tendon rupture: a meta-analysis of randomized trials. *J Bone Joint Surg*. 2012;94:2136-2143.

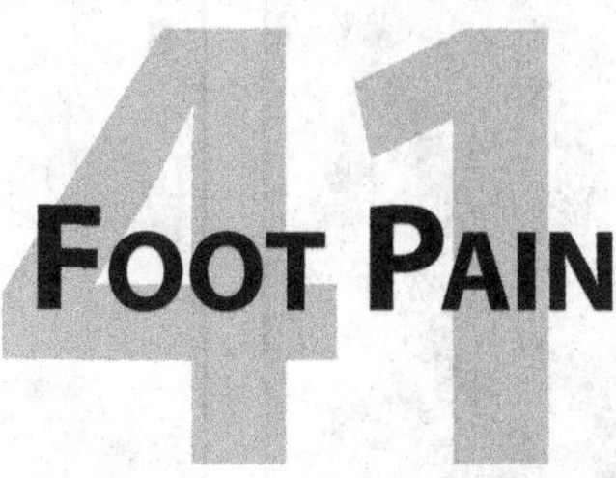

41 Foot Pain

Paul R. Stricker, MD, FAAP

1. What Is Flat Feet, or Pes Planus? Can It Cause Pain in Athletes?

Parents may present to an office setting due to concerns that their child may have flat feet, or worried about a familial pattern of flat feet. Pes planus describes the large plantar contact surface. The majority of children with flat feet have the normal "physiologic" variety, often accompanied by calcaneal valgum.[1] A flexible flat foot is an arch that flattens out with weight bearing (Figure 41-1A). The arch reappears when a child is nonweight bearing or rises up on his or her toes (Figure 41-1B). This description makes up the majority of people with flat feet, most of whom are also asymptomatic. This phenomenon is described as foot pronation. Even though foot pronation is usually pain-free, it has been implicated in contributing to ankle impingement, shin splints, iliotibial band pain, and patella maltracking, all of which can be painful. Feet that pronate do not require radiographs, and only require treatment if the flattening of the arch is contributing to other problems. An insert or orthotic may be recommended in these cases to help support the arch while the patient is in repetitive impact activities. Many over-the-counter orthotics can be used effectively at a minor expense. Custom orthotics are not often recommended in these cases involving children because they are expensive and will be outgrown relatively quickly and need to be replaced.

The abnormal flat foot is rigid, stiff, and often painful in the mid- or hindfoot during activity.[1,2] These painful flat feet make up the small minority of flat feet, and, unlike feet that pronate, do require radiographs. Rigid flat feet may be due to tarsal coalition (see question 2), congenital vertical talus, or a tight Achilles tendon. They may respond to casting or custom orthotics. Congenital vertical talus often requires surgery, whereas a tight Achilles may respond to appropriate stretching. If they remain painful, then surgical lengthening of the Achilles may be required. Patients with painful rigid flat feet should be referred to a pediatric orthopedic surgeon.

2. What Is Tarsal Coalition, and What Might Suggest This Condition? What Is Seen on Imaging Studies, and How Should the Health Care Provider Initially Manage and Refer Suspected Cases?

Tarsal coalitions are tarsal bones that are fused together. The two most common coalitions are between the calcaneus and tarsal navicular (calcaneonavicular [CN]), and between the talus and calcaneus (talocalcaneal [TC]).[1,2] Boys and girls are affected equally, and coalitions are often familial. Coalitions reduce the mobility of the foot, including inversion and eversion. These fusions may be asymptomatic, but usually become symptomatic with increasing levels of activity. If suspicious physical examination findings (which include inability to walk on the lateral edge of the foot or lack of calcaneal inversion on heel raise) are found, then foot radiographs are indicated. CN coalitions are usually apparent on routine oblique radiographs of the foot. TC coalitions may

Koutures C, Wong V.
Pediatric Sports Medicine: Essentials for Office Evaluation (pp 287-294)

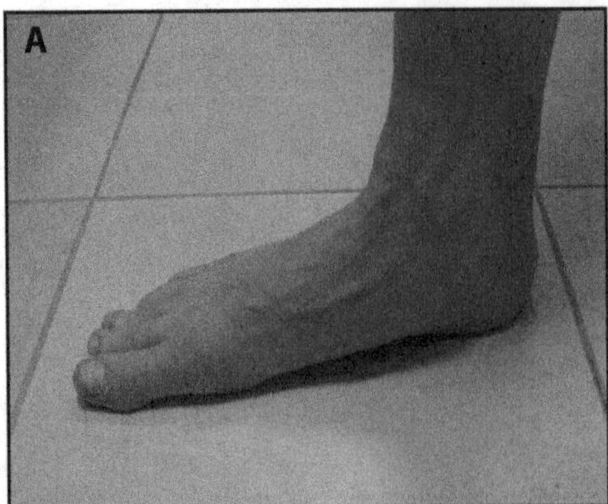

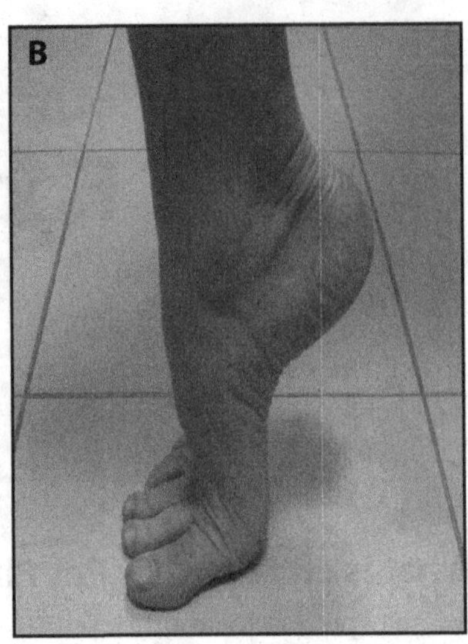

Figure 41-1. Demonstration of a flexible flat foot that on weight bearing has (A) flattening of the arch. (B) Arch reappears when going up on toes.

require a calcaneal view (Harris view), computed tomography (CT) scan, or magnetic resonance imaging (MRI) for proper imaging. Controversy exists as to the proper imaging for tarsal coalition. Reduction of radiation is always a legitimate concern, and since many young children with foot pain are not skeletally mature, an MRI may provide more meaningful imaging that could reveal cartilaginous or fibrous coalition along with intramedullary edema. Treatment of painful coalitions includes relative rest and a walking boot with an orthotic. A gradual return to weight bearing activity should be allowed after about 4 weeks. If pain recurs quickly, or if the child has recurrent significant painful episodes, then referral to a pediatric orthopedic surgeon should be made to discuss surgical resection of the coalition.

3. What Is an Accessory Navicular, How Does It Present, and What Associated Conditions May Occur? How Should It Be Imaged and Managed, and Which Cases Warrant Referral?

Accessory centers of ossification occur in bones throughout the skeleton. In the foot, the tarsal navicular bone is subject to an accessory center of ossification in about 4% to 21% of the population,[1] yet a smaller percentage remain unfused. This "accessory navicular" may appear as an incidental finding during radiographs for a foot or ankle injury, or it may be discovered when the child presents with a painful, swollen prominence on the medial aspect of the foot. The increased prominence may be asymptomatic, but the family may come to the clinic out of concern for a tumor. Routine anteroposterior (AP) and lateral radiographs of the foot are diagnostic, and the area should not be confused with a fracture.

Acute injuries to the accessory navicular can occur with direct trauma. A concern for a complete avulsion injury is failure to maintain the arch on heel raise—this mandates an immediate orthopedic referral. More commonly, the accessory navicular becomes painful as it is subject to repetitive stress. If the child has foot pronation (flexible flat foot) and is involved in running and jumping sports, the repeated stress on the arch and the opposing pull from the posterior tibialis tendon may cause irritation and inflammation of the fibrocartilaginous connection of the accessory bone to the parent navicular. Tendinitis of the posterior tibialis tendon can occur simultaneously.

Treatment consists of ice and reduction of activities, along with mechanical support of the arch with a semi-rigid orthotic. Good shoe wear along with the supported arch can be beneficial over the long-term without need for surgical excision, except in rare cases.

4. What Stress Injury Must Be Considered in Every Case of Either Diffuse or Focal Medial Midfoot Pain, Especially in Athletes Who Are Involved in Repetitive Jumping or Impact Sports? If Suspected, What Are Some Imaging Considerations? What Are the Most Common Management Recommendations?

Active youth involved in repetitive impact activities that present with progressive, interfering medial foot pain should alert the practitioner to the possibility of a tarsal navicular stress fracture. Although not as common as metatarsal stress fractures, navicular stress fractures due to overuse can occur and are a more significant injury. Examination may reveal an individual with a limp, point tenderness on the navicular bone, excessive pronation, limited dorsiflexion, or a rigid high-arched cavus foot, which increases the stress to the tarsal bones, especially the navicular. As with any overuse injury, there may be improper shoe wear or arch support, or a recent change or increase in activity.

Plain radiographs may be normal, and a navicular stress fracture often requires a bone scan or an MRI for diagnosis. If a stress fracture is found, a CT scan is often performed to determine the extent of the injury and can be used for follow-up imaging to assure that the fracture is healing correctly. Since nonunions of the navicular can occur due to its tenuous blood supply, it is imperative to document complete healing before the patient returns to sports or exercise activities.[3]

Treatment requires 6 weeks in a boot or cast and nonweight bearing with crutches, followed by 4 to 6 weeks of weight bearing in a boot. Interval CT scanning can follow the healing process. If healing has occurred, then a gradual introduction to weight bearing in a good supportive shoe with an orthotic can be initiated. Nonunions or persistently painful stress fractures that are unresponsive to treatment should be referred to an orthopedic surgeon for possible surgical fixation.

5. A Skeletally Immature Athlete Presents With Midfoot/Hindfoot Pain, and the Parents Are Concerned That the Patient Has Plantar Fasciitis. Is This Common in the Pediatric Population?

If a young athlete presents with heel pain, the diagnosis is most likely going to be calcaneal apophysitis (Sever's disease). If the child is skeletally immature, the combination of shearing forces from impact and increased tension in the Achilles tendon from inflexibility and/or accelerated growth can cause pain in the growth plate of the heel due to microfractures and inflammation. Since this process is not a "disease," the condition is more appropriately called apophysitis. There will be tenderness when "squeezing" the calcaneus. Plantar fasciitis is very rare in skeletally immature youth. A heel with a fused apophysis and point tenderness on the plantar surface is consistent with plantar fasciitis. Calcaneal stress fractures are also rare and quite painful when squeezing the body of the calcaneus, rather than just being painful at the apophysis.

Calcaneal apophysitis can cause an interruption or interference with activities, even to the point of limping/self-removal from activity. Calcaneal apophysitis occurs in younger athletes than tibial tubercle apophysitis, and is more common in individuals involved in impact activities such as soccer, whereas tibial apophysitis is more common in jumping/landing sports. Calcaneal apophysitis can be bilateral in about 60% of cases, and has an average age of appearance of 9 years in girls and 12 years in boys.[2]

As the long bones start to grow, increasing tension from the inflexibility of the Achilles contributes to the pain, along with the impact forces to the heel. Pain can wax and wane and can fluctuate over time. Since the growth process occurs over a few years, many youth with apophysitis need to be encouraged and informed that this condition may come and go over many months. Radiographs are rarely needed, unless the history and/or physical findings do not correlate with typical apophysitis. Acute treatment includes ice and rest with good supportive shoes and possibly a heel cushion or heel cup. Heel lifts should be used with caution since they decrease tension on the Achilles and can contribute to further inflexibility and tension. Heel cups, on the other hand, can be used during periods of pain. Frequent calf and Achilles stretching is required. Children should be encouraged to modify their activities to match their pain level. For example, if the child has reports of heel pain, then he or she can condition on a stationary bike or do a light practice of his or her sports drills for a couple of days before returning to his or her sport.

6. A Track Athlete Presents With Pain on Dorsiflexion of His or Her First Toe. What Could Be the Cause of This Pain?

Acute hyperflexion/extension of the first metatarsophalangeal (MTP) joint results in a ligamentous sprain referred to as "turf toe."[4] Swelling and pain are accompanied by an inability to toe-walk or push off with walking or running. In some cases, it can be a significant injury, with a prolonged loss of time from activity. Passive and active movements of the joint are painful and may require the use of crutches, ice, and nonsteroidal anti-inflammatory drugs. Fractures or avulsion fractures can occur, and radiographs should be obtained. Taping of the MTP joint, along with a steel shank or shoe with a rigid sole, can help reduce MTP motion once the athlete is able to bear weight. Surgery is not indicated unless a significant fracture/dislocation has occurred.

As symptoms improve, the athlete can maintain exercise that does not significantly stress the MTP joint (elliptical machine, rowing machine, strength training, stretching, and core strengthening). Upon the introduction to light impact activities and jogging, the joint should be taped and a stiffer shoe utilized until full pain-free range of motion has been restored.

7. A Young Teenage Girl Who Jumps Horses for Show in Competitions Is Reporting a New Pain at the Base of Her First Toe. What Is Occurring in This Patient?

The two sesamoid bones under the great toe MTP joint are incorporated into the flexor hallicus brevis tendon and help to increase the push-off force with which the muscle-tendon unit can contract—much like the patella enhances the forces generated by the quadriceps muscle. The first metatarsal head has concave facets with which the sesamoids articulate.[4] The sesamoid bones absorb much of the weight bearing force, and help to protect the flexor hallicus brevis tendon. Any activity that causes repetitive bending and/or impact of the first MTP joint on firm surfaces can irritate the surrounding soft tissues and the metatarsal-sesamoid articulation. Repetitive impact can also cause stress fractures of the sesamoids, manifested as increased uptake on a bone scan or increased edema on MRI. Acute injuries, such as jumping from a high surface, or severe turf toe injury can also cause acute inflammation or even frank fractures of one or both sesamoid bones. Acute fractures, especially with displacement, should be referred to a specialist.

Radiographs can be a bit confusing since sesamoids can have normal anatomic variations, such as a bipartite sesamoid. In addition to routine AP and lateral foot radiographs, a special sesamoid view is also helpful for optimal visualization.

Any activity that causes the athlete to spend significant time weight bearing on the ball of his or her foot causes an increased risk of sesamoiditis, including horseback riding in stirrups, equestrian activities, dance, running, and gymnastics, to name a few. Athletes will report pain with impact, going up on the ball of the foot, and push off. Initially, treatment may just require ice and nonsteroidal anti-inflammatory drugs, decreasing impact activities, and wearing a pad under the ball of the foot that unloads the sesamoids. Some individuals will benefit from taping the MTP joint to restrict dorsiflexion, similar to a turf-toe injury. Return to modified activities, followed by increasing exposure back to routine activities, allows the athlete to stay involved as much as tolerated.

More severe cases, or actual stress fracture of the sesamoid, require rest in a walking boot for 4 to 6 weeks, followed by the gradual return to nonimpact activities, then modified activities, and ultimately back to the sport.[3] Occasionally, a foot pad or a custom orthotic may be helpful for protection.

Sesamoiditis should not be confused with Freiberg's infarction, which is an osteochondrosis of the lesser metatarsal heads. Acute or chronic repetitive impact to the ball of the foot can be painful, and regular foot radiographs reveal lucencies in the metatarsal head, most commonly the second metatarsal. Staging of the process may be best accomplished with a 3-dimensional CT scan. Sesamoiditis is distinguished from Freiberg's infarction because the pain is on the plantar surface of the first metatarsal head.

8. A Football Player Was Tackled and Fell Awkwardly, Putting His Full Weight Onto His Plantar-Flexed Foot. He Had Pain, Swelling, and Edema at the Dorsum of the Base of His Second and Third Metatarsals, With an Inability to Bear Weight. What Is the Diagnosis?

A Lisfranc injury refers to a sprain, fracture, or fracture-dislocation of the second tarsometatarsal joint. The complex anatomy consists of the base of the second metatarsal and its articulation with the medial cuneiform by the Lisfranc ligament. The only articulation without a transverse ligament that joins the bases of the metatarsals is the articulation between the base of the first and second metatarsal.[1] This area can be injured by a direct crush-type blow, but more commonly with a longitudinal load placed on a plantarflexed foot along with rotation. Examples include a football player down on one knee and the foot is landed on by another player; falling backwards while the foot remains trapped; or a ballet dancer en pointe who falls forward.[1]

These injuries usually present with swelling, significant pain over the metatarsocuneiform area, and inability to bear weight or go up on toes. Shearing distraction force applied to the first and second metatarsal and squeezing the metatarsals may elicit pain in the area. Unfortunately, these injuries may be misdiagnosed as an ankle sprain or a minor injury, yet the ankle is usually pain free and the disability is disproportional to the physical findings. This should raise concern of a more substantial injury, and standing foot radiographs are required. AP, lateral, and oblique views should be ordered, and if possible, the AP and lateral views should be weight bearing with comparison views of the uninjured foot. If it is not possible to obtain weight-bearing views, the detail of a CT scan or MRI can help to define the extent of injury.

Diastasis between the first and second metatarsal, an abnormal lateral weight-bearing radiograph, or fracture may be visible. Injuries with no diastasis may be treated conservatively with a nonweight bearing cast for 4 to 6 weeks, followed by graduated weight bearing.[5] Fractures, dislocations, and diastasis require surgical fixation. Due to the complexity and morbidity of this injury, individuals with a suspected Lisfranc injury should be referred promptly to a sports medicine specialist or orthopedic foot surgeon.

9. What Is the Most Common Stress Fracture in the Foot?

Athletes involved in repetitive running and jumping sports are at risk for developing a stress fracture in the leg and foot. The most common stress fracture site is the tibia followed by the metatarsal shaft of the foot, with most occurring in the second, third, or fourth metatarsal.[3] Overuse, significant increase in activity, poor shoe wear, and pronation with inadequate arch support all contribute to increased stress in the metatarsals. Gradual onset of pain, with a reduction in speed and power, and eventual interference with activity is the usual history. Often, the pain is only associated with the high-impact activity, but over time it can become painful even with walking and other activities of daily living.

Limping may or may not be present, but there is usually subtle swelling seen in the area along with point tenderness on the metatarsal shaft. Squeezing the metatarsals, axial load pressure on the metatarsal head, and a bowing stress to the metatarsal has been described as means to elicit

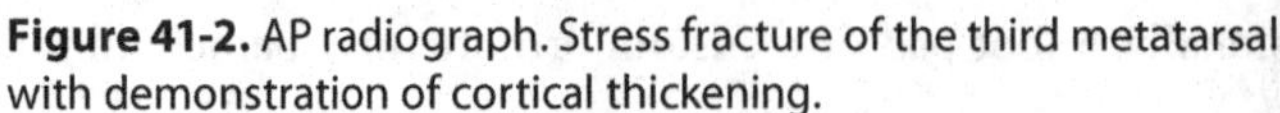

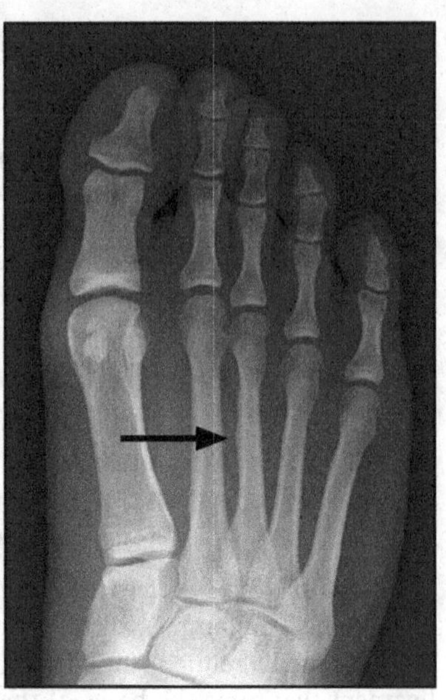

Figure 41-2. AP radiograph. Stress fracture of the third metatarsal with demonstration of cortical thickening.

pain. Often, simple point-specific pain with the history is adequate for moving forward with radiographs of the foot. After about 2 weeks of pain, radiographs may reveal early periosteal reaction (Figure 41-2). If the diagnosis is urgent based on the timing of an athletic event, a bone scan can be helpful for an earlier diagnosis.

If the individual is limping or has pain with simple walking, then the use of crutches for 1 to 2 weeks is helpful. However, since crutches can be difficult in the midst of a school campus with many kids and/or stairs, using a walking boot for 2 to 4 weeks with an orthotic to support the arch may be utilized more safely and efficiently. Nonimpact conditioning on a stationary bike or elliptical may be initiated after 4 weeks if there is no pain with palpation or the activity. Most metatarsal stress fractures require 6 weeks for healing, and after that point, gradual reintroduction to progressive-impact activities may be allowed. It is important for the athlete to understand that the new bone formation requires this gradual increase in load to adapt safely without the recurrence of the stress fracture.

10. Pain at the Outside of the Foot Is Common. What Are the Most Common Fractures Seen at the Fifth Metatarsal? How Can the Primary Health Care Provider Differentiate and Manage Each Type?

Both acute and chronic injuries can produce lateral foot pain on the fifth metatarsal.[3,5] It is important to determine the mechanism of injury and history of the onset of pain. There are different injuries that can occur to the proximal fifth metatarsal, so adequate history, physical evaluation, and radiographs are necessary to distinguish the true underlying problem and prescribe the appropriate treatment plan.[1]

Prepubertal youth with increased activity or who sustain an inversion injury can present with point tenderness to the proximal fifth metatarsal. This acute or chronic apophysitis usually appears during rapid growth and increased activity. Repeated traction from the peroneus brevis tendon attachment contributes to this uncommon condition. Radiographs reveal the apophysis with the line of separation parallel to the long axis of the metatarsal (Figure 41-3). Similar to other apophysitis conditions, Iselin's disease requires a temporary reduction of activity, ice, adequate shoe wear, and calf stretching. Return to activities is as tolerated.

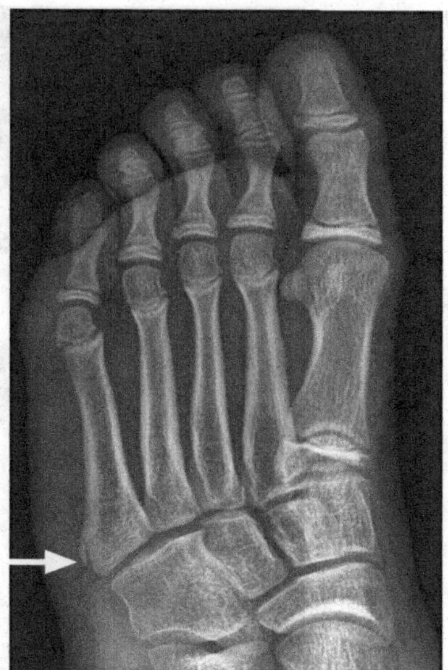

Figure 41-3. Oblique radiograph. Apophysis of the proximal fifth metatarsal (runs parallel to the long axis of the metatarsal).

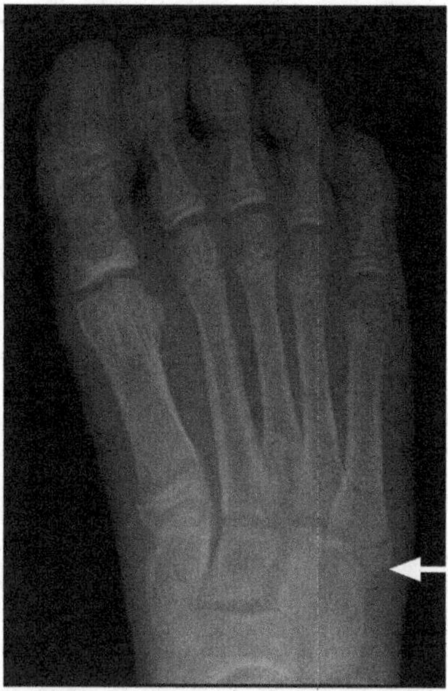

Figure 41-4. AP radiograph. Avulsion fracture of the proximal fifth metatarsal (runs perpendicular to the long axis of the metatarsal).

An acute inversion injury with the foot in plantarflexion can produce an avulsion fracture of the proximal fifth metatarsal. Controversy exists as to whether the injury is caused by the traction of the peroneus brevis tendon or by a lateral band of the plantar fascia.[1] Any ankle injury requires adequate physical evaluation of the ankle and the foot due to the tendon attachments on the foot. This history, coupled with point tenderness and swelling at the fifth metatarsal, warrants radiographs, including AP, lateral, and oblique foot films. These injuries produce a moderate-sized triangular fragment of bone, with the line of separation perpendicular to the long axis of the metatarsal (Figure 41-4). Most of these athletes will respond to 4 weeks in a weight bearing boot, followed by physical therapy and a gradual return to activities after 6 weeks. Fibrous unions can occur, yet individuals without symptoms can progressively return to activities unless the pain recurs. Rarely would any referral or surgical procedure be necessary.

In contrast to an avulsion fracture and a diaphyseal fracture, a different injury can occur transversely at the metaphyseal-diaphyseal junction, called a Jones fracture (Figure 41-5). This fracture usually occurs with running, jumping, and cutting maneuvers. This injury is critical to understand and diagnose due to the high incidence of nonunion (due to tenuous blood supply and reduced vascularity) and need for surgical fixation.[1,3,5] Being able to determine the radiographic location of the fracture is necessary to differentiate between other types of fifth metatarsal injuries. Initial treatment includes casting or boot with crutches, but referral to an orthopedic surgeon should be performed, as intramedullary screw fixation reduces the risk of nonunion and enables athletes a quicker return to activity.

Repetitive stress to the foot in running and jumping sports appears to cause stress fractures in the same area of the Jones fracture. The athlete may have had gradual increasing pain, and then has acute increase in pain upon landing from a jump. Radiographs reveal a fracture in the typical location of a Jones fracture, but already has pronounced increased calcific density along both sides of the fracture, denoting a chronic nonunion. Surgical consultation is indicated in this circumstance as well.

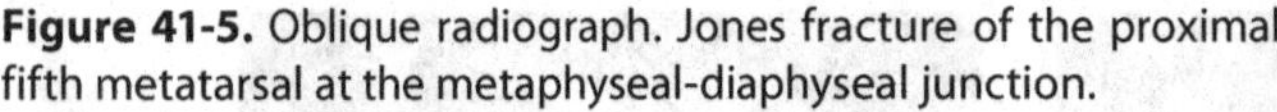

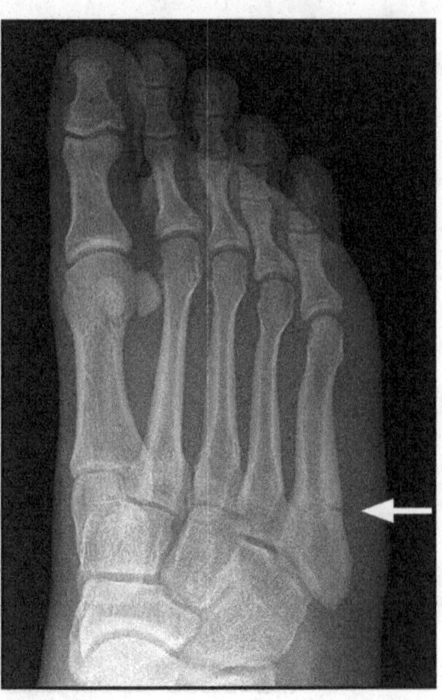

Figure 41-5. Oblique radiograph. Jones fracture of the proximal fifth metatarsal at the metaphyseal-diaphyseal junction.

Acute spiral fractures of the fifth metatarsal shaft usually occur from landing in plantarflexion with rotation and/or inversion. If there is minimal displacement without malrotation of the toe, these injuries can usually be treated conservatively with crutches and immobilization for 4 weeks, then progression to weight bearing and the gradual resumption of activities. If there is significant rotation of the fragment or shortening displacement, referral to an orthopedic surgeon should be performed.

11. What Is In-Toeing?

In-toeing is often referred to as being "pigeon-toed," and can be of concern to families primarily due to aesthetics. In some severe cases, it can cause tripping and can interfere with running. Children with severe cases should be referred to a pediatric orthopedist. The majority of cases simply require reassurance. Significant pronation, or flat feet, can sometimes be misdiagnosed as in-toeing, and should not require intervention, except for a possible arch support.

True in-toeing may occur due to metatarsus adductus, internal tibial torsion, or medial femoral torsion.[2] Most cases of mild metatarsus adductus correct spontaneously, and tibial and femoral torsions usually resolve to normal rotation by 8 to 10 years of age. Rarely does in-toeing require surgery, and most cases only need routine follow-up as the child grows. Significant rotations, pain, or persistent dysfunction require a referral to a pediatric orthopedist. In-toeing has not been found to impair physical performance in adolescents.

References

1. Simons SM, Sloan BK. Foot injuries. In: Birrer R, Griesemer B, Cataletto M, eds. *Pediatric Sports Medicine for Primary Care.* Philadelphia, PA: Lippincott Williams & Wilkins; 2002:431–455.
2. Sarwark JF, LaBella CR, eds. *Pediatric Orthopaedics and Sports Injuries.* Elk Grove Village, IL: American Academy of Pediatrics; 2010.
3. Kraft DE. Chronic foot and ankle injuries. In: Anderson SJ, Harris SS, eds. *Care of the Young Athlete.* 2nd ed. Elk Grove Village, IL: American Academy of Pediatrics; 2010:457–470.
4. Larson TD. Foot pain. In: Puffer JC, ed. *Twenty Common Problems in Sports Medicine.* New York, NY: McGraw-Hill; 2002:247–266.
5. Anderson SJ. Acute foot and ankle injuries. In: Anderson SJ, Harris SS, eds. *Care of the Young Athlete.* 2nd ed. Elk Grove Village, IL: American Academy of Pediatrics; 2010:443–456.

42 How to Guide Return to Play

Kenton H. Fibel, MD; Miriam G.S. Reece, MD, CAQSM; and Kenneth S. Taylor, MD

Lower Extremity Return to Play

1. What Are the Clinical Criteria for Allowing a Return to Running and Jumping?

- The recommended stages of recovery and rehabilitation include flexibility, strength, proprioception, endurance, and motor relearning, and finally, returning to full activity.[1]
  - Flexibility includes full joint range of motion (ROM) and muscle elasticity similar to the uninjured side.[1]
  - Strength should be comparable to the contralateral side. Early in an injury, isometric exercises are often well tolerated. Further strength training involving movement should be added when the patient's ROM is adequate.[1]
  - Proprioception includes reaction time, quickness, and agility of the injured side as it relates to the standard of play.[1]
  - Motor relearning is the act of performing all required activities/sports-specific drills at full speed, without pain or limitation, and with confidence.[1]
- One should base progression on the patient symptoms and his or her tolerance of advanced activity.[1]
- Recovery from an injury that requires surgical intervention will often have specific criteria that may differ from other return-to-play protocols.[1]
- A return to full training and sport occurs when the patient makes a full recovery of muscular and aerobic endurance and is able to perform sports-specific tasks without pain.[1,2]
- Rushing a return or inadequate rehabilitation can lead to further disability or injury.[1-3]
- Taping and bracing may help the patient during recovery; a rigid ankle brace or taping can help gain proprioception after ankle sprains, but they should not substitute for complete rehabilitation.[1,4]

2. What Type of Substitute Activities Can Be Considered as the Athlete Recovers From Injury?

- Commonly accepted alternate activities include cycling (adjusting resistance and seat positioning based on symptoms), swimming (tailored to the patient's tolerance), and other water-based exercises (including running in water with a vest for buoyancy).[3]

Koutures C, Wong V.
Pediatric Sports Medicine: Essentials for Office Evaluation (pp 295-300)

- It is best to start any alternative activity with a low resistance, and increase duration and resistance as tolerated.[1,3]
    - Integrate interval training (bike easy 30 seconds, harder for 30 seconds) later in the process.[1]
- Rehabilitation exercises can be used to maintain strength and endurance. Isometric exercises are often tolerated early in the injury rehabilitation process.[1]
- The goal is to maintain fitness, not to push the patient to the point of further injury.[3]

3. How Can Shoe Selection Assist in the Return-to-Play Process?

- Footwear should be well fitted and suited for the desired activity; it should be replaced at the appropriate intervals.[3]
    - The athlete should replace his or her running shoes after 250 to 500 miles.[3]
- The selection of a particular shoe is dependent on the injury and the sport.[3]
- Appropriate shoes can help correct underlying biomechanical and gait abnormalities that commonly cause overuse injuries and protect against subsequent injuries.[3]
- Shoes should be evaluated after the athlete sustains an injury for abnormal wear patterns.[3]
- Injury can also result from an athlete changing shoe types too quickly.[3]

4. How Can a Running Evaluation Be Helpful?

- A running evaluation is the most helpful from a prevention standpoint, but it can also enhance athletic performance, as correcting running form can increase efficiency.[3]
- It can often uncover potentially correctable mechanics that might lead to injury.[3]
- Such corrections may lead to a decrease in abnormal energy use and stress on the body.[3]
- It can approach an injury from a biomechanical standpoint, as the injured area may not be the root cause (ie, core weakness leading to knee-overuse injuries).[3]

5. What Are the Key Components of a Return-to-Running Program?

- Only scarce data exist about training progression after an athlete sustains an injury, but a gradual progression should be stressed.[1,3,5]
- If the athlete is in the middle of a growth spurt, emphasize a slower return to full running activity, allowing for adequate rest, and paying close attention to symptoms.[3,5,6]
- A good general guideline is the "10% rule," which is that total training should not increase more than 10% from one week to another. Total training includes intensity, duration, frequency, or any combination of these features.[3]
    - This can be modified for each individual athlete.[3]
- It is best to start with low-impact activity, and increase the impact as tolerated.[1-3]
    - Start with biking, then progress to walking, jogging, running, and then if necessary, can start participating in more intensive sport-specific skill development and practice drills.[1]
- The athlete should start on softer surfaces (grass or turf) before progressing to harder surfaces.[1]
- Speed work, hills, and track drills should be added later in the progression.[1,3]
- Periodization is a training technique that involves the systematic cycling of training loads over a period of time with set, well-defined resting periods.[3]
- Emphasizing rest time can help prevent overuse injuries that are more common with specializing in one sport at earlier ages and year-round participation.[3,6]

6. What Is the Difference Between Off-the-Shelf and Custom Orthotics (Insoles), and How Important Are They in Preventing or Treating a Lower-Leg Injury?

- An analysis of stance, gait, and biomechanics can be helpful in finding any functional imbalances might be correctable by orthotics.[3]
- There is a considerable cost difference between off-the-shelf and custom orthotics; therefore, many recommend starting with an off-the-shelf version.[4]
- If an off-the-shelf orthotic is deemed ineffective after allowing adequate time to adapt to the new biomechanics, then consider custom orthotics.[4]
- Some athletes have very asymmetric or unique feet and biomechanics, thus they may benefit from custom-fit orthotics over an initial off-the-shelf version.[3,4]

Upper Extremity Return To Play

7. What Are the Clinical Criteria for Starting Return to Overhead Activity After Sustaining an Injury?

- Factors to evaluate when deciding whether an athlete is ready to return to overhead activity include full ROM and strength, absence of pain, negative impingement and apprehension tests, minimal-to-no delayed-onset muscle soreness, prior performance level, and patient confidence.[7]
- Rehabilitation programs after operative management also focus on maximal expected ROM after the specific surgical procedure, period of time postoperative (physician- and injury-/procedure-dependent), and clearance from the surgeon when an athlete is making a return-to-play decision.[7]
- The throwing or functional interval program should consist of progressively greater force and faster throws (baseball), strokes (swimming), or hits (tennis).[7]

8. Are There Certain Strokes That Should Be Started When an Athlete Returns to Swimming After an Injury?

- The athlete should begin with the breaststroke and then progress to the crawl (freestyle) stroke, then the backstroke, and then finally the butterfly stroke.[8,9]
- One should focus on proper technique and increasing the distance with a slow and steady cadence. Swimming speed can be increased as long as the activity is pain-free. Once the athlete is up to full stroke speed, the next stroke in the progression can be added.[9]
- The interval program consists of progressively more forceful and faster strokes.[9]
- The athlete should begin twice-daily workouts only after having pain-free single-day swimming practices.[10]
- One should halt progression if he or she has any pain, especially if it lingers into the next training day.[9]

9. What Are the Key Components to a Baseball Return-to-Throwing Program?

- Since throwing a baseball involves the transfer of energy from the feet up to the trunk and ultimately out through the arm, it is important to emphasize strengthening the entire body when one is returning to throwing.[11]
- A proper warm-up prior to throwing is critical.[11]

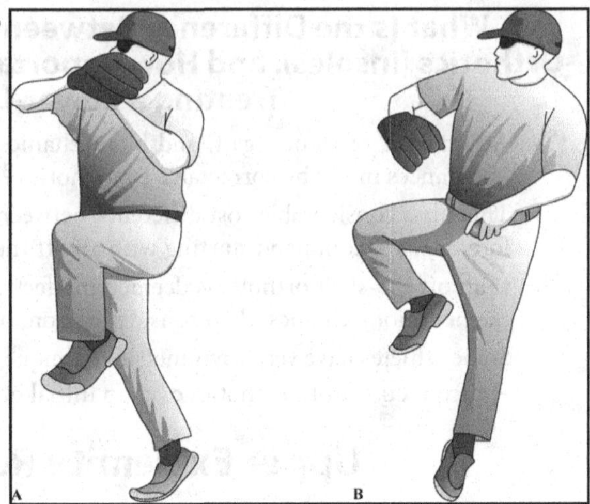

Figure 42-1. Crow hop. (A) Lifting left knee to (B) start right leg hop before skip and throw.

- Most injuries during rehabilitation occur due to fatigue.[11]
- Attention to proper throwing mechanics lessens the incidence of reinjury.[11]
- The minimum starting requirements include pain-free joint ROM (upper and lower extremities) and adequate muscle power and resistance to fatigue.[11]
- The chance for reinjury is lessened by a gradual progression of interval throwing.[11]
- An Interval Throwing Program consists of a specific number of throws, throwing distance, and intensity for each training session that varies based on the size of the field.
  - Phase I begins with throwing on flat ground, with a critical component of this phase being the use of the "crow hop," as it puts emphasis on proper mechanics.[11]
    - The "crow hop" is comprised of an initial hop, then a skip, followed by the throw (Figure 42-1).[12]
  - The ball's path should be in the trajectory of an arc and not on a flat line.[12]
  - One should avoid flat-foot throwing to prevent excess stress on the throwing shoulder.[12]
  - Position players should complete the entire program before attempting position-specific drills.[13]
  - Once a pitcher can perform phase I without experiencing symptoms, phase II can be initiated, which involves throwing from a mound.[13]
  - Additional information on this type of program can be accessed at the following link (specifically on pages 4 to 6)[11]: http://universityorthopaedic.com/pdf_files/IntervalRehabPrograms.pdf

10. Are There Certain Positions That Should Be Tried Earlier in a Return to Baseball? Can a Child With an Arm Injury Still Participate in Some Aspects of Baseball?

- Upper-extremity injuries in baseball players occur most frequently in pitchers and catchers due to the fact that they do more throwing. After pitchers and catchers, infield positions are at increased risk compared with outfield positions. First base typically is the least-risky infield position due to shorter and/or fewer required throws.[14]
- Appropriate time to return to batting varies depending on the type of injury.[11]
- The interval batting program should begin with dry swings, with a progression to hitting off of a tee, then a soft toss, and finally live pitching.[11]

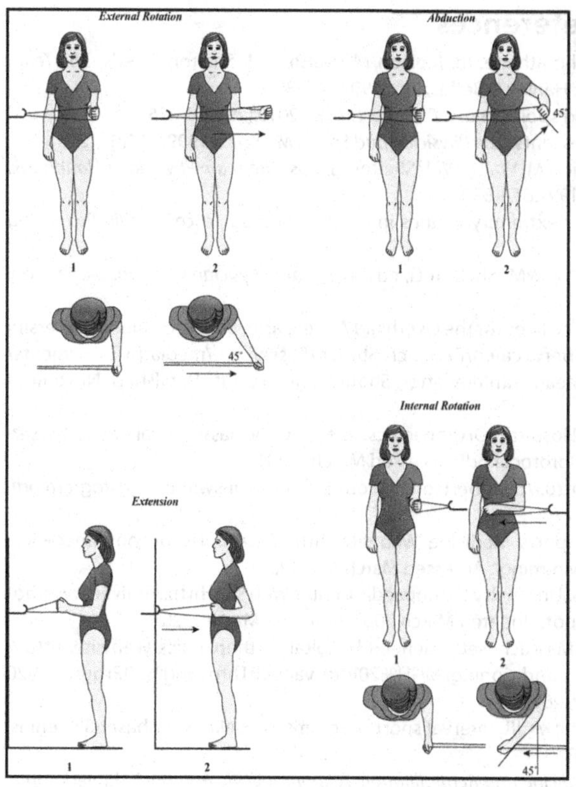

Figure 42-2. Band or cable exercises to strengthen the athlete's shoulder muscles (3 sets of 10 to 15 repetitions per exercise).

- Often, a player can successfully return to running, batting, and fielding drills (with ball underhand in place of overhead throws) while undergoing an arm rehabilitation program.[11]

11. Should Icing and Rehabilitation Exercises Continue While the Athlete is Starting His or Her Return to Sport?

- The athlete should continue with his or her rehabilitation exercises and using ice while starting his or her return to sport, as the benefits are just as important as at the beginning of the process.[8]
- Rehabilitation exercises are important to help prevent a recurrence of the injury (Figure 42-2).[8]

12. Once the Athlete Is Back to Full Participation, What Exercises Are Part of a Maintenance Program, and How Often Should They Be Done?

- A maintenance program (see Figure 42-2) involves rotator cuff and scapula stabilizer strengthening, flexibility and ROM exercises, along with lower-extremity and trunk strengthening.[13]
- The program should be designed to improve the strength, power, and endurance of the shoulder complex musculature.[15]
- Shoulder exercises are typically performed 3 times per week along with strength and conditioning programs that emphasize the entire body.[15]

References

1. Shelton G. Comprehensive rehabilitation of the athlete. In: Mellion M, Walsh WM, Shelton G, eds. *The Team Physician's Handbook*. 2nd ed. Philadelphia, PA: Hanley & Belfus, Inc.; 1997:371–390.
2. Clover J, Wall J. Return-to-play criteria following sports injury. *Clin Sports Med.* 2010;(29):169–175.
3. DiFiori J. Overuse injuries in children and adolescents. *The Physician and Sports Medicine.* 1999;27(1):1–12.
4. Fandel D, Frette T. Taping and bracing. In: Mellion M, Walsh WM, Shelton G, eds. *The Team Physician's Handbook.* 2nd ed. Philadelphia, PA: Hanley & Belfus, Inc; 1997:617–638.
5. LaBella C. Common acute sports-related lower extremity injuries in children and adolescents. *Clin Ped Emerg Med.* 2007(8):31–42.
6. Berg C. Youth sports issues. In: Mellion M, Walsh WM, Shelton G, eds. *The Team Physician's Handbook.* 2nd ed. Philadelphia, PA: Hanley & Belfus, Inc; 1997:67–72.
7. Pinsent C, Rae L, Palmer J. Return to Activity Guidelines for the Overhead Athlete after Shoulder Injury. University of Alberta Web site. www.physicaltherapy.ualberta.ca/en/Research/StudentResearch/~/media/pt/Documents/Return_to_Activity_Guidelines_for_the_Overhead_Athlete_after_Shoulder_Injury.pdf. Published November 2010. Accessed March 6, 2012.
8. Shoulder tendinitis. Massachusetts General Hospital, Orthopaedics. http://www.massgeneral.org/ortho/services/sports/rehab/Shoulder%20Tendinitis%20protocol.pdf. Accessed March 7, 2012.
9. Robertson WJ. Interval swimming program. http://billrobertsonmd.com/pdf/interval-swimming-program.pdf. Accessed March 6, 2012.
10. Functional Progression-Swimming. Missouri Sports Medicine Web site. http://northmissourisportsmedicine.com/uncategorized/functional-progression-swimming/. Accessed March 6, 2012.
11. Longobardi R. Interval rehabilitation programs. University Orthopaedic Center Web site. http://universityorthopaedic.com/pdf_files/IntervalRehabPrograms.pdf. Updated March 2007. Accessed March 7, 2012.
12. Interval Throwing Program for Little League. Massachusetts General Hospital, Orthopaedics Web site. http://www.massgeneral.org/ortho/services/sports/conditioning/MGH%20Interval%20Throwing%20Program%20for%20Little%20League.pdf. Accessed March 7, 2012.
13. Reinold MM, Wilk KE, Reed J, Crenshaw K, Andrews JR. Interval sport programs: guidelines for baseball, tennis, and golf. *J Ortho Sports Ther.* 2002;32(6):293-298.
14. Buschbacher R, Prahlow N, Dave SJ. *Sports Medicine and Rehabilitation: A Sport-Specific Approach.* Philadelphia, PA: Lippincott Williams and Wilkins; 2009.
15. Reinold MM. Little League Baseball Injury Prevention Program. Massachusetts General Hospital Web site. www2.massgeneral.org/sports/pdf/Injury%20Prevention/Baseball%20Tips/Little%20League%20Program.pdf. Accessed March 10, 2012.

43 The ABCs of Bracing and Taping

Monique S. Burton, MD

1. What Injuries/Situations Favor Taping, and Which Ones Are Better Served by Bracing?

- The desired objective of taping and bracing is to support the ligaments and the capsules of unstable joints by decreasing excessive/abnormal motion, support muscle-tendon units by compression/limitation of movement, and provide proprioceptive feedback from the affected body part, either following an injury or as to prevent a primary or secondary injury. There are specific taping techniques and bracing/braces that are appropriate for almost every body part.
- To determine whether a taping technique or a brace is more appropriate for a given injury or situation, the following factors need to be taken in consideration:
  - Comfort—There are some locations on the body where tape can be uncomfortable from the resulting pulling on the skin. Also, athletes with sensitive skin may find taping to be irritating, and a brace may be more suitable.
  - Convenience—If there is not an athletic trainer or other individual who is knowledgeable in taping techniques who is available to help an athlete, a brace may be more appropriate to ensure proper stabilization and the desired objective. On the other hand, some braces are challenging to find, and taping may be more accessible.
  - Cost—Some braces can be costly and not easily accessible to the athlete and family.
- Both tape and braces loosen with wear. Tape will need to be reapplied when this occurs; however, a brace may be readjusted quickly to improve the stability and therefore may help one make the decision of which is more appropriate given the individual's circumstances. Braces need to be replaced when they are overstretched and no longer able to provide an appropriate fit. Also, a new brace needs to be purchased when the athlete outgrows his or her old brace.
- Table 43-1 provides some examples of the areas that are commonly taped or braced and the type of brace that is most often used.

2. Can Taping or Bracing Take the Place of a Rehabilitation Program?

- A rehabilitation program is an essential component of injury management. Functional progressive rehabilitation allows the athlete to regain his or her strength, flexibility, and sports-specific goals. Taping and/or bracing may be included in a rehabilitation program to help provide stability, proprioception, or awareness to the injured body part, as well as proper dynamics for functionality.

Koutures C, Wong V.
Pediatric Sports Medicine: Essentials for Office Evaluation (pp 301-305)

Table 43-1. Indications for and Desired Goals of Bracing and Taping on Various Parts of the Body			
BODY PART	*TAPE/BRACE*	*INDICATIONS*	*DESIRED GOALS*
Fingers	• Taping injured finger to unaffected adjacent finger	• Finger sprain	• Finger stabilization
Wrist	• Wrist stabilization taping or brace	• Wrist sprain	• Stabilization of extension
Elbow	• Counterforce brace	• Medial or lateral epicondylitis/apophysitis	• Decrease stress at medial or lateral epicondyle
Ankle	• Ankle tape or ankle support brace	• Ankle sprain	• Ankle joint stabilization
Knee	• Patellar buttress brace • Patellar strap	• Patellar dislocation/subluxation, patellofemoral pain • Apophysitis/tendinitis	• Patellar stabilization • Relieve tension at apophysis or tendon

- Although taping and/or bracing may be used throughout the course of treatment, they are not intended to replace a thorough rehabilitation program.
- Ideally, at the end of a rehabilitation program, taping or bracing will no longer be necessary, and the athlete will have increased his or her strength, flexibility, and stability to provide the support needed to the affected body part.

3. What Is the Evidence for Prophylactic Bracing of the Knee to Reduce Either Medial Collateral Ligament or Anterior Cruciate Ligament Injuries?

- The use of prophylactic knee bracing for the prevention of medial collateral ligament (MCL) or anterior cruciate ligament (ACL) injuries is controversial.
- MCL injuries commonly occur from a valgus stress to the knee. An older prospective study demonstrated that bracing resulted in a nonstatistically significant trend toward the prevention of MCL injuries.[1] A 2005 review showed that a well-fitting, hinged knee brace may be helpful in decreasing the stress at the knee and, as a result, decreasing MCL injuries.[2] However, ACL injuries caused by an external blow did not appear to be protected by prophylactic bracing. In addition, there is some concern that there may be negative effects on performance level, leg cramping, and fatigue symptoms.[2]
- Insufficient scientific evidence exists to recommend prescribing prophylactic knee bracing at this time; however, further research is needed to clarify questions that surround this controversy, especially in the pediatric population.

4. What Types of Braces are Commonly Recommended for Anterior Knee Pain or Patellar Instability? What Is the Evidence for These Recommendations?

- Anterior knee pain is very common in the pediatric population, including patellofemoral pain syndrome, patellar tendinitis (Jumper's knee), patellar instability from a previous patellar dislocation/subluxation, and apophysitis at the distal patellar pole (Sinding-Larsen-Johansson syndrome) or tibial tuberosity (Osgood-Schlatter disease). The recommended brace varies depending on the underlying diagnosis.

- Although bracing may be a component of the treatment for anterior knee pain, a rehabilitation program that focuses on addressing strength imbalance, flexibility, core stability, and functional activities provides the most effective management for a complete recovery.
- A patellar stabilizer brace may be considered for athletes with patellofemoral pain syndrome or patellar instability following a patellar dislocation/subluxation. The intent of the brace is to provide stability in the patellofemoral joint. The brace is typically made of neoprene with a patellar cutout reinforced with a buttress, commonly C-shaped. The buttress is intended to help stabilize the patella in the femoral groove and prevent lateral movement. These braces are reasonably priced and can be obtained from orthopedic equipment suppliers or sporting goods stores.
- The patellar strap is another common brace/device that is used in anterior knee pain for patellar tendinitis, distal patellar pole apophysitis, and tibial tuberosity apophysitis. The objective of the patellar strap is to transfer the point of stress from the painful area to a different location, therefore decreasing tension and pain. Typically, the strap is placed between the distal patellar pole and the tibial tuberosity.
- Evidence to support the effectiveness of bracing for anterior knee pain is limited and inconsistent; however, patients often find comfort from a brace and like using it. It is important to caution them that braces have mixed reviews and stress that the most important part of a full recovery is the completion of a thorough rehabilitation program that progressively returns them back to their full physical activity level and sports-related goals.

5. Is There Any Evidence to Support Ankle Braces for Either Primary or Secondary Prevention of Ankle Sprains?

- Ankle braces and tape are commonly used for the prevention of primary and secondary ankle sprains.
- A systematic review of 14 randomized trials demonstrated that external ankle supports decreased the risk of ankle sprain. There was a greater reduction in risk amongst those with a previous ankle sprain than those with a primary injury.
- A 2000 meta-analysis of eight studies demonstrated that the use of tape or bracing reduced the incidence of ankle sprains; however, bracing was more effective than taping. It was not clear whether athletes with or without previous ankle injuries had more benefit.[3]
- A large, randomized controlled study of 1460 male and female high school basketball players demonstrated a reduction of incidence of acute ankle injuries in athletes with and without previous ankle injuries when using a lace-up ankle brace. The severity of ankle injuries, however, was not affected by the use of an ankle brace.[4] Another randomized controlled study of 2081 high school football players demonstrated similar findings of a decreased incidence of acute ankle injuries, but no reduction in severity with the use of lace-up ankle braces.[5]

6. Does Taping Help to Prevent Injuries for the Entire Game, Or Is Taping Beneficial for Only a Limited Time Period?

- Taping is only useful as long as the tape is providing proper stability. As the athlete participates in his or her sport, the tape naturally loosens over time. As the tape loosens, the intended benefit decreases to minimal or no benefit.
- Throughout the game/meet, athletes should reassess their tape and replace it as indicated to provide adequate support. This can present a challenge to find an appropriate time to

make the change during a competition or game. Planning for tape replacement in advance during scheduled breaks, such as half-time, will prevent frustration and urgency during a critical time of play.

7. Which Members of the Sports Medicine Team Are Well-Trained on How to Tape an Injury?

- If available, the most ideal person to tape the athlete's injury is the certified athletic trainer. His or her educational background includes extensive training and experience in taping.
- Other members of the sports medicine team may be able to provide assistance if they are adequately trained. Coaches are often required to have some training in taping, and they may be an appropriate resource if they have this background and regularly tape their athletes. In addition, the team physician may have experience in taping and may be able to assist as well.
- It is important that anyone that is applying tape be well-educated and experienced on what taping methods are best for the injured body part as well as on what techniques are needed to meet the intended purpose of the taping.

8. What Are Some Common Myths About Taping? Can Athletes Tape Their Injuries Themselves?

- Taping is extremely common in sports. Although reasons for taping stem from the desire to provide stability, control pain, and prevent injuries, myths and superstitions exist around taping. As we have seen on television and at various sporting events, taping is widely used by professional athletes, and the function is often hard to discern.
- Spatting, similar in appearance to ankle taping but external to the shoe, is commonly seen in football players. Football players feel that this may provide additional support, prevent their shoelaces from coming undone and getting in the way, improve ankle stability, and make their shoe feel tighter and as a result provide a better feel to their play; however, evidence does not currently exist to support this. Conversely, this type of taping makes removing the shoe difficult when an injury occurs and may also damage the shoe.
- Other common taping that may be seen is on the wrist, fingers, and elbows. Although taping in these locations can provide a stabilizing effect when applied by a trained individual, these are common locations that athletes may tape themselves for various other reasons. The use of tape may result from an injury and then became a trademark or "good luck" component when they performed well with the tape in place. Taping certainly is also stylish and trendy for athletes. It provides them with an opportunity to distinguish themselves or emulate other popular professional athletes. As long as the tape is not creating a harmful situation for the athlete and they understand the limitations of their taping technique, it is acceptable for them to continue.
- In most cases, taping to provide actual stability to an ankle or other joint should be performed by a certified athletic trainer or other individual trained and experienced in taping. In circumstances where an athletic trainer is not available, it may be useful to have another person, such as the coach, learn how to properly apply tape for the desired effect.

9. What Is Kinesio Tape? How Is It Best Used? What Is the Evidence Behind Its Use?

- Kinesio tape (KT) is an elastic therapeutic tape used for treating sports injuries. Dr. Kenzo Kase, an acupuncturist and chiropractor, developed the tape in the mid-1970s. KT claims to support injured muscles by lifting the skin microscopically, allowing improved blood and lymph flow to facilitate the body's natural healing process. KT was popularized during the 2008 Summer Olympic Games in Beijing when it was seen on many high-profile athletes.

- A 2012 meta-analysis reviewed 10 articles that met the inclusion criteria, of which only 2 investigated sports-related injuries. Researchers found that KT may have a small beneficial role in improving strength, range of motion in certain injured cohorts, and force sense error compared with other tapes.[6] Further studies are recommended to confirm these findings and to investigate the usefulness of KT in sports-related injuries.

10. What Is the Best Way to Order/Obtain Athletic Tape or Kinesio Tape for the Office or for an Athlete?

- Athletic tape can be ordered online. There are many different types of athletic tape, and therefore it is important to understand how and when to use the different types of tape for the various taping techniques. Although all athletic tape looks very similar, the quality can make a difference in the ease of its use. It makes sense to do a little investigating to find a tape that allows for ease of use and appropriate function, and fits within and an office's or an athlete's budget.
- KT is widely available and can be purchased online, at sporting goods stores, and at orthopedic supply stores.
- When making the decision to obtain tape for use, it is highly recommended that the person who will be assisting the athlete in taping take a course or apprentice himself or herself with an athletic trainer to ensure taping stability and quality, and that the taping is serving the intended purpose. It takes practice to maintain a certain level of expertise, so a person who wants to include taping as a regular part of his or her practice should make sure that there are many opportunities available to maintain his or her skill level.

References

1. Albright JP, Powell JW, Smith W, et al. Medial collateral ligament sprains in college football. Effectiveness of preventative braces. *Am J Sports Med.* 1994;22(1):12–18.
2. Najibi S, Albright JP. The use of knee braces, part 1: prophylatic knee braces in contact sports. *Am J Sports Med.* 2005;33(4);602–611.
3. Verhagen EA, van Mechelen W, de Vente W. The effect of preventative measures on the incidence of ankle sprains. *Clin J Sports Med.* 2000;10(4):291–296.
4. McGuine TA, Brooks A, Hetzel S. The effect of lace-up ankle braces on injury rates in high school basketball players. *Am J Sports Med.* 2011;39(9):1840–1848.
5. McGuine TA, Hetzel S, Wilson J, Brooks A. The effects of lace-up ankle braces on injury rates in high school football players. *Am J Sports Med.* 2012;40(1):49–57.
6. Williams S, Whatman C, Hume PA, Sheerin K. Kinesio taping in treatment and prevention of sports injuries: a meta-analysis of the evidence for its effectiveness. *Sports Med.* 2012:42(2):153–164.

44 Knowing Your Sports Medicine Resources

Alysha Taxter, MD and Teri M. McCambridge, MD, FAAP

1. What Is a Primary Care Sports Medicine Physician?

The majority of primary care sports medicine physicians have a background in family medicine or pediatrics. Some have backgrounds in emergency medicine, internal medicine, medicine-pediatrics, or physical medicine and rehabilitation. Most primary care sports medicine physicians have undergone 1 to 2 years of fellowship and have passed a sports medicine examination to obtain a Certificate of Added Qualification (CAQ). Some older physicians have been grandfathered into sports medicine without completing a fellowship if their practice focused on the care of sports conditions prior to the establishment of formalized sports medicine training. Although the majority of fellowship programs are affiliated with family medicine programs, there are an increasing number of pediatric-specific sports medicine programs. Because of their primary care background, they are proficient in caring for acute and chronic diseases in addition to fracture care, acute injuries, apophysitis, overuse injuries, eating disorders, concussions, and other medical conditions that are common in the athlete. It is not atypical for primary care-trained physicians to spend more time with their patients and to provide more education, as well as discuss prevention due to their training.

2. What Is a Certified Athletic Trainer? What Is a Physical Therapist? What Roles Do They Play on a Sports Medicine Team?

Although both care for athletes, there are many differences between a certified athletic trainer (ATC) and a physical therapist (PT). All ATCs must obtain, at a minimum, a bachelor's degree in athletic training from a program that is accredited by the Commission on Accreditation of Athletic Training Education. Its curriculum focuses on the following: (1) injury prevention, recognition, and evaluation; and (2) assessment of athletic injuries, treatment, rehabilitation, and reconditioning of musculoskeletal injuries. Most importantly, their work focuses on the care of athletes. After their training is complete, the trainers take a national examination that is sponsored by the "Board of Certification" for athletic trainers. The certification examination requires both a written test and a practicum. Once an athletic trainer passes both components, he or she is considered an "Athletic Trainer Certified," or "ATC." ATCs are required to meet recertification and continuing education requirements yearly. They commonly work closely with high school, college, and professional athletes. They can also work with hospitals, rehabilitation programs, and physician's clinics. They are skilled in basic emergency response and management and are competent in basic life support, automated external defibrillator use, and proper spine immobilization.

The ATC can assist the athlete and medical team beginning with the preparticipation examinations, where he or she can play a critical role in assessing an athlete's flexibility and vital signs, evaluating orthopedic conditions that require further rehabilitation, and determining an athlete's fitness level. An ATC can implement preventive strategies to decrease injury risk through

Koutures C, Wong V.
Pediatric Sports Medicine: Essentials for Office Evaluation (pp 306-312)

conditioning programs, equipment fitting, bracing, and taping. ATCs act as liaisons between athletes and the physician or other medical professionals. Finally, their training prepares them to develop the emergency action plan, maintain facility and equipment safety, and develop adverse weather recommendations for participants.

A sports PT specializes in the rehabilitation of musculoskeletal conditions. A PT typically has a bachelor's degree and a doctorate of physical therapy. Some institutions have combined programs that are completed in 6 years. A PT's curriculum includes the clinical application of foundation sciences, examination skills, differential diagnosis, intervention and therapeutic modalities, safety and protection, teaching and learning, and evidence-based practice.

PTs can subspecialize in cardiovascular and pulmonary therapy, clinical electrophysiology, geriatrics, neurology, orthopedics, pediatrics, sports medicine, and women's health. The ability to take a subspecialty examination requires 2000 hours of direct subspecialty patient care over 10 years or the completion of a post-professional clinical residency and a specialty practice examination. Eligibility to take the Sports Certification requires current basic life support certification or cardiopulmonary resuscitation for the professional rescuer in addition to the aforementioned training. The Sports Subspecialty Certification Examination tests the PT's skills of evaluation, diagnosis, prognosis, intervention, outcomes of rehabilitation, and when an athlete can return to activity. Additionally, PTs must be certified as a first responder by the American Red Cross, emergency medical technician or paramedic, or ATC by National Athletic Trainers Association Board of Certification.

An ATC's role includes being the first responder in athletic injury management, prevention, and rehabilitation for athletes on his or her team. The ATC has more day-to-day contact with both injured and noninjured athletes, whereas the PT has intermittent contact. The PT and the ATC help to assist those who have been injured, and can help rehabilitate the athlete and assist him or her with regaining the skills needed for return to play (RTP).

PTs and ATCs are not personal trainers. Personal trainers help design exercise and conditioning programs for clients and help athletes achieve fitness goals through the design of exercise programs and lifestyle modification.

3. What Are the Necessary Components on a Physical Therapy Prescription?

Table 44-1 includes the components that are recommended for a physical therapy prescription. Precautions for therapy include any special needs (eg, comorbid conditions that would influence therapy, such as hypertension, heart conditions, or position restrictions) or concerns (eg, limited weight bearing, limited joint range of motion, or closed chain exercises). Special requests such as the use of aquatic therapy, phonophoresis, and iontophoresis (which should not be done over an open physis), as well as providing the patient with braces, crutches, or custom orthotics, should be specified. The therapist should send reports about the patient's progress to the ordering physician. The majority of pediatric athletes have significant improvement with their pain and mobility after a short course of physical therapy.

4. How Can a Health Care Provider Connect With the School-Based/Local Certified Athletic Trainer?

Most high schools have an athletic director who can refer you to the school-based or local ATC, if available. Additional ways to make contact with a school-based ATC include asking other school officials. Establish a relationship with the principal, coach, or other parents. The National Athletic Trainers' Association is the organization that will have information about ATCs in your area.

Table 44-1. Sample Physical Therapy Prescription
Date: Patient Name: DOB: Date of Onset: Frequency and Duration:_number of visits a week for weeks
Reason for Referral: • Evaluate and Treat • Evaluate Only
Diagnosis:
Patient Exhibits Problems With: • Mobility • Pain Management • Range of Motion • Strength
Precautions for Therapy:
Special Requests: [ ] hand therapy [ ] aquatic therapy [ ] running program [ ] throwing program
Provide Patient With: [ ] orthotics [ ] braces [ ] crutches
Modalities to Be Used: [ ] iontophoresis [ ] phontophoresis [ ] whirlpool [ ] ultrasonography [ ] pulsed ultrasonography
Progression to Activity: [ ] per PT recs [ ] should be seen by physician for clearance

5. How Can a Sports Nutritionist Help With the Management of Young Athletes?

Nutrition is a highly specialized field. Most coaches, ATCs, athletes, and parents are not adequately trained or familiar with this specialty. Children have different nutritional and metabolic needs than adults. A sports nutritionist can help to improve exercise and sports performance by assisting with healthy eating choices. He or she can help an athlete gain muscle or lose fat, increase strength and power, and increase stamina and endurance. He or she provides assistance for hydration and optimum fluid intake before, during, and after sport. A sports nutritionist can address the specific needs of each individual athlete.

Additionally, sports nutritionists can be helpful for addressing food allergies or intolerances such as gluten sensitivity or lactose intolerance. They can design a program for vegetarians, vegans, fruitarians, and other unique diet choices. An athlete with diabetes will have different dietary requirements than other team members. Nutritionists address methods to resolve iron deficiency and provide ideal calcium and vitamin D intake for the prevention or treatment of stress fractures. They can also serve on multidisciplinary teams that provide services for athletes with eating disorders.

A sports nutritionist can address the misinformation athletes have about dieting and eating. He or she can provide athletes with education about protein use to gain muscle, as well as what carbohydrates are best for their sport and when the proper time is to consume them. A sports nutritionist can also address supplement and herbal use.

The use of a sports nutritionist is necessary when the nutritional needs of an athlete change. An injured/sick athlete has different caloric and nutritional needs than a healthy athlete. The needs of an athlete perioperatively are significantly different than the needs of an athlete during training; proper nutrition can promote healing and faster recovery. Additionally, nutritional needs change throughout the season and are also different during transition to off-season.

Sports nutritionists have a bachelor's degree in nutrition. They are credentialed to be a Board-Certified Specialist in Sports Dietetics. They work in a variety of settings, including athletic performance companies, collegiate/professional sports, sports medicine centers, student health, and Olympic training centers. They work with all sports, from dance and gymnastics to football and weight lifting. Sports nutritionists work with all athletes to help them be healthier and achieve their best athletic potential. (See the references at the end of this chapter for some recommended resources for pediatric nutrition for the athlete.)

6. Are all Orthopedists Specialists in Sports Medicine? How Can the General Pediatric Provider Tell If His or Her Orthopedic Colleague Has Knowledge in Sports Medicine Issues?

Not all orthopedists are specialists in sports medicine. In smaller communities without an excess of orthopedists, it is common for the orthopedist to practice general orthopedics without undergoing additional subspecialty training. Most orthopedists in large communities have additional subspecialty training and specialize in hand/upper extremity, joint replacement, foot and ankle, spine, trauma, pediatrics, or sports medicine. Sports medicine orthopedists are familiar with the management of orthopedic athletic injuries, but are not always familiar with the treatment of younger patients and nonorthopedic sports medicine conditions. Additionally, a pediatric orthopedist should be familiar with sports medicine orthopedic conditions such as anterior cruciate ligament (ACL) reconstructions and meniscus tears but will not be as familiar with nonorthopedic conditions or problems in the athlete that do not require surgery. Pediatric orthopedists will have varying levels of comfort concerning the management of pediatric sports medicine issues. It is not uncommon for patients referred to an orthopedist's office to see a midlevel provider such as a nurse practitioner or physician assistant who assists in the orthopedist's clinic. Due to a surgeon's heavy clinic schedule, patients may only spend several minutes with a surgeon to discuss their condition and future needs.

A general pediatric provider can tell if his or her orthopedic colleague has an interest in sports medicine if he or she is present at sporting events and actively participates in the care of athletes. Orthopedists can cover local high school teams; it is common for them to be on the sidelines of football games or on the bench basketball games. They can also provide coverage for local high school events such as camps, tournaments, and regional or state competitions. Additionally, they can provide medical services for city-wide events such as 5K races and marathons. Others are involved in mass preparticipation examinations at schools in their communities. An orthopedist interested in sports medicine can become a member of the American Orthopaedic Society for Sports Medicine and can pass a sports medicine examination to increase his or her knowledge in nonoperative care.

7. What Type of Cases Should Be Referred to a Pediatric Primary Care Sports Medicine Specialist Versus a Pediatric Orthopedic Sports Medicine Specialist?

A pediatric sports medicine specialist can care for all of the needs of a patient up until surgical management is required. Table 44-2 lists musculoskeletal issues that are commonly seen in a pediatric sports medicine clinic. Additionally, due to their primary care background, primary care sports medicine specialists can manage medical conditions that can affect athletic performance, such as asthma, vocal cord dysfunction (defined in Chapter 8), anemia, bone mineral density concerns, female athlete triad (defined in Chapter 17), and risk factors for stress fractures. They provide resources for dealing with RTP after injury and can also provide insight into sports psychology. They are knowledgeable about biomechanics and can provide recommendations to correct athletes' biomechanical misalignment. Primary care sports medicine physicians work closely with PTs, ATCs, and nutritionists to closely coordinate care for the athlete.

Appropriate referral to a pediatric orthopedist or a sports medicine orthopedist would be for the surgical management of a condition. Common orthopedic conditions that may need definitive

TABLE 44-2. COMMON MUSCULOSKELETAL INJURIES SEEN IN A PEDIATRIC SPORTS MEDICINE CLINIC	
ACUTE INJURIES	*OVERUSE INJURIES*
Burners and stingers	Apophysitis: Osgood-Schlatter disease, Sever's disease, etc
Concussions	Gymnast's wrist
Contusions	Hypermobility syndrome
Dislocations: finger, glenohumeral, patellar	Iliotibial band syndrome
Medial collateral ligament sprain	Little League shoulder and elbow
Nonoperative fractures (ie, buckle, Salter-Harris, clavicle)	Medial tibial stress syndrome (shin splints)
Osteochondritis dissecans	Patella-femoral dysfunction (anterior knee pain)
Sprains: acromioclavicular, wrist, finger, ankle, midfoot	Trochanteric bursitis
Turf toe	Spondylolysis and spondylolisthesis
Volar plate injuries	Stress fractures
	Tendinitis: rotator cuff, elbow, patellar, Achilles

operative management include ACL/meniscus injuries, osteochondritis dissecans lesions, complex fractures, joint instability (elbow, shoulder, and ankle) and labral tears.

Comanagement of certain musculoskeletal injuries (such as first-time patellar or glenohumeral dislocations) is often done by a primary care sports medicine physician and a sports medicine-trained orthopedic surgeon. Many high school, collegiate, and professional institutions utilize the talents of both primary care and surgical specialist.

8. How Can the General Health Care Provider Counsel Families on the Role of Alternative Medicine in the Treatment of Pediatric and Adolescent Sports Injuries?

The integration of alternative and complementary medicine with allopathic medicine is becoming more common. Many families will seek out alternative therapies on their own. Certain chiropractors have sought out additional training in sports injury care with an emphasis on soft-tissue management. Thus, when counseling families on the role of chiropractic care for sports injuries, it is essential to identify and refer to chiropractic practitioners, like with any other health care professional, who have demonstrated comfort and experience working with pediatric athletes.

Acupuncture stems from traditional Chinese medicine with the goal to relieve pain and other symptoms through the use of small needles to pressure points in the skin. It is used throughout the world for pain management. A systematic review of the safety of acupuncture in children estimated that 150,000 children use acupuncture. The most common adverse events reported were mild and included pain, bruising, bleeding, and worsening of symptoms.[1] Serious adverse events were caused by substandard practice. Acupuncture is safe in children when performed by appropriately trained practitioners. There is a low risk for serious adverse events. Its low cost and ease to perform make it a favorable alternative or complement to other therapies.

There is no definitive evidence to recommend or decline the referral to alternative medicine specialists for the pediatric population.

9. What Is Prolotherapy, and What Type of Injuries May Benefit From Its Use?

Prolotherapy involves injecting a hyperosmolar glucose solution into a ligament or tendon to cause inflammation, increase blood flow, and stimulate tissue repair. There is no standard technique or recipe for glucose preparations, solution concentrations, or injection techniques.[2] Hyperosmolar dextrose (typically 15% dextrose once diluted with other additives), phenol-glycer-in-glucose, and morrhuate sodium are the most common. The dextrose solution is also combined with saline and lidocaine. A volume of 2 to 5 mL is injected into a tender ligament and tendon attachment and adjacent joint spaces in a "peppering" fashion monthly for 3 months. There is no definitive explanation for why this provides pain relief and healing. It is thought that the local irritation from the needle and the glucose causes inflammation, which will stimulate the release of growth factors, thereby promoting healing.

Prolotherapy is commonly used in chronic, degenerative, or overuse conditions such as osteoarthritis, tendinopathy, and low-back pain. The most evidence-based medicine regarding the use of prolotherapy is in the treatment of lateral epicondylitis and Achilles tendinosis.[3]

Prolotherapy is contraindicated if there is overlying cellulitis or concerns for a septic joint. Side effects include mild pain, bleeding, and a flare at the injection site.

Prolotherapy is usually coupled with other alternative therapies such as manipulations or steroid injections. This adjunctive therapy has not been well studied despite being practiced for over 10 years, and lacks definitive evidence for use in children. It is typically considered when traditional therapies fail.

10. What Is Platelet-Rich Plasma Therapy, and What Types of Injuries May Benefit From Its Use?

Platelet-rich plasma (PRP) is a newer therapy for the treatment of ligamentous and tendon injuries. It has been used in plastic and maxillofacial surgery since the 1990s. PRP is obtained by the centrifugation of autologous whole blood. The buffy coat, which contains cellular plasma and platelets, is mixed with thrombin and calcium salt for injection into injured tissue. The plasma contains growth factors that theoretically promote healing by the site-specific delivery of growth factors and platelet-released cytokines. It is proposed that local injection and higher concentration of factors than would otherwise be endogenously produced promotes more rapid healing. The stimulation of reparative cells and the inhibition of proinflammatory cytokines are also provided by PRP. However, there is a lack of quality randomized control trials, and the majority of the literature has been provided by case reports.[4] Animal models show conflicting results regarding accelerated healing. There is no standard preparation or delivery of PRP. The platelet concentrations and function are variable based on the preparation technique. Risks include infection and failure of improvement. This therapy has commonly been used in elbow tendinopathy, rotator cuff surgery, patellar tendinopathy, and ACL reconstruction.[5] PRP is typically not covered by insurance and is usually paid out of pocket. Estimated costs are from several hundred to several thousand dollars.

11. What Is Active Release Therapy, Who Can Perform It, and What Types of Injuries May Benefit From Its Use?

Active release therapy (ART) began in the 1980s by a chiropractor to provide additional therapy for athletes who had failed other modalities. This technique utilizes a type of myofascial release that uses active motion to break down scar tissue in overused or injured muscles. The important part of this therapy is finding the scar tissue; this is done through feeling the differences in a tissue's texture, tension, and movement. Although similar to massage, ART uses active movement and pressure applied to muscles and deep tissues. It is painful, and the goal is to mechanically break up scar tissue. Patients can have bruising and pain after undergoing ART. It is believed that the disruption of the scar tissue allows the muscles, nerves, fascia, and soft tissues to freely glide over one another more easily. Most people will respond within the first or second session if they are going to have any effect from this therapy. The number of necessary sessions depends on the condition; acute injuries can see improvement after one visit, whereas chronic injuries may require multiple visits.

Multiple health care providers who work with soft-tissue conditions, including chiropractors, PTs, massage therapists, ATCs, and physicians, are able to take the ART course and become certified in the ART technique.

Overuse injuries may benefit from this technique. The ART Web site (www.activerelease.com) recommends that ART can be helpful in the management of headaches, back pain, carpal tunnel, shin splints, shoulder pain, sciatica, plantar fasciitis, knee problems, and tennis elbow. There has been some literature as to the effectiveness of this technique in rehabilitation literature; however, the majority of literature is case reports.[6-9] There is a lack of strong research or evidence that ART is beneficial for the care of athletes.

References

1. Adams D, Cheng F, Jou H, Aung S, Yasui Y, Vohra S. The safety of pediatric acupuncture: a systematic review. *Pediatrics*. 2011;128(6):e1575–e1587.
2. Rabago D, Yelland M, Patterson J, Zgierska A. Prolotherapy for chronic musculoskeletal pain. *Am Fam Physician*. 2011;84(11):1208–1210.
3. Distel LM, Best TM. Prolotherapy: a clinical review of its role in treating chronic musculoskeletal pain. *PMR*. 2011;3(6 Suppl 1):S78–S81.
4. Taylor DW, Petrera M, Hendry M, Theodoropoulos JS. A systematic review of the use of platelet-rich plasma in sports medicine as a new treatment for tendon and ligament injuries. *Clin J Sport Med*. 2011;21(4):344–352.
5. Paoloni J, De Vos RJ, Hamilton B, Murrell GA, Orchard J. Platelet-rich plasma treatment for ligament and tendon injuries. *Clin J Sport Med*. 2011;21(1):37–45.
6. Robb A, Pajaczkowski J. Immediate effect on pain thresholds using active release technique on adductor strains: Pilot study. *J Bodyw Mov Ther*. 2011;15(1):57-62.
7. Yuill EA, Macintyre IG. Posterior tibialis tendonopathy in an adolescent soccer player: a case report. *J Can Chiropr Assoc*. 2010;54(4):293-300.
8. Durante JA, Macintyre IG. Pudendal nerve entrapment in an Ironman athlete: a case report. *J Can Chiropr Assoc*. 2010;54(4):276-81.
9. Howitt S, Wong J, Zabukovec S. The conservative treatment of Trigger thumb using Graston Techniques and Active Release Techniques. *J Can Chiropr Assoc*. 2006;50(4):249-54.

Suggested Readings

American Academy of Pediatrics Committee on Nutrition. *Pediatric Nutrition Handbook*. 6th Edition. Elk Grove Village, IL: American Academy of Pediatrics; 2009.

Clark N. *Nancy Clark's Sports Nutrition Guidebook*. 4th Edition. Champaign: Human Kinetics; 2008.

Suggested Web Sites

Active Release Techniques (ART): www.activerelease.com
American Board of Physical Therapy Specialties (ABPTS): www.abpts.org
American College of Sports Medicine (ACSM): www.acsm.org
American Medical Society for Sports Medicine (AMSSM): www.amssm.org
The American Orthopaedic Society for Sports Medicine (AOSSM): www.sportsmed.org
American Physical Therapy Association (APTA): www.apta.org
Board of Certification for the Athletic Trainer: www.bocatc.org
National Academy of Sports Medicine (NASM): www.nasm.org
National Athletic Trainers' Association (NATA): www.nata.org
Sports, Cardiovascular, and Wellness Nutrition: www.scandpg.org
The Federation of State Boards of Physical Therapy (FSBPT): www.fsbpt.org

Financial Disclosures

Dr. Suraj Achar has no financial or proprietary interest in the materials presented herein.

Dr. Suriti Kundu Achar has no financial or proprietary interest in the materials presented herein.

Dr. Holly J. Benjamin has no financial or proprietary interest in the materials presented herein.

Dr. David T. Bernhardt has no financial or proprietary interest in the materials presented herein.

Dr. Kate E. Berz has no financial or proprietary interest in the materials presented herein.

Dr. Terra Blatnik has no financial or proprietary interest in the materials presented herein.

Dr. Joel S. Brenner has no financial or proprietary interest in the materials presented herein.

Dr. Susannah Briskin has no financial or proprietary interest in the materials presented herein.

Dr. Paul D. Brydon has no financial or proprietary interest in the materials presented herein.

Dr. Monique S. Burton has no financial or proprietary interest in the materials presented herein.

Dr. Kelly Chain has no financial or proprietary interest in the materials presented herein.

Dr. Philip J. Cohen has no financial or proprietary interest in the materials presented herein.

Dr. Yasmin D. Deliz has no financial or proprietary interest in the materials presented herein.

Dr. Rebecca A. Demorest has no financial or proprietary interest in the materials presented herein.

Dr. Emanuel Elias has no financial or proprietary interest in the materials presented herein.

Dr. Emelynn J. Fajardo has no financial or proprietary interest in the materials presented herein.

Dr. Kenton H. Fibel has no financial or proprietary interest in the materials presented herein.

Dr. Katherine M. Fox has no financial or proprietary interest in the materials presented herein.

Dr. Matthew Grady has no financial or proprietary interest in the materials presented herein.

Dr. Andrew J.M. Gregory has no financial or proprietary interest in the materials presented herein.

Dr. Mark Halstead has no financial or proprietary interest in the materials presented herein.

Dr. Tho Brian Hang has no financial or proprietary interest in the materials presented herein.

Dr. Quynh B. Hoang has no financial or proprietary interest in the materials presented herein.

Dr. T.J. Howell has no financial or proprietary interest in the materials presented herein.

Dr. Mary M. Hung has no financial or proprietary interest in the materials presented herein.

Dr. Phuong N. Huynh has no financial or proprietary interest in the materials presented herein.

Dr. Amanda Weiss Kelly has no financial or proprietary interest in the materials presented herein.

Dr. Chris Koutures has no financial or proprietary interest in the materials presented herein.

Dr. Austin Krohn has no financial or proprietary interest in the materials presented herein.

Dr. David Kruse has no financial or proprietary interest in the materials presented herein.

Dr. Cynthia R. LaBella has no financial or proprietary interest in the materials presented herein.

Dr. Michele LaBotz has no financial or proprietary interest in the materials presented herein.

Dr. Greg Landry has no financial or proprietary interest in the materials presented herein.

Dr. Christopher Lynch has no financial or proprietary interest in the materials presented herein.

Dr. Teri M. McCambridge has no financial or proprietary interest in the materials presented herein.

Dr. Megan Groh Miller has no financial or proprietary interest in the materials presented herein.

Dr. Rob Monaco has no financial or proprietary interest in the materials presented herein.

Dr. Mohammed Mortazavi has no financial or proprietary interest in the materials presented herein.

Dr. Kirk Mulgrew has no financial or proprietary interest in the materials presented herein.

Dr. Kyle B. Nagle has no financial or proprietary interest in the materials presented herein.

Dr. Jeremy Ng has no financial or proprietary interest in the materials presented herein.

Dr. David Olson has no financial or proprietary interest in the materials presented herein.

Dr. Kentaro Onishi has no financial or proprietary interest in the materials presented herein.

Dr. Neesheet Parikh has no financial or proprietary interest in the materials presented herein.

Dr. Byron Patterson has no financial or proprietary interest in the materials presented herein.

Dr. Miriam G.S. Reece has no financial or proprietary interest in the materials presented herein.

Dr. Stephen G. Rice has no financial or proprietary interest in the materials presented herein.

Dr. William O. Roberts has no financial or proprietary interest in the materials presented herein.

Dr. Anthony Saglimbeni has no financial or proprietary interest in the materials presented herein.

Dr. John A. Schlechter has no financial or proprietary interest in the materials presented herein.

Dr. Charmaine Sekona has no financial or proprietary interest in the materials presented herein.

Dr. Robby S. Sikka has no financial or proprietary interest in the materials presented herein.

Dr. David V. Smith has no financial or proprietary interest in the materials presented herein.

Dr. Paul R. Stricker has no financial or proprietary interest in the materials presented herein.

Dr. Alysha Taxter has no financial or proprietary interest in the materials presented herein.

Dr. Kenneth S. Taylor has no financial or proprietary interest in the materials presented herein.

Dr. Nate Waibel has no financial or proprietary interest in the materials presented herein.

Dr. David Wang has no financial or proprietary interest in the materials presented herein.

Dr. Valarie Wong has no financial or proprietary interest in the materials presented herein.

Dr. Tracy L. Zaslow has no financial or proprietary interest in the materials presented herein.

INDEX

Printed in the United States
by Baker & Taylor Publisher Services

Printed in the United States
by Baker & Taylor Publisher Services